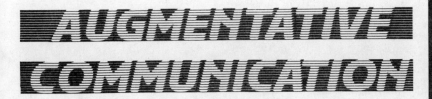

# AN INTRODUCTION

# AUGMENTATIVE COMMUNICATION:
## *An Introduction*

Editor
Sarah W. Blackstone

Technical Editor
Deborah M. Bruskin

December 1986

AMERICAN SPEECH-LANGUAGE-HEARING ASSOCIATION
Rockville, Maryland

## General Information

Development of *Augmentative Communication: An Introduction* was supported in part by Grant Number G008400718 from the U.S. Department of Education, Washington, DC. Information presented in this narrative is intended to provide resource material. The contents do not necessarily represent the policies or opinions of the American Speech-Language-Hearing Association or the U.S. Department of Education.

*Augmentative Communication: An Introduction* and the *Curriculum Guide for an Introductory Course in Augmentative Communication* are published by the American Speech-Language-Hearing Association. Copies may be obtained by writing to:

**Publications Sales Office**
American Speech-Language-Hearing Association
10801 Rockville Pike
Rockville, Maryland 20852
(301) 897-5700

ISBN 0-910329-36-2
Library of Congress catalog number 86-72931
Printed in the United States.

*Dedicated to individuals
with severe expressive communication disorders and their families
and to the professionals who are committed to improving
the quality of their lives*

# CONTRIBUTING AUTHORS

David R. Beukelman, Ph.D.
Barkley Memorial Center
University of Nebraska
Lincoln, Nebraska 68583-0732

Sarah W. Blackstone, Ph.D.
American Speech-Language-Hearing Association
10801 Rockville Pike
Rockville, Maryland 20852

Andrea Blau, Ph.D.
4901 Henry Hudson Parkway
Riverdale, New York 10471

Joan Bruno, M.S.
Communication Technology Center
Children's Seashore House
4100 Atlantic Avenue
Atlantic City, New Jersey 08404

E. Lucinda Cassatt-James, M.A.
American Speech-Language-Hearing Association
10801 Rockville Pike
Rockville, Maryland 20852

Carol G. Cohen, M.S.
Schneier Communication Unit
Cerebral Palsy Center
Syracuse, New York 13208

Barbara Collier, LCST
Augmentative Communication Service
Hugh MacMillan Medical Centre
Toronto, Ontario M4G 1R8

Sharon Crain, M.S.
Sparks Center for Developmental and Learning Disorders
University of Alabama at Birmingham
Birmingham, Alabama 35233

Patricia Dowden, M.S.
Augmentative Communication Center
Rehabilitation Medicine, RJ-30
University Hospital
Seattle, Washington 98195

Judith R. Frumkin, M.S.
Schneier Communication Unit
Cerebral Palsy Center
Syracuse, New York 13208

Carol Goossens', Ph.D.
Sparks Center for Developmental and Learning Disorders
University of Alabama at Birmingham
Birmingham, Alabama 35233

Jayne Higgins, M.A.
191 Calle Magdalena
Encinitas, California 92024

George Karlan, Ph.D.
Special Education
South Campus Court E
Purdue University
West Lafayette, Indiana 47907

Louise Kent-Udolf, Ph.D.
Education Service Center
Region II
209 North Water
Corpus Christi, Texas 78401

Arlene Kraat, M.A.
Morton Roberts Center for
  Augmentative Communication
Speech and Hearing Center
Queens College
City University of New York
Flushing, New York 11367

Janice Light, M.A.
Augmentative Communication Service
Hugh MacMillan Medical Centre
Toronto, Ontario M4G 1R8

Lyle L. Lloyd, Ph.D.
Audiology and Speech Sciences
Purdue University
West Lafayette, Indiana 47907

Pamela Mathy-Laikko, M.A.
S-153 Trace Center
Waisman Center
1500 Highland Avenue
University of Wisconsin-Madison
Madison, Wisconsin 53705

Jane Mills, M.A.
191 Calle Magdalena
Encinitas, California 92024

Pat Mirenda, Ph.D.
Department of Special Education
  and Communication Disorders
Barkley Memorial Center
University of Nebraska
Lincoln, Nebraska 68583-0732

Adriana L. Schuler
San Francisco State University
1600 Holloway Avenue
San Francisco, California 94132

Howard Shane, Ph.D.
Communication Enhancement Clinic
The Children's Hospital
300 Longwood Avenue
Boston, Massachusetts 02115

Sheela Stuart, M.A.
Crippled Children's Hospital and School
2501 West 26th Street
Sioux Falls, South Dakota 57105

Gail Van Tatenhove, M.S.
Communication Systems Evaluation Center
434 N. Tampa Avenue
Orlando, Florida 32802

Gregg Vanderheiden, Ph.D.
Trace Research and Development Center
University of Wisconsin-Madison
Madison, Wisconsin 53705

Patricia Wasson, M.A.
Education Service Center
Region 20
1314 Hines Avenue
San Antonio, Texas 78208

David E. Yoder, Ph.D.
Medical Allied Health Professions
School of Medicine
Wing E, 222H, Room 234
University of North Carolina
Chapel Hill, North Carolina 27514

Kathryn M. Yorkston, Ph.D.
Department of Rehabilitation Medicine
University of Washington
Seattle, Washington 98195

# PREFACE

Augmentative communication is a relatively new area of clinical practice that combines the knowledge and skills of professionals from many disciplines. To serve the many needs of individuals with severe expressive communication disorders, specialized theoretical and practical preparation, in addition to discipline-specific education, is required. The *Leadership Training in Augmentative Communication Project* (Grant Number G008400718), funded in part by the U.S. Department of Education and carried out at the American Speech-Language-Hearing Association (ASHA) from October 1984 to July 1986, has addressed this need for preservice education in speech-language pathology and audiology. The educational materials that have been developed as part of this project include a curriculum guide for a graduate course in augmentative communication and this narrative, which is based on and enhances the curriculum guide.

The need for improved professional education in the area of augmentative communication was recognized at ASHA almost 10 years ago. The project and this narrative were a result of the dreams and plans of the Ad Hoc Committee on Augmentative Communication and members of the National Office staff, particularly Charles Diggs, who wrote the proposal to fund the project. This narrative reflects not only the dedication of professionals in the augmentative communication area, but also commitment on the part of two agencies, the U.S. Department of Education and the American Speech-Language-Hearing Association, to improving the lives of individuals with severe communication disorders.

Specific recognition and thanks to the following groups and individuals for their significant contributions to this narrative.

*President's Committee on Mental Retardation.* Every project has a beginning. The ideal model of the curriculum was developed by an interdisciplinary group of professionals (Shirley McNaughton, Michael Rosen, Howard Shane, Barbara Sonies, Bonnie Thornton, David Yoder, and Charles Diggs) in January 1982. The President's Committee on Mental Retardation, under the direction of Fred Krause, provided the funds to bring these experts together.

*External Advisory Groups.* We are indebted to the members of the project's *technical advisory group* (David Beukelman, Fromma Cummings, George Karlan, Arlene Kraat, Richard Luftig, and Gregg Vanderheiden). Their help in the initial phases of the project was invaluable. Each individual brought a high level of knowledge and skill to this project. They helped to define the format and the content areas for all of the project's materials, reviewed selected materials, and provided continuing advice, support, and counsel throughout the project.

Members of the *consumer advisory group* (Thomas Burns, Patricia Cashdollar, Kenneth Jaffe, Barry King, Mary Louise Ortenzo, Penny Parnes, Barry Romich, Gil Schiffman, Fran Schreiber, David Smith, Lana Warren, Larry Weiss, David Yoder, and Susan Yim) contributed significantly to the success of the project by reviewing and making valuable recommendations on materials that were sent to them by the project staff.

*Internal Advisory Group.* This group (Patricia Larkins, James Lingwall, Stan Dublinske, Alfred Kawana, Peggy S. Williams, and Dennis Lavery) contributed its support, suggestions, and the broad perspective of the fields of communication sciences and disorders, special education, and publications. These individuals were always available to help out when we needed it.

*Workshop Participants.* One hundred university faculty and manufacturers of augmentative communication aids and materials participated, with the project staff and the authors, at a workshop in Orlando, Florida, in January 1986. The purpose of the workshop was to impart state-of-the-art information, to further develop the educational materials, and to facilitate a network among individuals who teach in the area. The first draft of each chapter in the narrative was reviewed by more than 50 of these participants, whose valuable suggestions were incorporated into subsequent chapter revisions.

*Authors.* The contributing authors have brought their unique experiences and perspectives to this narrative, in addition to their special knowledge of augmentative communication. I believe that these individuals have contributed to each other's growth during the development of this narrative. They are a very special group of professionals; each is committed to imparting his/her knowledge and skills to others. I would like to give special thanks to them for contributing to my understanding of the area of augmentative communication. These individuals are willing to share, to grow, to change, to consider, and to challenge. That is, I believe, why they are among the leaders in this area.

*Project Staff and Significant Others.* Very special thanks to the staffs of both of the augmentative projects that I have directed at ASHA. To Thomas Davis, who provided expertise in word processing and who is largely responsible for the production of this narrative. His work has allowed us to reduce the cost of the narrative and to make it readily available to those who wish to use it. James Gelatt, the project's administrator, has provided guidance and unending support during all phases of the project. E. Lucinda Cassatt-James, a colleague and friend for many years, was always available to discuss ideas. Her valuable contributions to the augmentative communication area are well known. And thanks to Janis Froehlich, who helped us in preparing for and running the workshop in Orlando.

I would also like to thank Alfred Kawana and Anne Sundermann, as well as Joanne Weiner and her staff.

My greatest thanks go to Deborah Bruskin, the technical editor. Deborah had no background in the area of augmentative communication prior to joining this project. She could now teach a graduate-level course in her sleep. She has taught us all how to write more clearly and concisely, and her skills, dedication, and professionalism are unsurpassed. This narrative is largely a reflection of her talents.

There are other individuals whose love, encouragement, patience, and understanding were of great personal support to me this past year. Thank you.

This narrative is not an attempt to rehash the way it was; rather, it represents a new look at the augmentative communication area, a new attempt to make sense out of what we do, have done, and should be doing. In fact, development of this narrative was based upon a reexamination of what we do and why, when, and how we do it. For the opportunity and time to reflect and rethink, we are indebted to the U.S. Department of Education, and particularly our project officer, Martha Bokee. We sincerely hope that the goals of the Department (i.e., to improve the educational opportunities of children and youth in educational settings) will be realized, in part, because of the educational experiences now available to professionals who will provide services to these severely speech/language-impaired individuals.

The goal of the narrative is to create awareness and to impart knowledge. We have attempted to use consistent terminology, which is not always easy in an area as new as this. Even the contributing authors, many of whom have "been around for a long time," feel that we, as professionals, are just beginning to identify the pertinent questions. It will be years before we have some of the answers, and then, of course, there will be other questions that we have not yet thought about. The reader should not expect a cookbook approach. The narrative offers some different perspectives; we encourage you to form your own.

Contributors to this narrative hope to inspire and to challenge you. The future offers great promise for augmentative communication, and each of us can play a part. It is our sincere hope that ultimately, our hard work will improve the quality of life and the opportunities available to communicatively impaired individuals.

*Sarah W. Blackstone*

Project Director
*Leadership Training in*
*Augmentative Communication*

# TABLE OF CONTENTS

# CHAPTER 1

## OVERVIEW

GREGG C. VANDERHEIDEN

*Trace Research and Development Center*
*University of Wisconsin, Madison*

DAVID E. YODER

*Department of Medical Allied Health Professions*
*University of North Carolina at Chapel Hill*

## OBJECTIVES

- Introduce students to the area of augmentative communication.

- Introduce students to persons for whom augmentative communication is necessary.

- Discuss the various augmentative components that are used to improve the communication competencies of severely speech/ language- and writing-disabled individuals.

- Provide students with a chronology of events regarding the evolution of augmentative communication.

- Discuss major issues that professionals in augmentative communication must be acquainted with and knowledgeable about.

- Provide a glossary of some terms used throughout the text.

# INTRODUCTION

## *Augmentative Communication and Normal Communication*

Augmentative communication refers to all communication that supplements or augments speech.  Everyone uses augmentative communication aids and techniques.  Long before able-bodied children have access to speech, they interact with their caregivers by means of nonverbal augmentative techniques, such as smiles, eye gaze behavior, and differential vocalizations.  Such communication is evidence of early intentions and is powerful in its communicative effect.

After speech is acquired, we continue to use both verbal and nonverbal augmentative communication techniques extensively.  Birdwhistell's research (1955), for example, indicates that transmission of social meaning during conversational exchange is expressed more through nonverbal behavior (65%) than through speech (35%).  In some cases, augmentative techniques are used in combination with speech; in other cases, the augmentative techniques themselves are more effective than speech for some purposes or environments.  For example, written communication may be used for independent work, homework, and tests, on the job, and in many other applications where spoken communication would not be as effective or where permanence is required.  Writing may also be used as a "cognitive amplifier" when organizing thoughts, creating outlines, doing mathematical calculations, and so on.  Nonverbal behaviors, such as gestures, are often much better than speech at communicating certain thoughts or emotions.  If someone is sad or angry, it is often much easier to express those feelings through body movement or vocalization than through words.  The same is true for delight, fascination, surprise, interest, and many other moods or attitudes that must be conveyed.  Similarly, a quick gesture can be used to call people, to ask them to leave, or to express one's opinion or choice.

It is also quite natural for able-bodied individuals to rely heavily on augmentative aids and techniques in situations where speech is not effective.  In a noisy environment where comprehension is difficult, speech is often augmented with gestures, exaggerated facial expressions, pantomime, pointing to objects or actions in the room, or even written communication, all of which are augmentative communication techniques.  In a situation such as scuba diving, where speech is temporarily not possible, gestures or writing (via grease pencil and slate) may be used to communicate.  When one is unfamiliar with a language, or where a message is poorly organized, writing out the message often makes it easier to decipher and understand.  Thus, the overall communication system of an able-bodied individual consists of both speech and a wide range of augmentative aids and techniques.

## *Augmentative Communication and Disabled Individuals*

Just as able-bodied individuals must rely heavily on augmentative communication techniques in certain situations where speech does not work well for them, speech/language-impaired individuals must also rely heavily upon augmentative techniques. The more severe the speech/language impairment, the more a person will rely on augmentative aids and techniques to supplement residual oral communication.

It is important to note, however, that for most speech/language-impaired individuals, speech is not the only communication channel that is affected. The ability to use many of the standard augmentative communication techniques (gestures, facial expressions, writing) is also usually impaired. Thus, it is not just their speech, but also their nonvocal and nonverbal communication channels that are impaired. In addition, physical, sensory, and cognitive impairments can change the way an individual communicates and can change the individual's overall communication needs. In attempting to develop effective communication systems for severely impaired individuals, therefore, it is important to realize that just about every aspect of communication may be affected. Conceiving of the problem as just being one of providing the individual with an alternate way to speak does not take into account the many implications of the disability on the other nonspeech aspects of communication. Table 1-1 contains a list of some of the many factors that must be taken into consideration in developing an overall communication system for an individual.

## *Special Augmentative Components*

When communication needs cannot be met through speech and standard augmentative techniques (e.g., writing, gestures, facial expressions), special augmentative aids and techniques that have been developed specifically for use by individuals with severe expressive communication disorders must be employed. They have generally been developed for two basic reasons. Although some individuals are able to use them, standard augmentative techniques are not comprehensive enough to meet the full range of their communication needs. Because these individuals must rely very heavily or completely on their augmentative communication channels, more systematic and comprehensive forms of the standard augmentative channels were required. Specialized gesture systems and sign language systems evolved in this manner.

Other individuals are unable to use standard augmentative techniques at all due to their physical, sensory, or cognitive impairments. Special augmentative components were therefore required that could be used with their residual skills. For example,

**TABLE 1-1. COMMUNICATION**[*]

## REASONS FOR COMMUNICATION

Give Information

Get Information

Express:

    Intentions

    Beliefs

    Feelings

Get Listener To:

    Do

    Feel

    Believe

Solve Problems

Describe Events

Entertain

Learn New Behavior

Interact

Converse & Dialogue

## SITUATIONS

Setting:

    Home

    Neighborhood

    Work

    Recreation

    School

Communication Partners:

    Caregiver/Parent

    Teacher

    Friends

    Extended Family

    Employer

    Strangers

    Acquaintances

## REPRESENTATIONAL BEHAVIORS

*Verbal Behavior*

Spoken:    Written:

    Phonemes    Letters

    Morphemes

    Words

    Sentences

    Syntax

*Nonverbal Behavior*

Kinesics

Paralinguistics

Proxemics

Chronemics

(Based upon adaptations of separate works of Chapman, 1981; Brown et al., 1979; Higginbotham & Yoder, 1982.)

---

[*] The process by which meanings are exchanged between individuals through verbal and nonverbal behavior.

individuals unable to produce vocal, written, or signed symbols may be able to point to special preprinted graphic or orthographic symbols on a communication chart in order to communicate. Individuals unable to point with their hand may use special lightbeam pointers attached to their head. Individuals unable to point at all may use scanning techniques, where items are presented one at a time for their selection. Those who are also blind may use a scanning system where the items are presented auditorily for their selection. Special strategies are also required and have been developed to compensate for loss of facial and body gesture, intonation, and other components of the normal communication system that have been lost.

## *Multi-Component Nature of Communication Systems*

Whether we are talking about the normal communication system of an able-bodied individual or a special system for someone with a disability, an individual's communication system will contain both speech and a variety of augmentative components that are used together to meet the individual's needs. The major difference for individuals with severe speech/language and/or writing impairments is that they must rely heavily on augmentative communication components, including specially developed aids and techniques.

In developing expressive communication systems for severely speech/language-impaired individuals, therefore, the systems should not be thought of as being essentially different, but rather as being basically the same as those systems used by able-bodied individuals. The fundamental principles of communication apply, and professionals in the augmentative communication area must be well versed in (a) normal child development and language acquisition with all of its complexities, (b) adult language characteristics and impairments (aphasia), and (c) nonverbal communication. The difference between the communication system of a normal speaker and of an individual who utilizes special augmentative techniques is more one of form than of substance. Our perception of the complexity of the disabled person's overall communication system is due more to our lack of familiarity with the components than its actual complexity (McNaughton, 1975). The need to be more sensitive to the difference in communication form of individuals with disabilities is also evidenced in a study by Staudenbauer (1985). Staudenbauer reported that 2-year-old children with cerebral palsy were found to interact with their caregivers in a manner similar to that of able-bodied children. The parents were described as being very sensitive to their children's form of communication, and effective communication exchanges between the parent and child were observed. Although parents recognized differences between interactions with their earlier-born, able-bodied children and interactions with their disabled children, these differences related to the type of behavioral output (mode of expression) used by the children rather than to the quantity of the output. This study is important because the professional community has often assumed that young, severely motor-impaired individuals do not engage effectively in early communicative behaviors with their caregivers. Staudenbauer's results suggest that researchers who are usually unfamiliar with the atypical motor responses and vocalizations of their subjects may categorize the communication attempts of subjects as a *disordered* rather than a *different* type of expression. Further, the study suggests that if parents utilize different and expanded interaction strategies that are within the capabilities of their children, even more effective interaction patterns might be possible.

Emphasis should not be placed on the development of an augmentative communication system, but on the development of an *effective overall communication system*, one that includes speech and standard and special augmentative communication techniques as components of the system. In addition, a communication system should also include a wide range of communication skills (developed abilities) and strategies (tricks and methods for more effective use of techniques). Hymes (1972) defines communication competence as "the knowledge of when to speak [communicate], when not, and what to talk [communicate] about, with whom, where, and in what manner." This knowledge is as essential to effective communication as the communication components themselves. Training or development of such knowledge must be provided as part of the evolution of the individual's communication system.

## *The Study of Augmentative Communication*

Study in the augmentative communication area, therefore, refers to the investigation and refinement of less frequently used modes or channels of communication in our society and the application of these symbols, aids, and techniques with individuals whose specific disabilities prevent them from using speech and/or writing as effectively as able-bodied persons. It focuses upon all communication components, including speech. Study in the augmentative communication area includes:

- examination of various disabling conditions (cerebral palsy, mental retardation, amyotrophic lateral sclerosis, stroke, etc.) and their impact on an individual's ability to use primary communication techniques, such as speech and writing;

- development of specific strategies to facilitate the use of speech (i.e., speech approximation, electrolarynx);

- development of specific techniques and strategies to facilitate the use of standard augmentative modes (gesture, pointing, etc.);

- study and development of special augmentative communication components, such as signing, communication boards, etc.;

- study of the impact of using special augmentative communication components;

- development of strategies for reducing the negative impact of using augmentative components;

- development of evaluation procedures to determine unmet needs and the most effective augmentative strategies for individuals having a wide range of physical, perceptual, and cognitive disabilities (varying in both type and degree);

- development of strategies for more effective use of augmentative communication components; and

- development of appropriate teaching materials and training procedures for mastery of these techniques.


## POPULATION


Although everyone uses standard augmentative communication components, there are many individuals who, because of accident or illness, cannot meet their communication and interaction needs through standard modes of communication, including speech. These individuals must rely more heavily upon less frequently used communication techniques or must use special symbols, aids, or techniques. This includes individuals with a wide range of different disabilities that may leave them unable to communicate through the use of speech or writing. This condition may be permanent or it may be temporary. It may have occurred later in life, through accident, injury, or illness, or be a condition beginning at birth. If occurring early in life, the condition may also interfere with the development of language and cognitive skills unless intervention is done early. Table 1-2 summarizes the disabilities that can result in sufficient impairment of speech and writing capabilities as to necessitate heavy reliance on augmentative modes of communication.

It is important to note that the degree of disability may vary widely. For example, one individual with cerebral palsy may be totally unable to speak, while

## TABLE 1-2.  DISABLING CONDITIONS THAT MAY REQUIRE INCREASED RELIANCE ON AUGMENTATIVE COMMUNICATION

### CONGENITAL CONDITIONS

Cerebral palsy
Mental retardation
Severe profound hearing impairment
Deaf/blindness
Autism
Developmental apraxia
Developmental aphasia

### ACQUIRED DISABILITIES

Closed head injury
Cerebral vascular accident
Spinal cord injury
Laryngectomy, glossectomy
Asphyxia

### PROGRESSIVE NEUROLOGICAL DISEASES

Amyotrophic lateral sclerosis (ALS or Lou Gehrig's Disease)
Multiple sclerosis (MS)
Muscular dystrophy (MD)
Parkinson's disease
Huntington's chorea
Acquired immune deficiency syndrome (AIDS)

### TEMPORARY CONDITIONS

Shock/trauma/surgery
    (Accidents, intubation, weakness, concussion, tracheotomy, laryngectomy,
    severe burns to the face, etc.)
Guillain-Barré (may become a chronic condition)
Reyes Syndrome (may become a chronic condition)

another may have speech that is very intelligible. Still a third individual may have speech that is useable only with familiar individuals or when talking about predictable topics. It may be possible to use speech for 30 to 40 percent of an individual's communication, relying on other augmentative techniques for more complicated topics, with strangers, or in situations where the individual cannot be understood. There are also individuals who have little or no difficulty in speaking, but who are unable to write legibly or with sufficient speed to keep up in their educational or employment settings. Specialized augmentative aids and techniques may be required for these individuals as well.

The course of the disability can also vary greatly. Children with congenital conditions, such as cerebral palsy or mental retardation, will continually acquire new skills and abilities through the course of their communication program and their lives. Initially, they may need to rely heavily on augmentative components; however, as they develop and receive appropriate therapy and management, their speech and/or writing skills may improve. Individuals with temporary communication impairments, such as Guillain-Barré or postsurgical patients with temporary tracheotomies, will also see improvement in their communication capabilities over time. In this case, special augmentative components are needed during the critical trauma period, or until it is possible to reestablish fully functional communication through speech.

In contrast, in individuals with progressive conditions, such as amyotrophic lateral sclerosis or multiple sclerosis, communication skills will degenerate and will follow quite a different pattern. Traditional modes of communication will progressively become less available to them, and they will need to rely more heavily on standard augmentative communication techniques, such as gesture, eye gaze, and pointing, to augment speech and writing. As their condition progresses further, however, they may need to use more specialized techniques and aids that will allow them to continue to communicate and write despite their physical impairments.

Individuals who become speech impaired as a result of accidents and diseases that affect the brain and spinal cord are increasing. This is partially due to the increase in automobile accidents, the repeal of helmet laws for motorcycle drivers, drug and alcohol abuse, and increased longevity. Medical science has found ways to provide emergency care to save lives and to sustain life; this, in turn, has resulted in the need for special communication techniques for many individuals. Surgery for the removal of cancerous tumors from the oral facial region and the larynx may also result, in some cases, in the need for augmentative communication.

Thus, the evaluation and intervention procedures for severely speech/language- and/or writing-impaired individuals will differ depending upon the age of the person, the cause of the disability, the course of the disability, and the demands of the environment. As a consequence, it is necessary for one studying the area of augmentative communication to master the wide diversity of intervention procedures that have been developed in order to accommodate the range of physical, perceptual, sensory, linguistic, and cognitive disabilities represented by this population.

## HISTORICAL PERSPECTIVE

A detailed history of the development of augmentative communication is probably impossible to assemble, since it involves many disciplines as well as concurrent but independent efforts from different parts of the world. Much of the early work was informal and undocumented; as a result, many of the early pioneers will remain unrecognized. However, the area of augmentative communication seems to have grown out of three primary areas of effort that have converged in the last 15 years.

The first of these areas involves the use of communication and language boards. Work in this area was carried out in a number of countries, and evidence of the use of communication boards can be found in very early literature. The first documented systematic work may have been done by F. Hall Roe (cited in Goldberg & Fenton, 1960) on the development of his own communication boards. More recently, general documentation of communication board work has been done by Dixon (1965), Feallock (1958), McDonald and Schultz (1973), Sayre (1963), Sklar and Bennett (1956), and Vicker (1974), among others. From these efforts (largely clinically based) came many of the fundamentals about communication and interaction using communication boards and symbols, as well as some basic augmentative techniques.

The second area reflects efforts coming out of the work being done with hearing-impaired individuals. Sign and gesture systems originally developed for this population were later applied with physically handicapped, aphasic, mentally retarded, and autistic individuals (Creedon, 1973; Larson, 1971; Shaeffer, 1980). They were also used as the basis for developing other special gestural and modified signing systems for physically handicapped individuals. Research in language acquisition in primates also provided input to this area. Additionally, within the past 20 years, research related to speech and language needs of the mentally retarded person has focused on functional communication and the manner in which their ideas can be expressed. Signing (Fristoe & Lloyd, 1977; Kopchick & Lloyd, 1976; Reichle, Williams, & Ryan, 1981), gesture codes (Duncan & Silverman, 1977; Topper, 1975), and graphic, nonelectronic aids (Hodges & Schwethelm, 1984; Mirenda, 1985) have all been shown to be effective augmentative communication techniques for mentally retarded persons. Most of these nonspeech techniques have been in use for many years. This early work with mentally retarded individuals has influenced our more recent advances in vocabulary selection, as well as our investigation of the application of electronic technology with this population.

The third area of effort was originally based chiefly in Europe, and dealt with special typing and environmental control systems for vocal but physically handicapped individuals. The best known of these efforts were those of Maling, Jefcoate, and colleagues at Possum, Inc., in England, although work in this area was by no means confined to this group (Copeland, 1974). From this work came the early fundamentals for providing clients with access to communication aids and devices. Many of these interfaces and selection techniques are described in chapter 3. This work was first brought to America by the Canadians, who continued the work of the Europeans for some time before the United States became heavily involved.

In the United States, the different areas of effort came together and began to receive serious attention with the passage of P.L. 94-142 (Education for All Handicapped Children Act) in 1975, which guaranteed all handicapped children equal educational opportunities. For many years prior to passage of P.L. 94-142, the emphasis for individuals with dysarthria and other severe speech impairments was largely restricted to oral language. Communication boards were viewed more as a last resort than as a technique that a clinician would employ to assist a child or adult in the acquisition of language and/or facilitation of a full communication system. Sign language was rarely, if ever, used with nonspeaking individuals except for the severely hearing-impaired.

One might speculate that the negative attitude toward the use of special augmentative communication components in the early years was greatly influenced by the oralist movement in the United States. The philosophical arguments among educators concerning the appropriateness of teaching oral language versus manual systems for hearing-impaired individuals were widely debated for a number of years. The idea of total communication (i.e., the use of signs to accompany oral language) was introduced and seemed to result in a somewhat more relaxed attitude toward the use of nonoral language for communication purposes. However, since the advent of P.L. 94-142, and more recently the availability of high technology, attitudes toward introducing augmentative communication techniques at an early point in the intervention process have been much more positive.

P.L. 94-142 makes it mandatory to devise plans tailored to the intellectual capabilities of severely disabled individuals. This requires new techniques and strategies that enable severely speech-impaired individuals to benefit from all educational opportunities. Speech-language pathologists who had previously been told that the use of communication boards was unethical, and who had sometimes been fired for applying them, suddenly found such approaches to be the only rational mechanism for helping severely speech-impaired individuals communicate effectively. For ambulatory, mentally retarded individuals, various sign systems were introduced with real success.  This was also true with autistic children.  There were efforts to find different graphic symbols that would improve the efficiency of communication in nonreading, cognitively, and perceptively disabled children.  In an attempt to take some of the burden off classroom teachers and aides, more automated and electronic means for communication were also sought, particularly for physically handicapped individuals.  Aids and techniques developed previously to assist in writing were brought in and applied to other communication problems in order to provide independence in conversing and writing (Vanderheiden & Grilley, 1975).

An interesting trend occurred during this process, particularly with regard to electronic aids.  Although initial work focused on writing systems, later applications, especially with regard to portable aids, tended to focus more on the conversational aspects of communication.  This may be partly attributed to the fact that speech-language pathology played an important role in this phase and because, in most cases, conversation precedes writing in normal child development.  As a result, aids that had voice output only were often provided to individuals who also needed a writing mechanism in order to be able to participate in their educational programs.  More recently, however, the focus has broadened, and the total communication needs of these individuals are being considered.  We now recognize that there is a full spectrum of communication needs, including:

- quick phrases, expletives, and interjections;

- messages;

- interactional conversation;

- written communication (to others and self); and

- access to and use of computers and information systems in the environment.

The advent of high technology, and particularly the microprocessor, is facilitating intervention in all of these areas.  Individuals with more advanced skills are being provided with fully functional communication aids that can address all of the above functions.  Text-to-speech technology provides individuals with a "voice" and a level of intelligibility that continues to improve with advances in speech synthesis.  Voice output is also allowing younger children and retarded individuals to use aids.  Modern display technology now permits the representation of special symbol systems.   Animated  graphics,  when  combined  with  speech,  facilitate  both  the acquisition and use of gestures and signs. One can only speculate on the many additional ways that technological advances will continue to improve both the communication system components and the skill development programs for individuals using special augmentative communication techniques. It should be remembered, however, that some of the most powerful and effective advances have been and continue to be in such "nontechnical" areas as assessment techniques, training approaches and materials, and the development and documentation of better interaction strategies for individuals using different communication aids and techniques.

Other key events that have had a major impact on the area of augmentative communication in the United States were the ASHA position paper on "nonspeech" communication (ASHA, 1981), the founding of the International Society for Augmentative and Alternative Communication (ISAAC) in 1983, and the founding of *Augmentative and Alternative Communication*, the first journal in this area, in 1985.

## TERMINOLOGY

This text contains a number of terms that have sometimes been used differently by different individuals in the past. The lack of consistency in using these terms has made it difficult for new readers in the field, and has also made it difficult for experienced readers to understand and interpret the results of research and other writing. In an attempt to provide a more standardized terminology, the following terms and definitions will be used within the scope of this book. They are presented in logical rather than alphabetical order to facilitate understanding. A more comprehensive listing of terms is provided in the glossary at the end of the text.

*Communication*: This term refers to the process by which information is exchanged between individuals through verbal and nonverbal behaviors.

*System*: A system is an integrated group of components that works together as a whole. Within this book, the term will be used in several different contexts. The most common context will be in discussing an individual's communication system. A *communication system* refers to the integrated network of symbols, techniques, aids, strategies, and skills that an individual uses to communicate. For example, an individual system would be comprised of an integrated set of components, including facial and manual gestures, speech and other vocalizations, graphic symbols, conversation and writing aids, as well as specific strategies and skills for using these various modes successfully in a variety of communication contexts. An electronic communication aid would *not* be a communication *system*, but rather one *component* of an individual's overall system.

*Augmentative*:  The term augmentative means supplemental.  In this context, it means supplemental to speech.  Everyone uses different augmentative techniques (writing, gestures, facial expression, etc.) when communicating and interacting with others.

*Standard augmentative components*:  Those techniques and aids used by able-bodied persons to supplement speech.  These include ordinary gestures, facial expression, typing, and writing.

*Special augmentative components*:  Special augmentative components refer to those methods of communication that have been specially developed or refined for use by severely handicapped persons who have more limited abilities.  The use of special gestures, signing, graphic symbols, communication aids, and special selection techniques are examples of special augmentative components.

*Alternative*:  Used in conjunction with augmentative (e.g., augmentative and alternative communication), the term alternative acknowledges that there are some individuals whose speech is so impaired that they must rely completely on standard and special augmentative techniques--which for them do not augment speech but are alternatives to speech.  Because most severely speech/language-impaired individuals produce some meaningful vocalizations under some conditions, the term alternative is rarely used in this text.

*Mode*:  The term mode is used to distinguish between the different major channels or forms of communication, such as speech, gesture, and writing.

*Technique*:  A technique is a particular method for doing something.  In this text, the term refers to methods for the transmission of ideas.  Linear scanning, row-column scanning, two-movement encoding, signing, common gestures, facial expressions, and oral speaking are examples of different transmission techniques.  Techniques may or may not involve the use of a physical aid.

*Communication aid*:  This type of aid is usually a physical object or device that helps an individual communicate.  Communication boards, charts, and mechanical or electrical aids are considered communication aids.

*Strategy*:  A strategy is a specific way of using aids or techniques more effectively for specific purposes.  For example, there are strategies for communicating with an impatient person, strategies for stabilizing the hand for more accurate pointing, strategies for participating in group discussions, and so on. Strategies are perhaps the most important and least attended to component in the individual's overall communication system.

*Skill*: Skills are abilities that are developed over time and usually with practice. Pointing and spelling are two examples of skills. An individual's competence in using augmentative components is usually a function of both the number and quality of the strategies that have been taught (or learned independently) and the skills that have been developed.

*User interface*: Switches, touch panels, joysticks, lightbeams, and sensors are some of the physical means that an individual uses to control a communication aid. To "interface" an individual means to find the anatomical site and control mechanism or technique that the individual can use most effectively to operate an aid or device.

*Symbol*: A symbol is something that stands for or represents something else. A Rebus, picture, Blissymbol, word, ASL sign, gesture, or speech sound are all examples of symbols.

*Nonverbal*: Nonverbal communication refers to communication that does not involve the use of words in any form (spoken, written, or signed). Examples include communicative information exchanged through body movements, facial expressions, and eye contact (kinesics); vocal sounds accompanying verbal messages (paralinguistics); the way we position ourselves in relation to other persons (proxemics); and the amount of time it takes to express an idea (chronemics).

*Verbal*: Verbal refers to communication through words--spoken, written, or signed.

Two terms have appeared in the literature to describe severely speech-impaired persons, but are rarely used now. *Nonvocal* was abandoned with the advent of speech synthesizers and the realization that nonvocal downplayed the importance of vocalizations, speech approximations, and speech in individuals with partially functional speech. *Nonoral* also has negative implications with regard to the importance and usefulness of residual speech or vocalizations by severely speech-impaired individuals. Most individuals who require special augmentative components can produce some intelligible vocalizations.

## MAJOR ISSUES IN AUGMENTATIVE COMMUNICATION

*Effect of Augmentative Communication Techniques on the Development of Speech*

For many years, a controversy existed regarding the appropriateness of using augmentative communication techniques with individuals who were thought to have some potential for developing speech.  Concerns arose with regard to taking an "either/or" approach to the topic and the belief that use of augmentative aids and techniques would impede or prevent the development and use of speech.  Clinical experience has shown this not to be the case.  No research to date has documented a decrease in functional speech potential as a result of the use of augmentative techniques; in fact, studies have documented increases in functional speech potential (McDonald & Schultz, 1973; McNaughton, Kates, & Silverman, 1978).  The use of augmentative communication components has been shown to increase both the intelligibility and number of vocalizations for many individuals (Harris & Vanderheiden, 1980; McNaughton et al., 1978).  Two causes have been cited for the increase in speech intelligibility when using augmentative communication components.  In some cases, individuals may use their communication board to cue the message receiver into the general topic or idea, after which their partially intelligible speech is more understandable.  In other cases, individuals are reported to be more relaxed when they have a communication board that they know they can fall back on should their speech not be understood.  Being more relaxed, they are more fluent and more intelligible in their speech.  When they are not understood, they can simply turn to their slower but clearer communication aid.  For many individuals who do not yet have any intelligible speech, augmentative communication components often provide greater motivation to work toward effective speaking skills.  Through the use of communication aids and techniques, these individuals learn that they can communicate successfully; they also experience the meaning, pleasure, and power of effective communication and the feeling of being able to control their environment.  The slower rate of augmentative communication aids and techniques and their reduced flexibility in comparison to speech, however, is frustrating, providing great motivation for individuals to develop and use their speech capabilities whenever possible.

The above discussions, of course, presume that the individuals with speech potential continue to receive speech and language therapy.  Removal of an individual from speech therapy when an augmentative technique is provided will have negative effects on both the development of communication skills using augmentative components and on any potential for developing more functional speech and language capabilities.

## High versus Low Technologies

The application of high and low technologies is often presented as if they were mutually exclusive. From the discussions in this book, it should become clear that both are essential components of the individual's communication system. In the past, the use of higher technologies was limited primarily to individuals with higher cognitive abilities and advanced communication needs, such as writing and computer access. With advances in our understanding and application of technology, communication aids are now being developed that can be used effectively with younger and more severely cognitively impaired individuals. For example, aids that can provide immediate and consistent vocal (and sometimes visual) feedback help younger or more retarded individuals develop initial communication and interaction skills. Higher technology, however, does not necessarily mean higher function. Some of the most powerful communication techniques do not involve the use of any technology (e.g., speech, signing, facial expression, yes/no headshakes, and gesture). Even individuals with the most advanced electronic communication aids still rely heavily upon standard augmentative components. Thus, the need for lower-technology communication aids and techniques does not decrease when electronic aids are brought in to meet advanced communication needs. Coupled with the fact that electronic aids are very often not available due to maintenance, convenience, or hostility of certain environments, the need for a balanced system of low- and high-technology communication aids, techniques, and strategies can be seen. In short, "you never outgrow your need for low."

## Total Costs for Specific Communication Techniques

Cost is one of the key factors in the prescription of communication system components. In many cases, individuals are not provided with aids because of the perceived high cost of the aids. However, less expensive communication aids require the same amount of training time and more frequent assistance from others, thus raising the costs of these aids. In looking at the cost of a communication system, therefore, it is important to examine the costs related to:

- purchase;

- training;

- use (e.g., time for assistant or interpreter if one is required); and

- maintenance.

For example, in comparing the costs of a manual communication board to an electronic, conversational communication and writing aid, it is obvious that the purchase cost for the manual communication board ($15 to $100) is much less than the purchase cost for the advanced electronic aid ($2,500). If it is assumed that the training time for both, including vocabulary development, overlay preparation, and individual training time, is about the same, it can be estimated that training would take approximately 20 to 100 clinical hours. Even for a $15,000-per-year clinician, this results in a cost of $287 to $1,436, taking into account normal productivity and overhead factors. The cost to use the aids, however, differs sharply. The cost per year for the electronic aid will be limited to the electricity to charge the batteries and paper for its printer (estimate $50 to $70). However, the cost of operating the communication board could range from $5,000 to $16,000 *per year* for a user enrolled in a regular educational program. These costs reflect the length of time that teachers or paraprofessionals will need to spend helping an individual complete classroom and independent assignments. (The time spent in conversation is not included in these costs, since it is assumed that a second person will be present anyway.) At this point, the cost of the communication board is between $5,300 and $17,536, and the independent electronic aid is between $2,787 and $3,936.

It is also important to look at the maintenance and repair costs of the aid, as well as the cost to maintain and revise the vocabulary of the aid. Whereas communication boards require very little physical maintenance, the cost of maintaining an electronic aid is roughly 5 to 10 percent of the purchase price per year ($125 to $250 per year for our example). The time required to revise the vocabulary and layout of a communication board, however, would be approximately 20 to 50 hours. If done just once a year, this would cost between $287 and $718. The cost for updating an electronic aid can vary widely. If it, too, must be changed, updated, and redrawn by the therapist, the cost would be approximately the same. If the aid is user-programmable, allowing the individual to update and change the vocabulary (including the display, as is possible with some of the newer aids), there is no intervention required on the part of other individuals, and there would be no cost involved.

A comparative summary of the costs of purchasing and maintaining a communication board and an electronic aid is contained in Table 1-3.

In looking at the costs of providing an individual with a communication aid, therefore, there are two important principles to remember:

1. The acquisition cost of an aid is not the total cost. If funding is
   secured for the acquisition cost only, then it is extremely unlikely

**TABLE 1-3. COMPARATIVE COSTS OF COMMUNICATION AIDS (1985-1986)**

|  | *Wooden Communication Board* | *Electronic Communication Aid* |
|---|---|---|
| Purchase | $   50 ($15-100) | $2,500 |
| Initial programming/ training | $  800 ($300-1,500) | $   800 |
| Use (per year) | $8,000 ($5,000-16,000) | $    75 |
| Maintenance (aid) (per year) | $   10 ($5-50) | $   175 ($125-250) |
| Maintenance (vocabulary) (per year) | $  400 ($300-700) | $   200 ($0-400) |
| TOTAL | $ 850 initially + $8,410/year | $3,300 initially + $ 450/year |

that the individual will end up with an aid that can be used effectively, since neither the training nor the support necessary to use the aid are provided.

2. Communication aids with low acquisition costs may in fact be much more expensive overall.

Finally, it is important to note that the education of a severely or multiply disabled individual can cost between $60,000 and $200,000 over the individual's educational years, depending upon the type of educational placement. Without an effective expressive communication system that addresses a range of changing communication needs, it is unlikely that this individual will receive much benefit from this investment.

## *Aids as Tools*

Many augmentative communication techniques involve the use of an aid. It is important to remember that aids are tools that may be part of an augmentative communication technique, and not the solution in themselves. It is not uncommon to hear of individuals who have been provided with a communication aid and then removed from speech and language therapy, since they now "have a way to communicate." This would be equivalent to providing somebody with a piano and then removing him from music lessons, since he now has the ability to make music. An excellent discussion of this issue is provided by Rodgers (1984). For a communication aid to provide any benefit at all, it must be utilized as part of an overall training and skill development program.


## *Skills versus Strategies*

Two of the most important yet most commonly overlooked components of a communication system are the skills and strategies that go along with the aids, techniques, and symbols. Skills refer to those abilities that the individual acquires through practice and continual use. Strategies refer to specific techniques that are discovered by or taught to the individual. "Tricks of the trade," for example, would be examples of strategies, not skills. A carpenter knows many strategies for properly driving a nail, but must develop skills in swinging the hammer in order to hit the nail properly. Similarly, when learning to play golf, there are many strategies that can be taught to facilitate hitting the ball ("Keep your head down," "Line up the ball off your left heel," etc.). These are not skills that are developed, but rather strategies or tricks that are taught. An individual must practice using these different strategies in order to develop the skills involved in using them successfully.

Similarly, in communication there are many skills that must be developed. Many of these are motoric in nature, but others are conceptual, social, and linguistic. There is a very large number of communication strategies that people learn and that are responsible for the effectiveness of most of our communication. Yelling to get attention, the pointed use of a pause, the use of facial expression, and almost all of our expressions of speech are learned from other individuals. In some cases, these strategies have been taught directly in order to make us more effective communicators. For the most part, however, these strategies are acquired by watching other individuals use them effectively. This process of acquiring communication strategies begins at infancy and continues throughout life. Because this process is so natural to us, we do it unconsciously and do not realize the importance or impact of the acquisition of these communication strategies.

The importance of the distinction between skills and strategies in augmentative communication stems from the fact that professionals have little or no knowledge about which skills or strategies facilitate the effective use of special augmentative communication techniques, symbols, and aids under various circumstances with a variety of clients. Moreover, there is very little documentation of strategies. Physical disability, or even the nature of the aids and techniques themselves, may preclude the use of strategies that are normally used by able-bodied persons. Because of these physical and time constraints, different strategies are called for with most of the special augmentative components. Unfortunately, we are unfamiliar with such strategies because we do not use them in our everyday communication (they are as unsuitable for our communication systems as many of our strategies are for use with many augmentative communication aids and techniques). As a result, persons who use augmentative components have no good source for acquiring strategies, nor any good models of their effective and appropriate use. Effective strategies do exist and good role models can be found. There are severely impaired communication aid users who, because of physical disability, are quite slow, yet can still captivate an audience, tell jokes, and hold their own in an argument. They are genuinely interesting people with whom to converse. On the other hand, there are other individuals with much faster communication systems who seem to take all day to communicate, are unable to make their needs or desires known, and have difficulty in expressing themselves effectively using their communication systems. Some of these differences may be chalked up to the charisma of some users. However, the real difference in effectiveness is more correctly attributable to the use of strategies.

To emphasize the difference between skills and strategies, it should be noted that effective operation of an aid and/or technique is primarily a function of skills. Effectiveness in using augmentative components to actually communicate is probably more a function of the strategies that the individual has discovered or been taught (either directly or through modeling).

In training individuals to effectively use augmentative communication components, greater attention needs to be paid to the identification and teaching of effective strategies that help to overcome some of the constraints introduced by the use of special symbols, aids, and techniques. These strategies also need to facilitate the incorporation of augmentative components into an individual's overall communication system. Modeling is essential to this process. The effective use of aids and techniques by both the clinician and the disabled individual is important. Some of these strategies are described in this book.

## *The Interdisciplinary Team and the Role of the Speech-Language Pathologist*

Depending upon the particular needs of the client, the interdisciplinary team may include any or all of the following: speech-language pathologist, physical therapist, occupational therapist, educator, medical specialists, audiologist, psychologist, seating and fitting specialist, engineer, social worker, vocational counselor, vendors, third-party agents, extended family and friends, and, of course, the primary caregivers and the client.

The central role in initiating and coordinating the services of this team should be taken by the person most likely to initiate the recommendation for an augmentative communication assessment, based on this person's evaluation of the client's oral motor performance, language competence, and communication needs.  Further, this person needs to possess the knowledge of language development and communication interaction that will be essential to the client's success in augmentative communication. In most cases, the speech-language pathologist would be the person who best meets these requirements.

Therefore, the role of the speech-language pathologist in providing services to persons with severe expressive communication disorders (especially when serving as the team coordinator) may include:

1. assessing, describing, documenting, and continually evaluating the communication/interaction behaviors and needs of individuals with severe expressive communication disorders;

2. evaluating and assisting in the selection of the various communication aids and techniques in order to develop an effective repertoire of augmentative components;

3. developing speech and vocal communication to the fullest extent possible;

4. evaluating and selecting the symbols for use with the selected techniques;

5. developing (and evaluating the effectiveness of) intervention procedures to teach the skills and strategies necessary to utilize augmentative components in an optimal manner;

6. integrating assessment and program procedures with family members and other professional team members;

7. training persons who interact with the speech/language- and/or writing-impaired individual; and

8. coordinating augmentative communication services.

In addition to the above, another primary role of the speech-language pathologist is that of client advocate.  Although the use of augmentative communication is continually increasing, there remains, for the most part, a knowledge/experience gap in terms of the general public's acceptance and understanding of the area.  Successful communication development programs necessitate that speech-language pathologists help clients develop effective skills with which to interact with both speaking and other speech-impaired persons in their community. To achieve this, and to help clients secure financial support for needed communication prostheses, clinicians must be able to serve as client advocates-- educating their coworkers and communities about augmentative communication in general and their client's needs in particular.[1]

## *Personnel Preparation*

Current training should provide speech-language pathologists with competency in the areas of basic speech, language, and hearing processes. Training in competency areas specifically related to the development and use of augmentative communication components has not, at present, been incorporated into most programs. This latter training should include the development of competencies specifically related to:

1. assessment procedures for determining augmentative communication candidacy and selection of system components;

2. assessment of prelinguistic communicative interaction;

3. currently available aided and unaided techniques;

4. available symbol options;

5. the nature of augmentative communication interaction between unimpaired and severely speech/language-impaired persons;

6. development and evaluation of communication intervention programs specifically designed to teach individuals with severe expressive communication disorders those skills needed to achieve communication competence using augmentative communication components;

7. knowledge of the effect of appropriate seating and positioning on the user's control of the speech mechanism and on a particular communication technique; and

8. advocacy and funding procedures.[2]

---

[1] (Adapted from ASHA Position Paper on Nonspeech Communication, 1981)
[2] Op. cit.

Similar special training efforts are also needed for the other disciplines that participate in the augmentative communication service delivery team.

### *Interaction/Conversation versus Respondent Behavior*

Initially, we believed that our major responsibility for persons who did not use speech as primary means of communication was simply to "fit" them with a special augmentative aid or technique; everything else would fall into place. This meant that individuals who had not used speech as interactive tools for any part of their life would intuitively know not only how to use their special communication components, but also how to engage their peers and significant others in rather sophisticated conversation.

The early work of Harris (1978, 1982) demonstrated that this was not so. Children who had access to sophisticated communication aids did not automatically begin to use those devices as conversational tools. For the most part, individuals who had used augmentative communication for academic purposes, or to interact with family and friends, were being taught to do so in a respondent manner. Questions were asked of the user, and a single picture, word, or statement was made in response. Few individuals who used augmentative techniques were encouraged to initiate communication, and, if they were, it was to initiate simple requests. Only recently (Kraat, 1985) has there been a concerted study of interaction/conversation and the repair mechanisms necessary for successful communication between augmentative communication users and their speaking peers.

## SUMMARY

In closing, there are several major points that should be emphasized:

1. There are no augmentative communication systems--only augmentative communication techniques, aids, symbols, and strategies that are components of the individual's overall communication system.

2. Functional speech is always a component in the individual's system, even if it is limited to certain words, topics, people, or environments.

3. Speech is never the sole component of a person's communication system. Even fully able-bodied people have, need, and use a wide variety of standard augmentative communication techniques and aids.

4. Nonverbal communication plays a large role in normal communication. Some research suggests that, in some situations, nonverbal communication conveys more social information than verbal behavior. Nonverbal communication techniques are frequently underutilized in the intervention programs designed to develop communication systems for individuals with severe expressive communication disorders.

5. Special augmentative communication symbols, aids, and techniques have application with individuals who are temporarily without use of speech (e.g., in intensive care units), as well as with individuals with permanent speech and/or writing impairments.

6. Intervention must include teaching individuals how to effectively interact using the aids and techniques, not just how to operate them. The emphasis should be on spontaneous and interactive use rather than respondent behaviors.

## STUDY QUESTIONS

1. Name several standard augmentative communication components that are used by both disabled and able-bodied persons.

2. What special augmentative communication components for disabled persons were cited in the chapter that were extensions or elaborations of standard augmentative components?

3. Name 10 different functions or uses of communication.

4. In describing an individual's communication system, we said that it is composed of many different communication aids, symbols, and techniques, as well as skills and strategies. What is the difference between skills and strategies? Which is most often left out of our communication development programs?

5. Why it is important that a communication system for an individual include both high and low technology and both aided and unaided techniques?  List the many different communication aids and techniques that you personally use (for yourself, not your client.

## REFERENCES

American Speech-Language-Hearing Association.    (1981).    <u>Position statement on nonspeech communication</u>.  <u>Asha</u>, <u>23</u>, 577-581.

Birdwhistell, R. (1955).  <u>Background to kinesics</u>.  <u>ETC.</u>, <u>13</u>, 10-18.

Brown, L., Branston, M., Hamre-Nietupski, S., Pumpean, I., Certo, N., & Gruenewald, L. (1979).    A strategy for developing chronological-age-appropriate functional curricular content for severely handicapped adolescents and young adults.  <u>Journal of Special Education</u>, <u>13</u>, 81-90.

Chapman, R. (1981).  Exploring children's communicative intents.  In J. Miller (Ed.), <u>Assessing language production in children</u> (pp. 111-136).  Baltimore: University Park Press.

Copeland, K. (1974).  <u>Aids for the severely handicapped</u>.  London:  Spector Publishing.

Creedon, M.    (1973, March).    <u>Language development in nonverbal autistic children using a simultaneous communication system</u>.  Paper presented to the Society for Research in Child Development, Philadelphia.

Dixon, C. (1965).  Some thoughts on communication boards.  <u>Cerebral Palsy Journal</u>, <u>26</u>, 12-13.

Duncan, J., & Silverman, F.  (1977).  Impacts of learning Amer-Ind on mentally retarded children:  A primary report.  <u>Perceptual and Motor Skills</u>, <u>44</u>, 1138.

Feallock, B. (1958).  Communication for the non-verbal individual.  <u>American Journal of Occupational Therapy</u>, <u>12</u>, 60-63.

Fristoe, M., & Lloyd, L.  (1977).  Manual communication for the retarded and others with severe communication impairment:  A resource list.  <u>Mental Retardation</u>, <u>15</u>(5), 18-21.

Goldberg, H., & Fenton, J. (1960). <u>Aphonic communication for those with cerebral palsy: Guide for the development and use of a conversation board</u>. New York: United Cerebral Palsy of New York State.

Harris. D. (1978). <u>Descriptive analysis of communication interaction processes involving nonvocal severely handicapped children</u>. Unpublished doctoral dissertation, University of Wisconsin-Madison.

Harris, D. (1982). Communicative interaction processes involving nonvocal physically handicapped children. <u>Topics in Language Disorders</u>, <u>2</u>, 21-37.

Harris, D., & Vanderheiden, G. (1980). Augmentative communication techniques. In R. Schiefelbusch (Ed.), <u>Non-speech language and communication intervention</u>, (pp. 259-301). Baltimore: University Park Press.

Higginbotham, D., & Yoder, D. (1982). Communication within natural conversational interaction: Implications for severe communicatively impaired persons. <u>Topics in Language Disorders</u>, <u>2</u>(2), 1-19.

Hodges, P., & Schwethelm, B. (1984). A comparison of the effectiveness of graphic symbol and manual sign training with profoundly retarded children. <u>Applied Psycholinguistics</u>, <u>5</u>, 223-252.

Hymes, D. (1972). On communicative competence. In J. Pride & J. Holems (Eds)., <u>Sociolinguistics</u>. Baltimore: Penguin Books.

Kopchick, G., & Lloyd, L. (1976). Total communication for the severely language impaired: A 24 hour approach. In L. Lloyd (Ed.), <u>Communication assessment and intervention strategies</u> (pp. 501-521). Baltimore: University Park Press.

Kraat, A. (1985). <u>Communication interaction betweeen aided and natural speakers: A state of the art report</u>. Toronto: Canadian Rehabilitation Council for the Disabled.

Larson, T. (1971). Communication for the nonverbal child. <u>Academic Therapy Quarterly</u>, <u>6</u>, 305-312.

McDonald, E., & Schultz, A. (1973). Communication boards for cerebral palsied children. <u>Journal of Speech and Hearing Disorders</u>, <u>38</u>, 73-88.

McNaughton, S. (1975). <u>Symbol secrets</u>. Toronto: University of Toronto Press.

McNaughton, S., Kates, B., & Silverman, H.  (1978).  Handbook of Blissymbolics. Toronto:  Blissymbolics Communication Institute.

Mirenda, P.  (1985).  Designing pictorial communication systems for physically able-bodied students with severe handicaps.  Augmentative and Alternative Communication, 1(2), 58-64.

Reichle, J., Williams, W., & Ryan, S. (1981).  Selecting signs for the formulation of an augmentative communication modality.  Journal of the Association for the Severely Handicapped, 6, 48-56.

Rodgers, B.  (1984).  The holistic application of high technology for conversation, writing, and computer access aid system.  Discovery '84:  Technology for Disabled Persons Conference Papers (Christopher Smith, Ed.).  Menomonie, WI: Materials Development Center, Stout Vocational Rehabilitation Institute, University of Wisconsin-Stout.

Sayre, J.  (1963).  Communication for the non-verbal cerebral palsied.  Cerebral Palsy Review, 24, 3-8.

Shaeffer, B.  (1980).  Spontaneous language through signed speech.  In R. Schiefelbusch (Ed.), Nonspeech language and communication:  Analysis and intervention (pp. 421-446).  Baltimore:  University Park Press.

Sklar, M., & Bennett, D.  (1956).  Initial communication chart for aphasics.  Journal of the Association of Physical and Mental Rehabilitation, 10, 43-53.

Staudenbauer, T.  (1985).  An on-line analysis of communicative intention displayed by young children with severe physical handicaps while interacting with various partners.  Unpublished master's thesis, University of Wisconsin-Madison.

Topper, S.  (1975).  Gesture language for a nonverbal severely retarded male.  Mental Retardation, 13, 30-31.

Vanderheiden, G., & Grilley, K.  (1975).  Nonvocal communication techniques and aids for the severely physically handicapped.  Baltimore:  University Park Press.

Vicker, B.  (1974).  Nonoral communication system project 1964/73.  Iowa City: Campus Stores Publishers, University of Iowa.

# CHAPTER 2

## GOALS AND USES

HOWARD C. SHANE

*Communication Enhancement Clinic*
*The Children's Hospital*
*Boston, Massachusetts*

## OBJECTIVES

- To discuss the characteristics of individuals with severe expressive communication disorders.

- To discuss the goals of augmentative interventions.

- To determine which factors should be considered when recommending augmentative communication interventions.

## INTRODUCTION

It is difficult to determine the prevalence of individuals with severe expressive communication disorders in our society. These persons can be found in all age groups and at all levels of intellectual ability. They have a variety of disabilities and use many different augmentative aids and techniques to address a range of communication needs. In addition, the number of individuals who benefit from augmentative intervention has increased as augmentative communication has become an expanding area of clinical practice. Previously unserved populations are now being provided with opportunities to communicate that had not been available until recently. As the application of communication technologies continues to expand, costs are dropping and the quality of available options is improving. This is particularly obvious in the area of portable computers, graphics, and speech technologies (speech synthesis and voice recognition). Because of these advances, a wider range of communication needs can now be addressed using special augmentative aids and techniques.

In this chapter, characteristics of individuals with severe expressive communication disorders are discussed with regard to how their disabling conditions are affected by augmentative communication interventions (e.g., time of onset, length of disability, and etiology). Although the goals of augmentative interventions vary depending on the needs of clients, some common goals are presented and discussed along with other factors that should at least be considered by professionals prior to initiating the augmentative communication intervention process. Clinical management of individuals with severe expressive communication disorders should include initial and follow-up assessments, recommendations for intervention programs, prescriptions for communication aids and assistive devices, development of vocabulary displays, procurement of funding for aids and treatment services, and the implementation and evaluation of individualized training programs for clients and their communication partners.

## POPULATION CHARACTERISTICS

It is estimated that more than 2 million people in the United States, or about one percent of the total population, have a speech impairment. Between 200,000 and 1,000,000 of these individuals are estimated to be so severely speech disabled that they may require communication augmentation (Diggs, 1983; Montgomery & Hanson, 1984). Included in these estimates are individuals with mental retardation, cerebral palsy, traumatic brain injury, amyotrophic lateral sclerosis, dystonia musculorum deformans, Huntington's chorea, Parkinson's disease, head and neck cancer, spinal cord injuries, cleft palate, developmental language disorders, autism, apraxia of speech, hearing impairment, the deaf-blind, and the multihandicapped (Aiello, 1980; Blackstone & Isaacson, in press; Fristoe & Lloyd, 1978; Green & Hopkins, 1985; Kiernan, Reid, & Jones, 1982; Matas, Mathy-Laikko, Beukelman, & Legresley, 1985). Excluded are individuals who are deaf, and who are not otherwise multihandicapped. Surveys indicate that between .3 to .6 percent of the total school-age population and from 3.5 to 7.0 percent of students receiving special education services in California (Aiello, 1980) and Washington State (Matas et al., 1985) are severely speech impaired and may benefit from the use of augmentative communication components. To date, prevalence information about the adult population is lacking or based on conjecture. Also lacking is information about the prevalence of individuals who are writing impaired and who require special augmentative techniques to enable them to produce text, draw, or access data-based systems.

Unlike chapter 1, which presented an overview of the population, this chapter will give the reader a greater understanding of the diversity and complexity of problems associated with severe speech and/or writing impairments. The areas discussed include the onset of the disabling condition in an individual's life, the duration of the disability, and the etiology of the impairment. There is some overlap across the areas, but each profoundly affects the intervention process and should be taken into consideration.

## *Time of Onset*

Expressive communication disorders can begin at birth (congenitally based) or can occur later in life as a result of either disease or accident (adventitiously based). The time of onset affects both the course of treatment and the impact the condition has on the individual and the individual's family. Congenitally based problems, which are present in fetal life or early childhood and which preclude or impede normal physical and/or mental development (Scheiner & McNabb, 1980), necessitate long-term training aimed not only at providing a host of expressive communication approaches commensurate with developmental levels, but also at facilitating speech and language growth. Acquired forms of severe expressive communication disorders constitute a substantial handicap and are rarely completely remediated. Acquired conditions generally result from trauma or surgical removal or alteration of parts of the speaking mechanism, or from a trauma to or a gradual deterioration of the central or peripheral nervous system. Neurological trauma can result from an external agent, such as a forceful strike to the head or puncture of the cranium (e.g., gunshot wound). It can also arise from an internal event, such as a cerebral vascular accident. With acquired disabilities, the onset of an expressive communication disorder often occurs after the attainment of language, including literacy skills. Of course, if a language disorder coexists with a speech motor disorder (either acquired or adventitiously based), rehabilitation would include reestablishment of viable language or symbolic processes, as well as the provision of special aids and techniques. Rehabilitation teams recommending augmentative components should make selections based on the residual language available to these individuals.

In the advanced stages of several degenerative conditions (e.g., multiple sclerosis, amyotrophic lateral sclerosis), the speaking mechanism is severely affected. Because of the progressive nature of these conditions, the deterioration of speech intelligibility may be gradual. The best time to discuss the availability of augmentative communcation remains an unstudied problem. For some individuals, knowing that effective communication, albeit through augmented techniques, will always be available is comforting. For others, contemplating total speech loss while still dealing with the realization of the presence of the disease itself can represent a psychologically overwhelming prospect.

As intelligibility problems increase, management of the communication disorder changes. While speech therapy may be used initially, the use of augmentative and then alternative methods are eventually implemented. For example, a client that initially uses slurred speech may become unintelligible under some conditions and begin to indicate desired messages directly through finger pointing. Because motor control generally deteriorates in other areas at the same time that oral motor problems worsen, the client may decide to use an electronic aid because of an inability to point. Scanning techniques that allow single switch input and that permit communication to continue may be used. Later, the client's control site may change as a function of a deteriorating neurological status. For example, the client may become unable to depress a switch with a finger movement, but may use the blink of an eye to activate switches to produce desired messages.

## *Length of Disability*

The inability to speak is not necessarily a permanent condition; individuals can be temporarily speechless. Because conditions resulting in severe expressive communication disability can be related to medical or physical/structural factors, it is possible to be temporarily unable to speak even with an otherwise normally functioning speech system. Such is the case with intubated or tracheotomized patients. Further, patients who have had laryngectomies (or other structures important to speech production surgically removed) are often temporarily unable to speak. Additional surgeries and speech therapy may or may not enable these individuals to speak once again.

There are individuals whose speech cannot be understood regardless of listener familiarity or the context in which information is communicated. For them, the inability to communicate is a 24-hour condition. Other individuals are unable to communicate only when interacting with new listeners or when discussing technical or novel information. For them, time spent at home or in familiar environments with familiar people often results in productive speech interaction. An individual who is capable of communicating in this manner should be considered an "8-hour nonspeaking person," and interventions should be planned accordingly.

*Etiology*

Damage to the central and/or peripheral nervous system represents the most common etiology of severe speech impairment. For purposes of this text, mental retardation, cerebral palsy, speech motor disorders, and language disorders are all disorders that can result in severe speech impairments. Since many individuals who experience these disorders do speak, these labels cannot be equated with being nonspeaking. Severe speech and writing impairments fall into four general etiological categories: sensory (hearing and visual impairments), cognitive (mental retardation, language disorders, behavioral/emotional disorders), structural (craniofacial abnormalities, including a lack of anatomical structures necessary for speech and/or writing), and motor (speech motor impairments, paralysis or paresis of upper extremities).

*Sensory*. Hearing impairment is frequently associated with significant receptive and expressive communicative disabilities. Intervention with the deaf is not the focus of the augmentative communication area (see ASHA Position Statement, 1981). However, some augmentative techniques used with the severely to profoundly hearing impaired, such as American Sign Language, have been applied successfully with persons who hear but are unable to speak. Some individuals who are hearing impaired have other multihandicapping conditions that affect their ability to understand or to express thoughts and ideas beyond what could be expected solely on the basis of their sensory loss. These individuals can benefit from the use of special augmentative communication components other than sign. For example, low- and high-tech communication aids with graphic symbols may be required for individuals with mild to moderate hearing impairments, as well as those with more severe sensory impairments, if physically handicappping conditions are present.

Visual impairments do not interfere with speech production; however, they may preclude individuals from reading and writing in standard ways. Thus, augmentative communication aids and techniques are commonly used in educational and vocational settings to accomplish a variety of paper and pencil or keyboarding tasks for the blind. In addition, visually impaired individuals with multihandicapping conditions also may be severely speech impaired, thus requiring the use of specialized augmentative communication techniques to augment speech and to allow conversation to occur. Fortunately, several communication choices for this group of speech-impaired individuals are available.

*Cognitive*. Individuals with cognitive impairments represent a widely diverse and often multihandicapped population whose disordered processes of speech and language vary. Many cognitively disabled individuals are severely speech impaired. In fact, the severity of mental retardation seems to be directly related to the occurrence of speech impairment. The etiologies of speech impairments will depend more on the individual's other handicapping conditions (i.e., cerebral palsy, sensory impairment) than on the degree of cognitive impairment.

Because of the developmental and neurologic relationship between speech and language, a language disorder may underlie and be accompanied by severe speech problems. Similarly, disordered cognitive and/or social development may disrupt language acquisition because of the interrelationships among linguistic, cognitive, and social factors (Bates, Benigni, Bretherton, Camaioni, & Volterra, 1979; Prutting, 1982, cited in Wetherby, 1985). Severe receptive and expressive language impairments can be either congenital or acquired. For example, individuals with autism, which often occurs in conjunction with severe mental retardation (Ritvo & Freeman, 1978), have severe language and communication impairments. Nearly half the children with autism are described as semimute (Fay & Schuler, 1980), despite their intact articulation skills. Some respond favorably to augmentative communication aids and techniques. Adults with acquired language disorders (aphasia) also may benefit from augmentative interventions, but generally do not respond as favorably as children who experience language/learning disabilities.

Finally, emotional factors can contribute to an individual's inability to communicate (Cohen & Shane, 1982). The appropriateness of using augmentative communication techniques in this situation is unclear. For an individual experiencing elective mutism, for example, the principal communication goal should be speech production. Whether augmentative techniques can facilitate the attainment of speech or actually impede speech output or recovery remains an unstudied problem.

*Structural.* Congenital malformation, physical trauma, as well as surgical alteration or excision can result in impairment of the oral mechanism and a severe speech disability, and may necessitate the use of augmentative techniques. Some congenital anomalies are so extreme that speech output seems questionable. However, compensatory strategies are often needed only until successful speech production is possible. Johnston, Ferrier, and Shane (1984), for example, studied the speech development of a child born with severe microglossia. Results over a 12-month period showed a normal progression of phonological development with a mildly diminished phonemic repertoire. Some congenital malformations, such as those experienced by children born with severe midfacial clefts, may be so structurally incapacitating that various augmentative components will be needed to supplement speech production throughout the individual's life.

Trauma or surgery can lead to severe damage of important areas of the speaking mechanism, including the larynx, the tongue, and the soft/hard palate. For some individuals, surgical reconstruction will result in intelligible speech. For others, alternative voicing methods, such as esophageal speech, leads to "acceptable" although altered speech output. When speech is not a viable option, augmentative techniques, such as artificial/mechanical larynges, communication aids, and gestural communication methods, become useful.

  *Motoric*. Severe speech motor disorders, including dysarthria and apraxia of speech, are most commonly associated with augmentative communication interventions. Dysarthria and apraxia (or dyspraxia) of speech are recognized clinical entities in both adults and children and will not be discussed here. Individuals with speech motor disorders have varying amounts of difficulty controlling the muscles involved in speech production. Depending on the extent of their impairment and communication needs, they benefit from augmentative interventions.

## INTERVENTION GOALS

  The goals of augmentative interventions are varied and complex, but the primary goal is to enable an individual with severe speech and or writing impairments to communicate effectively enough to enter or return to society as a contributing member. This section contains a discussion of the important goals or expectations of interventions in the augmentative communication area.

### *Equalize the Gap between Comprehension and Production*

  Individuals with severe expressive communication disorders typically exhibit a notable discrepancy between their level of comprehension and their ability to speak and/or write. This discrepancy often cannot be measured by standard tests and is sometimes determined through systematic observations. Shane and Bashir (1980) suggested that a discrepancy between understanding and production contributes significantly to the decision to use augmentative techniques. Blackstone (in press) states that "communication augmentation should be considered in addition to more traditional speech and language therapy if an individual experiences or is at some risk for experiencing 'communicative dissonance,' a dissociation between communication needs and capabilities." Communicative dissonance may be observed in very young children, as early as 18 months of age, or in older children whose cognitive functioning has reached at least the 12- to 18-month level. It occurs when intelligible speech fails to develop, when the ability to speak is lost, or when physical or cognitive disabilities preclude the use of written language in educational programs or vocational settings. The degree of communicative dissonance experienced depends on the disparity between an individual's communication needs and capabilities. Thus, a major goal of augmentative communication interventions is to employ compensatory interventions that will result in enhanced expressive capabilities and a reduced level of discrepancy. The greater the communicative dissonance, the greater the potential contribution of augmentative interventions.

A number of factors can interfere with the attainment of this goal: (a) insistence on oral speech or writing by hand when it is unattainable; (b) an unwillingness to implement or use augmentation by the client or communication partners (which may be related to limited confidence in the aid or technique); (c) low motivation in learning to use an augmentative aid, technique, or strategy; and (d) the unavailability of aids or the services necessary to train individuals to use the aids effectively.

## *Promote Greater Participation in the School Setting*

P.L. 94-142 mandates that all students, regardless of handicapping condition, be educated in the least restrictive academic setting. The student with a severe expressive communication disorder is at greater risk than other disabled students of not benefitting from an educational experience. Normally, students are expected to participate in school through frequent speaking interactions, such as responding orally to questions, participating in spelling contests, reading aloud, asking questions, participating in groups, requesting clarification, and so on. The student who is writing impaired is less likely to be able to complete paper and pencil tasks. Performing mathematical calculations, taking notes, completing homework, or writing classroom assignments are but a few of the many instances where the ability to write is needed in order to fully participate in school. The ability to write underlies a successful school experience.

Communication aids, especially hi-tech aids based on advanced microprocessors, significantly increase the likelihood that these students can be educated in the same educational setting as unimpaired children. Educational opportunities are likely to increase if individuals can both speak and write, albeit through electronic means. As professionals realize the full potential of the computer, equal participation and fully mainstreamed educational opportunities can be made available to a greater number of these students. The computer can be a great equalizer--a tool that allows the nonspeaking student to compete with speaking, able-bodied peers.

For many severely speech/language-impaired children, full participation in a normal classroom is not always possible. Nevertheless, successful use of augmentative aids and techniques can permit inclusion in the least restrictive educational setting and allow for varying amounts of interaction and participation with able-bodied and handicapped peers and a more normalized educational experience.

*Enhance Vocational Opportunities*

More and better work opportunities are becoming available to persons with severe speech and writing impairments. Underlying these opportunities are improved communication technologies, the availability of positions that utilize technology in the workplace, and supportive work environments. Communication skills are very important within most work settings. Because of the availability of technology that can help impaired individuals to write, to access a computer, and to engage in conversation, the prospect of competitive employment is becoming more of a reality. However, even though individuals may be able to perform employable tasks, they must also demonstrate good work habits and be able to communicate effectively with employers and others. For individuals with mentally handicapping conditions, the ability to access or interact with a computer may be less important than the existence of effective communication skills or their ability to perform tasks efficiently (either independently or with supervision). Augmentative interventions should focus not only on teaching the mechanics of various aids and techniques, but more importantly on teaching the strategies and skills that will insure the successful utilization of augmentative components in various communication environments. Thus, interventions should teach individuals a range of communication skills (over time) that are transferable and will increase their future vocational opportunities.

*Promote Interpersonal/Social Interaction*

A principal aim of augmentative interventions is to provide individuals with the tools necessary to converse effectively. It is the ability to request goods and services, to comment on current, past, and future events, to specify preferences and emotions, or to simply "chat" that facilitates social and emotional involvement. Given the constraints of most communication aids and augmentative techniques (see chapters 3 and 5), meeting the conversational needs of these individuals is very difficult. However, the development of skills and special strategies does allow this critical goal to be addressed.

*Reduce Frustrations Associated with Communicative Failure*

Individuals whose language comprehension and intellectual development exceeds their ability to express themselves are predictably at risk for behavioral and emotional difficulties secondary to their communication problems. For some, frustration is expressed as a mild degree of annoyance, while for others, anger and temper tantrums frequently accompany the inability to reveal thoughts and needs. Depression and/or behavior outbursts, such as self-abusive behaviors, can result from persistent communicative failure. Augmentative communication techniques, when applied early, can lessen these frustrations and, in some cases, can lead to increased speech output (Shane, 1981).


## *Enhance Language Comprehension*

Augmentative communication components can also be used to enhance language development and comprehension.  This reflects a "total communication" approach, as advocated for the hearing impaired.  For persons who are severely speech impaired, there is a tendency to view augmentative communication aids and techniques exclusively as expressive communication tools.  However, augmentative communication components can facilitate the development or return of language comprehension. Interventions that focus in this area often include receptive language training for clients and instruction for parents, teachers, and other significant persons (e.g., how to highlight symbols that are signed or selected on an aid while simultaneously speaking the message).


## *Facilitate Speech Development*

Parents, spouses, and other professionals associated with nonspeaking persons frequently express the fear that utilization of augmentative communication components will inhibit or retard speech development.  A typical presumption is that reduced attention to speech improvement, or less encouragement to speak, will reduce the client's interest in learning how to speak.  Others fear that a communication aid will become a "crutch" that could be relied upon forever.

Clinical evidence to date, however, supports the position that the use of augmentative communication aids and techniques seem to facilitate, not inhibit, speech development, growth and recovery (see chapter 1).  Coupled with the natural process of speech maturation and articulation therapy, persons with poor speech intelligibility who use augmentative communication aids and techniques may become intelligible under some circumstances (see Silverman, 1980, for a comprehensive listing of clinical evidence).  In a personal communication, P. Parnes (1983) cautions that an initial reduction of speech may occur when an aid is first introduced, but that reduction is not permanent.  This writer has observed many instances of a lasting improvement in speech once the user gains proficiency with a communication aid.  Further, it is not uncommon to note that the spoken communication first heard actually mirrors those messages most often expressed through the communication aid itself.

## *Serve as an Organizer of Language*

Once augmentative communication aids and techniques are introduced, a language production problem may be noted. Apparent difficulty with symbol use, syntax, or the use of language may reflect the individual's lack of experience and skills or may be indicative of a specific language production disorder. In many cases, the use of visual-spatial symbols, such as those displayed on a communication aid or manual signs, seems to improve expressive language performance. For example, the "Fitzgerald Key" has been adapted widely as the organizing format for assistive communication aid displays. It was originally introduced by Fitzgerald (1949), who advocated the key as an organizational format for teaching grammar to the hearing impaired. The key, as well as other organizational formats, may be helpful to some individuals because of organizational benefits derived from the visual representation of a message (Vicker, 1974).

## *Enhance Speech Intelligibility*

Speech intelligibility, which varies across the population of persons who are classified as severely speech impaired, is not only a function of the message sender's articulation skills, but also the message receiver's ability to interpret messages. In addition, intelligibility is usually a function of listener familiarity with the speaker or topic, the type of communication environment, and the novelty of the message or amount of information contained in a message. For some, augmentative components provide the primary means for an individual to converse or write. For others, an augmentative communication aid, technique, or strategy serves as an occasional backup to speech. In this case, a well-planned augmentative technique can enhance speech intelligibility because the listener is provided with simple cues that contribute to overall understanding. Beukelman and Yorkston (1975), for example, report that speech intelligibility of some severely dysarthric speakers improved when the first letter of an intended word was signaled just prior to that word being spoken. Cueing a listener about intended topics or signaling (e.g., by spelling or gesturing, etc.) the occasionally difficult word can lead to an overall improvement in speech and/or message intelligibility. In both cases, by augmenting speech, a severely speech-impaired individual is able to use residual speaking abilities as the principal expressive mode and to use augmentative components as a backup mode.

## FACTORS TO BE CONSIDERED IN DETERMINING CANDIDACY FOR
## AUGMENTATIVE INTERVENTION

It is not possible to have generalized candidacy requirements for augmentative intervention because each intervention must be individualized.  The communication needs and abilities of individuals differ and must be developed before the application of certain aids and techniques can be considered.  A person with amyotrophic lateral sclerosis (ALS), for example, who becomes incapable of speaking and writing, can be provided with augmentative techniques that allow full access to  expression of ideas, wants, and needs.  To master the operation of special augmentative techniques, such an individual would take advantage of previously acquired linguistic skills (i.e., reading and expressive writing) in order to generate messages--albeit at a reduced rate and in a different manner than employed before the onset of the disease.  On the other hand, a child with cerebral palsy, in addition to learning how to operate assistive devices, learning  the pragmatics of conversation, and adjusting to atypical interaction styles, must also learn a linguistic system in order to generate intelligible messages. Finally, a multihandicapped adult with severe mental retardation may need to learn a small number of signals/symbols that are recognizable to those in his day program in an attempt to decrease the frequency of disruptive behaviors observed.  In each case, management of the communicative disorder is different because of the diversity of the needs, problems and future expectations of the individual, and the environments within which the individual needs to function.

Thus, requisite skills and capabilities will depend on the individuals and the environments in which they work, socialize, and reside.  The very nature of severe expressive disorders, as well as the nature of the instruments available to evaluate the person who is speech/language and/or writing impaired, makes it difficult to determine prerequisites to initiating intervention.  One reason is that communication technologies are providing more options for speech-impaired individuals.  Thus, skills once thought to be requisite are no longer essential to a particular augmentative aid or technique.  Furthermore, the population of persons with severe expressive speech and writing disorders includes many individuals who have little or no speech and/or writing competence.   One cannot equate this lack of ability with communicative incompetence.   Many persons labeled nonspeaking also carry other labels, such as severely or profoundly retarded, schizophrenic, or autistic, or have experienced brain damage as a result of a trauma, accident, or degenerative disease.  In any case, the real abilities of such persons are not well understood.   To insist that they meet this requisite or these prerequisites before beginning treatment may result in no treatment at all.   The severely speech- and writing-impaired population is replete with individuals who are "locked in their bodies" and for whom augmentative intervention may represent the only viable communication option.  To adhere to rigid prerequisite principles may impede trial and error intervention approaches, which are often necessary when little or no documental data about performance exists. The irony of the use of prerequisites, then, is that while we "require" or expect certain behaviors or abilities to be achieved before we begin a particular intervention or move from one approach to the next, the very nature of the disability often masks or prevents adequate or realistic appraisal of actual abilities. By suggesting requisite skill accomplishment, professionals may, in fact, prevent themselves from gaining insight into a person's true capabilities and skills.

## *Need to Communicate*

Not all people with severe expressive communication failure are enthusiastic about using an augmentative communication system. Acceptance, in fact, often varies as a function of the etiology of the severe expressive speech and/or writing conditon, the time of onset, the encouragement of others, and the perception of, or anticipation about, speech recovery or development. It seems to hold true that the more motivated a person is to use an augmentative approach, the greater their communicative success is likely to be. Persons who are newly nonspeaking as a result of accident or trauma are often less motivated to employ an augmentative approach to communication, particularly the use of communication aids and assistive device that have synthetic voice output. For many nonspeaking persons, the recovery or return of their own voice represents the only acceptable option. Nevertheless, these individuals may eventually accept a communication aid with written output once they resign themselves to their own inability to speak. For these individuals, when the motivation to communicate exceeds their desire to speak, they will utilize assisted output.

Severely speech/language-impaired children may also appear to be unmotivated to communicate using the aids and techniques that have been selected for them. Closer analysis often reveals, however, that their apparent unwillingness to use an augmentative technique may be related more to poor vocabulary selection, inappropriate ways of selecting messages, or a limited display layout than to a low motivational level. Thus, altering component characteristics of the individual's communication system may accelerate motivation. In summary, what appears to be low motivation may actually reflect an inappropriate selection of augmentative components and/or the need to train strategies and skills that will enable the individual to use a particular aid and/or technique effectively and efficiently.

As discussed in chapter 1, the decision to use an augmentative method can be influenced by the belief that such an approach will have a dilatory effect on speech recovery (in the case of acquired speechlessness) or speech development (in the case of congenital speechlessness). As described earlier, however, individuals should be reassured that use of an augmentative approach does not mean that there will be no further speech recovery or improvement.

*Motoric Factors*

Motoric factors to consider prior to recommending the use of augmentative components have been separated into three areas:  (a) sign-production; (b) selection techniques; and (c) seating/positioning.

*Sign formulation.*  Competent use of gestures and signs (see chapter 3) requires sufficient upper extremity motor control to formulate sign/signals that are comprehensible to the communication partner.  As a general rule, the more ideas and concepts an individual needs to represent through signs, the greater the motoric skills that will be necessary to represent that vocabulary.  Intelligibility of sign production is dependent upon coordination of *handshapes* in conjunction with certain *movements* within precise *locations* (Shane & Wilbur, 1980).

*Sufficient motor control to specify targets.*  The ability to specify target areas on a communication aid underlies the capacity to express oneself.  The techniques for selecting messages (e.g., direct selection or scanning) will vary as a function of the client's cognitive and motoric abilities and  preferred methods of control.

The ASHA position statement on augmentative communication specifies that no person is too physically handicapped to benefit from an augmentative communication system (ASHA, 1981).  It is possible to make this statement because of the technologies available to the nonspeaking individual for selecting messages and performing other communication tasks (i.e., ranging from direct selection to scanning).  For example, the availability of scanning allows a person to access targets and, therefore, to specify vocabulary regardless of physical disability.

Thus, an important motoric prerequisite to employing a communication aid is determining the optimal control site for a client.  A preferred transmission technique may change over time as a function of maturation, instruction, and rehearsal. However, at all times the selection technique should allow the client access to the greatest number of target areas in the shortest amount of time.  In addition, the technique should permit consistent, reliable, and nonfatiguing selection of targets (see chapters 3 & 4 for further discussion).

*Seating and positioning.*  The seating and positioning of a person with a severe speech motor impairment affects overall motor control, as well as the quality of speech production and the manner and precision of selecting targets on a communication aid. It is inappropriate, therefore, to evaluate motor speech production or to administer speech therapy unless a client's positioning is adequate.  Furthermore, assessing range of motion, a method of indication including control site for switch or joystick operation, needs to be coordinated with adequate seating and positioning.  It is not uncommon, for example, for the modification of a patient's positioning to actually change that patient's ability to use a particular selection technique.

### Communication Factors

Communication factors need to be considered in deciding whether to introduce an augmentative intervention. These include information relating to preferences, cause/effect behaviors, and signaling or indicating behaviors.

*Preferences*. Individuals who recognize and/or indicate preferences for items, activities, or persons from the environment are more likely to benefit from augmentative interventions. The incentive to communicate usually grows out of a desire to request preferred goods and services. It is also fun to communicate. However, when an individual shows little overt preference, little success at communication intervention will take place. Generally, relevant information on preferences of individuals with severe expressive communication disorders is gained through careful interviews with informed caregivers or familiar observers and during environmental observations. When little data on preferences is derived, it may be necessary to present a variety of items and to observe favorable reactions over time to determine an individual's preferences.

*Cause/effect*. The awareness of causal relationships between an individual's behavior and its effect on the environment is especially relevant. Early intervention for young, nonspeaking children, as well as intervention directed at older nonspeakers, therefore, often needs to begin with teaching the association between one's behavior and its effect on the environment. This behavior is especially critical to observe in nonspeaking persons who are physically handicapped. For them, the learning that occurs from interacting with the physical environment is severely restricted. Further, because of restricted spoken output, there is little opportunity to realize the effect or to learn the importance of speech on controlling the environment. At the outset, this training might entail the use of toys or other age-appropriate devices that can be activated easily by the operation of a switch. Later on, the power of communication, as the result of expressing a desire through aided or unaided methods, becomes an important tool in teaching an individual how to control the environment.

*Signal behavior*. An individual can indicate preferences through some observable or demonstrable actions. Signal behavior is intimately related to the motoric skill required for indication, that is, being able to signal through gesture, sign, pointing, scan signal alignment, and so on, is critical to the development of either aided or unaided communication. The signal behavior actually used by an individual is selected following careful evaluation. As a general rule of thumb, the signal behavior of choice is one which is least cumbersome to use and requires the least amount of interpretation.  Further, it is not unusual for a signal behavior to change over time as a result of maturation, instruction, and practice.  An infant with cerebral palsy for example, may initially be best able to specify information through eye gaze.  This method, although physically easy to control, does require another individual to interpret the intended message.  Eventually, as the child matures, he may develop the ability to point, thus reducing the need for interpretation and increasing his independence.

## SUMMARY

This chapter has attempted to further the reader's understanding of the population of persons considered nonspeaking; to detail benefits that result from the use of augmentative communication components; and to discuss certain skills and behaviors deemed important to augmenting the communication of individuals with severe expressive communication disorders.

Perhaps the most notable feature of the population is its diversity.  It includes both children and adults, some of whom have normal intellectual and language processes, and some of whom are born with significant handicapping conditions that render them severely speech/language and writing impaired.  Some individuals have speech that is sometimes understood while others have no functional speech.

Augmentative communication symbols, aids, and techniques offer many and varied opportunities for these individuals.  For some, a facilitation of speech sometimes occurs and an organization of language processes seems to result.  For others, intervention offers temporary expressive communication while they recover from surgery or await other compensatory or more permanent communication solutions.  Most importantly, however, augmentative techniques provide for enhanced communication opportunity in the face of severe writing and speech impairment

Because of the extreme diversity of this population and the range of augmentative communication intervention options, it has been suggested that determining requisite skills prior to intervention might impede rather than foster the development of enhanced communication.  Nevertheless, several motoric and language-related factors relating to decisions to introduce augmentative communication are discussed.

## STUDY QUESTIONS

1. The nonspeaking population has been characterized as diverse. Please explain.

2. The concept of the "8 hour" and "24 hour" nonspeaking person has been discussed. Keeping this concept in mind, please outline the principal goals of an augmentative communication intervention approach for a 9-year-old, dysarthric child whose speech is understood with 90 percent accuracy at home and 20 percent accuracy at school. Be sure to include goals for both the home and school settings.

3. Clarify and elaborate on the following statement: The establishment of obligatory prerequisite skills and behaviors prior to initiating intervention for the nonspeaking individual is often inappropriate. Give one example of how prerequisite skills might negatively interfere with communication growth of a person who is nonspeaking. How might they be a benefit?

4. Discuss your rationale for providing detailed information on augmentative techniques and aids to a person who has been recently diagnosed as having amyotrophic lateral sclerosis. At this time, the individual's speech is only mildly impaired and he can write. Also discuss your rationale for not informing this individual.

5. Accurate incidence and prevalence statistics on the nonspeaking population are unavailable. How might you gather such infomation. Be specific, taking into account the diversity of the population.

## REFERENCES

Aiello, S. (1980). <u>Non-oral communication survey: A summary report</u>. Paper presented at the annual convention of the American Speech-Language-Hearing Assoication, Detroit, MI.

American Speech-Language-Hearing Association, Ad Hoc Committee on Communication Processes and Non-speaking Persons. (1981). Non-speech: A position paper. Asha, 23, 267-272.

Bates, E., Benigni, T., Bretherton, I., Camaioni, L., & Volterra, V. (Eds.). (1979). The emergence of symbols:  Cognition and communication in infancy. New York: Academic Press.

Beukelman, D., & Yorkston, K. (1977).  A communication system for the severely dysarthric speaker with an intact language system.  Journal of Speech and Hearing Disorders, 42, 265-270.

Blackstone, S. (in press).  Augmentative communication:  A clinical management process model.  In L. Bernstein (Ed.)  The vocally impaired.  New York: Academic Press.

Blackstone, S., & Isaacson, R. (in press).  Service delivery in augmentative communication.  In L. Bernstein (Ed.)  The vocally impaired.  New York: Academic Press.

Cohen, C., & Shane, H. (1982).  An overview of augmentative communication. In N. Lass, L. McReynolds, J. Northern, & D. Yoder (Eds.), Speech, language, and hearing (pp. 875-890).  Philadelphia:  W. B. Saunders.

Diggs, C. (1983).  Leadership training in augmentative communication.  Proposal submitted to the U.S. Department of Education, Personnel Preparation. Rockville: American Speech-Language-Hearing Association.

Fay, W., & Schuler, A. (1980).  Emerging language in autistic children.  Baltimore: University Park Press.

Fitzgerald, E. (1949).  Straight language for the deaf. Washington, DC:  The Volta Bureau.

Fristoe, M., & Lloyd, L. (1978).  A survey of the use of non-speech systems with the severely communication impaired. Mental Retardation, 16, 99-103.

Green, J., & Hopkins, B. (1985).  The communications and telecommunications needs of the cerebral palsied population in Canada.  Government of Canada.

Johnston, J., Ferrier, L., & Shane, H. (1984). Phonological development of a child with microglossus. Paper presented at the American Speech-Language-Hearing Association, San Francisco.

Kiernan, C., Reid, B., & Jones, L. (1982). Signs and symbols: Use of non-vocal communication systems. London: Heinemann Educational Books.

Matas, J., Mathy-Laikko, P., Beukelman, D., & Legresley, K. Identifying the nonspeaking population: A demographic study. Augmentative and Alternative Communication, 1(1), 17-31.

Montgomery, J., & Hanson, R. (1984). Augmentative communication advocacy 1984. Presented at the Third International Conference of the International Society for Augmentative and Alternative Communiction, Boston.

Prutting, C. (1982). Pragmatics as social competence. Journal of Speech and Hearing Disorders, 47, 123-134.

Ritvo, E., & Freeman, B. (1978). NSAC definition of syndrome of autism. Journal of Autism and Childhood Schizophrenia, 8, 162-167.

Scheiner, A., & McNabb, N. (1980). The deaf population of the United States. Silver Spring, MD: National Association of the Deaf.

Shane, H. (1981). Decision making in early augmentative communication. In R. L. Schiefelbusch & D. D. Bricker (Eds.), Early language: Acquisition and intervention (pp. 389-425). Baltimore: University Park Press.

Shane, H., & Bashir, A. (1980). Election criteria for the adoption of an augmentative communication system: Preliminary considerations. Journal of Speech and Hearing Disorders, 45, 408-414.

Shane, H., & Wilbur, R. (1980). Potential for expressive signing based on motor control. Sign Language Studies, 29, 331-347.

Silverman, F. (1980). Communication for the speechless. Englewood Cliffs, NJ: Prentice-Hall.

Vicker, B. (1974). Non-oral communication system project 1964-1973. Iowa City: Campus Store.

# CHAPTER 3

# COMMUNICATION SYSTEMS AND THEIR COMPONENTS

GREGG C. VANDERHEIDEN

*Trace Research and Development Center*
*University of Wisconsin - Madison*

LYLE L. LLOYD

*Audiology and Speech Sciences (and Special Education)*
*Purdue University*
*West Lafayette, Indiana*

## OBJECTIVES

- Discuss the role of augmentative communication components in the lives of individuals with and without expressive communication disorders.

- Profile the breadth of requirements that a communication system must meet in order to be effective.

- Provide terminology that can be used to categorize the relative strengths and weaknesses of different augmentative components.

- Provide a theoretical framework and overview of current symbol systems and transmission techniques.

- Highlight the importance of strategies in the communication system.

- Demonstrate the need for multiple communication components within the overall communication systems of all individuals.

## INTRODUCTION

This chapter contains a discussion of the many different techniques and strategies that have been developed and described to date for communication. This includes both standard communication components, such as speech and common gestures, and special augmentative components that have been developed specifically for individuals having different types of impairments.

Before listing and describing the many symbols, aids, techniques, and strategies available for constructing an individual's communication system, it is useful to establish the context in which these components will be used and to develop a common vocabulary for discussing the techniques and their relative strengths and weaknesses. The chapter will, therefore, begin with an examination of normal communication systems and a listing of the functions and constraints they must meet. Discussion will then focus on a set of dimensions along which the various component solutions can be examined, followed by a description of symbols, transmission techniques, and communication strategies. Finally, some examples of communication system components for a specific individual will be given.

This chapter is designed to be read more than once--especially by those not already familiar with most of the concepts and information covered. The interrelationship of the topics makes it necessary to have some knowledge of all of the topics before entering into a detailed discussion of any. A first, straight-through reading is therefore recommended, followed by more detailed study. The chapter is divided into the following sections: system requirements, system dimensions, and system components (symbol systems, transmission techniques, and strategies for increasing the speed and effectiveness of communication). Study questions are provided after some of the sections. These questions should be answered before proceeding to the next section.

## *Normal Communication Systems*

As discussed previously, the communication systems of normal, nonhandicapped individuals consist of many different communication components. Although speech is used extensively by the general population, it is not always the most effective communication technique; other techniques, such as writing, facial expression, gestures, and symbols or signs, are used regularly to supplement speech. We switch back and forth between the different communication techniques (speech, gesture, etc.) depending upon which techniques we think would be most effective for the particular message, individual, and environment. Thus, we all need and use many different modes of communication to meet our daily communicative needs.

Different communication strategies are also used to meet communicative needs in different situations. Even when using a single technique, such as speech, we employ many different strategies, depending upon the topic, the environment, and the people with whom we are communicating. For example, when speaking with close friends and family, we often employ a shorthand form of communication, using small gestures or single words to convey what would otherwise require complete sentences or paragraphs. When we are with people who are familiar with the topic and concepts being discussed, we may substitute pronouns much more freely than we would with someone who is having difficulty in following what we are saying. If our message receiver is in a hurry, we also tend to shorten our communication and may not use complete sentences. In noisy environments, we are apt to speak more slowly, use simpler sentences, choose our words more carefully, and accompany our speech with gesture whenever possible. In fact, whenever our communication rate is slowed down, the entire form of our communication is likely to change.

A study by Chapanis, Ochsman, Parrish, and Weeks (1972) involved the comparison of two groups of normal individuals engaged in problem-solving activities. In these experiments, two individuals sat at a table with a partition between them so they could not see each other. One was given a problem to solve, while the other was given the solution to the problem. The study examined how each individual attempted to transmit the solution to the other. With one group, the individuals communicated by speaking to each other; in the other group, they communicated by writing to each other. Although the speaking group communicated eight times faster than the writing group, the writing group took only twice as long to solve the problems. The writing group also used only 118 unique words in their communication, while the speaking group used 1,564 unique words. The handwritten communication also exhibited drastically modified linguistic structure, including informally adopted rules for "telegraphing," abbreviating, and otherwise modifying the message while allowing the content to be understood.

Thus, what is "normal" varies greatly depending upon the rate of communication, environmental constraints, the communication partner, and the task at hand. Unfortunately, individuals who communicate using shortened or telegraphic sentences are perceived as having inferior language and cognitive skills (Creech & Viggiano, 1981) even though that is considered "normal" for anyone communicating at a slower rate. This paradox leaves many individuals who must rely on slower communication techniques, such as an alphabet board, in a "Catch-22" situation. The abbreviated form is normal for very slow communication channels, yet, when used, is viewed as abnormal by the general public. Specific strategies, however, can be employed to circumvent this, even for individuals who must rely on slower than normal communication techniques.

## *Multi-Component Communication System for Disabled Persons*

People generally do not use one technique exclusively for communication. In designing a communication system for individuals with communicative disabilities, it is important to remember that their systems, too, must be composed of many symbols, aids, techniques, and strategies if they are to effectively address a multitude of communication needs and situations.

The communication system for a disabled individual, therefore, should not consist of a single technique or aid, but rather a collection of techniques, aids, symbols, and strategies that the individual can use interchangeably. For example, an individual using an electronic communication aid may also have a manual communication board to use in hostile environments (rain, beach); may use signing or limited vocal communication for expressing basic needs to familiar individuals; may use signals (for bathroom and other important needs) that can be seen easily across a room and can be sent and received with little or no concentration or time commitment; and may employ a battery of skills and strategies for gaining and maintaining listener attention, communicating with total strangers, talking about topics not represented on the communication board or aid, and so forth. Provision of the system includes not only provision of the techniques (and any specific symbols and aids needed to implement them), but also the development of the *skills* in the individual and the teaching of *strategies* that promote effective use of aids and techniques in varying situations and environments. Such a system is referred to as the Multi-Component (MC) communication system. The following sections contain a discussion of the various techniques, symbols, and strategies that are necessary in order to provide an MC communication system, beginning with a look at the basic requirements of a fully functional system of communication.

## REQUIREMENTS OF A MULTI-COMPONENT COMMUNICATION SYSTEM

The diversity of daily communication situations results in a large and diverse set of constraints or requirements on an individual's communication system. In examining these requirements, it will be noted that many of them are mutually exclusive, or seem impossible to meet simultaneously. However, if one remembers that different components can (and must) be incorporated into an individual's system, and that it is the combination of these components that must meet the requirements, the task seems less formidable.

The list in Table 3-1, although not exhaustive, provides a good profile of the requirements that an individual's communication system *must* fulfill. Each of these requirements is discussed below.

### *Provides Full Range of Communicative Functions*

The individual's overall communication system must provide for more than just communication of basic needs. It must address the full range of an individual's communication needs, including:

1. communication of basic needs
2. conversation
3. writing and messaging
4. drawing
5. access to computers and information systems

*Basic needs* include requests for food, drink, water; requests to be moved, toileted, positioned; and basic statements regarding the state of the individual (hot, cold, sick, etc.). Often, these basic needs can be communicated in a very simple and straightforward fashion, such as gestures, vocalizations, or signals.

*Conversational needs* are much more complex and involve providing the individual with a means of expression in more complex and interactive fashions. Questions, discussions, arguments, jokes, explanations, and story-telling are some examples of the conversational functions that the individual's communication system must be able to provide (see chapter 1). Some needs can be met with limited vocabulary systems or prestored sentences. The bulk of our conversation, and that which is most interesting, is composed of novel sentences that are constructed on the

## TABLE 3-1. REQUIREMENTS OF AN OVERALL MULTI-COMPONENT COMMUNICATION SYSTEM: A CHECKLIST.

A multi-component system is a system of different symbols, techniques (with aids as required) and strategies that are used together to meet an individual's overall needs and constraints. The following checklist is useful in evaluating the systems of individual clients. Remember that the questions apply to the overall system of symbols, techniques and strategies, not just to a single symbol/technique.

Checklist for
Client's System

| Yes | No | MULTI-COMPONENT COMMUNICATION SYSTEM REQUIREMENTS |
|---|---|---|

A. PROVIDES FULL RANGE OF COMMUNICATIVE FUNCTIONS
- Communication of basic needs
- Conversation
- Writing and messaging
- Drawing
- Computer access (electronic communication, learning, & information systems)

B. COMPATIBLE WITH OTHER ASPECTS OF INDIVIDUAL'S LIFE
- Seating system & all other positions
- Mobility
- Environmental controls
- Other devices, teaching approaches, etc., in the environment

C. DOES NOT RESTRICT COMMUNICATION PARTNERS
- Totally obvious yes/no for strangers (from 3-5 feet away)
- Useable/understandable with strangers and those not familiar with special techniques or symbols
- Promotes face-to-face communication
- Useable with peers/community
- Useable with groups

D. USEABLE IN ALL ENVIRONMENTS AND PHYSICAL POSITIONS
- Always with the person (always working)
- Functions in noisy environments
- Withstands physically hostile environments (sandbox, beach, travel, classroom)

E. DOES NOT RESTRICT TOPIC OR SCOPE OF COMMUNICATION
- Any topic, word, idea can be expressed
- Open vocabulary
- User definable vocabulary

F. EFFECTIVE
- Maximum possible rate (for both Quicktalk & Exacttalk)
- Very quick method for key messages (phatic, emergency, control)
- Yes/no communicable from a distance
- Basic needs communicable from a distance
- Ability to interrupt
- Ability to secure and maintain speaking turn (e.g., override interruptions)
- Ability to control message content (e.g., not be interpreted)
- Ability to overlay emphasis or emotion on top of message
- Low fatigue
- Special superefficient techniques for those close to individual

G. ALLOWS AND FOSTERS GROWTH
- Appropriate to individual's current skills
- Allows growth in vocabulary, topic, grammar, uses
- New vocabulary, aspects easily learned

H. ACCEPTABLE AND MOTIVATING TO USER AND OTHERS
- Individual
- Family
- Peers/friends
- Education or employment environment

I. AFFORDABLE
- Purchase
- Maintenance

spot in response to the situation and conversation of others. The diversity of topics and uses of conversation, combined with the requirements for speed, make conversation the most challenging and difficult of communication needs to satisfy.

Most individuals will also require some means for *written communication*. Any individual functioning at or above the first-grade level will need some mechanism for producing written work in order to participate in the educational process. For example, a mechanism for writing is mandatory for anyone expected to develop math skills, or to take part in a regular educational program. For educational testing and assignments, it is important for the individual to have a mechanism for writing that is completely independent of another individual. Otherwise, it is difficult to secure an accurate assessment of the individual's abilities, since an assistant almost always inadvertently cues the communication aid user. Clinical experience suggests that when interpreters are used, there may be discrepancies of as great as two years between test performance scores and actual performance levels. An independent means of writing is also important for fostering individual creativity and achievement in the arts and sciences.

*Drawing* is a form of communication that is often overlooked, yet there are many times when we must revert to drawing in order to convey our meaning. Artistic expression is one example. However, drawing is used far more commonly for other purposes in daily life. For many areas of education and employment, the ability to draw, chart, or sketch is critical. These activities include geometry, fashion design, business, almost all forms of engineering, architecture, and even giving directions to one's home.

*Computer access* is a need that did not exist in the past and has just recently become a communication need. Computers are becoming an integral part of many school systems, and soon individuals who cannot use computers will not be able to participate in many educational programs. Computers are being incorporated even more rapidly in industry. By 1990, only a very small portion of the nonmanual labor jobs will not involve and require individuals to operate computers (Naisbitt, 1982). Similarly, libraries, shopping malls, and banks are increasingly using electronic information systems to replace their card catalogs, store directories, and tellers. This does not mean that disabled individuals will need to understand or know how to program computers, any more than we must be able to understand or repair a motor vehicle in order to use one. However, they must be provided with the means to access computers used in electronic communication, learning, and information systems.

*Compatible With Other Aspects of Individual's Life*

Components of an individual's communication system must be integrated into all aspects of that individual's life.  For example, augmentative aids and techniques must be compatible with a person's special wheelchair, the easy chair or couch at home, the floor, the bed, the prone stander, and any other place the individual may be. A communication aid must not interfere with the individual's mobility controls, such as controls on the electric wheelchair, or with the individual's ability to move and to communicate simultaneously.  Similarly, the components of the communication system should be coordinated with the environmental controls that the individual requires and should be compatible with other devices and teaching approaches in the individual's environment.  For example, a device that has voice output only (no printer) may be disruptive in a regular classroom when used for taking a test or doing independent work.  It may also be a requirement that aids be capable of handling existing worksheets, books, and other standard pre-printed educational materials if individuals are to join a mainstream educational program or classroom where these materials are used.

*Does Not Restrict Communication Partners*

The system should provide some technique that can be used with and understood by strangers and those not familiar with special techniques or symbols.  A totally obvious yes/no indication for strangers is essential.  This can be in addition to a less obvious but perhaps more convenient yes/no indication used with those familiar with the individual.  Since strangers may often come no closer than three to five feet from the impaired individual, they must be capable of interpreting the yes/no indication from this distance.

The individual's system should also permit independent interactions to occur with peers and persons in the community.  The individual's system should not restrict communication to those who can read and write or who know the individual's special symbols.  The system should promote or allow "face-to-face" communication and should provide a mechanism for communicating with groups of individuals.

*Useable in All Environments and Physical Positions*

The ability to communicate should always be possible.  Although it is not possible to have all components of an individual's communication system available in all environments (e.g., an electronic communication aid will not be used in the bathtub), enough functional components of the system (e.g., a manual board, gestures, etc.) should be available and operating at all times to permit effective communication. The system should allow communication in noisy environments, as well as in physically hostile environments (sandbox, beach, travel).

## *Does Not Restrict Topic or Scope of Communication*

If an individual can spell, it is fairly easy to provide a communication system that can be used to express any topic, word, or idea. However, for those who are limited to a closed vocabulary consisting of a small number of words (100 to 500), the provision of an open communication system (i.e., one in which any word/thought/idea could be expressed) becomes extremely difficult. A system should be as open as possible and, ideally, should also allow individuals to define and expand the vocabulary themselves.

## *Effective*

For a communication system to be truly effective, it must provide many capabilities, including:

- Communication at the maximum possible rate. This includes both a quick method for communicating phatic, emergency, predictable or often-used messages ("quicktalk"), as well as novel, spontaneous, and unpredictable communication that is more detailed and explicit ("exacttalk").

- A mechanism for communicating "yes" and "no" from a distance to allow the individual to interact with family members and others engaged in other activities.

- The ability to communicate basic needs from a distance, so that even when no one is willing and/or able to offer assistance, the individual can still communicate these needs.

- The ability to interrupt.

- The ability to secure and maintain speaking turns. This includes not only the ability to finish messages, but also the ability to avoid having people interrupt and/or "interpret" sentences without the individual being able to rebut.

- The ability to supplement linguistic content with nonverbal communication (e.g., kinesics, paralinguistics, proxemics, chronemics).

The system must involve low fatigue techniques, especially for individuals in educational or employment situations where long communication or work sessions are required. There should also be special, superefficient techniques that are useable by those who are close to and familiar with the individual.

### *Allows and Fosters Growth*

The system should not only be appropriate to the individual's current skills, but should also be capable of expanding as the individual's skills and abilities increase. The components of the individual's current system should either allow for growth (in vocabulary, topic, grammar, and functions or uses of communication), or should provide for a logical transition to more advanced components.

### *Acceptable and Motivating to User and Others*

The recommended aids, symbols, and techniques must be both acceptable to and motivating for the individual. Lack of use, or the unwillingness of the individual to utilize the components in certain environments, may otherwise result. Similarly, they must be acceptable to the family, to peers and friends, and to those in the individual's educational or work environments, or the offending components may be ignored or not made available to the individual. The system should also be motivating or interesting to others. Some incentives must exist if partners are going to expend the necessary time and energy required to implement and use augmentative communication techniques. A motivating system can also encourage partners to assist in improving the individual's system by developing strategies, increasing the individual's vocabulary, and so on.

### *Affordable*

Although cost should not be a primary consideration, it is, unfortunately, a major constraint. Different techniques have a variety of associated costs for purchase, training, use, and maintenance. Attention should be paid to the relative costs of alternatives that may provide the same or similar functions. Often, the funding for purchase of the aid is the easiest to secure, since it is a one-time cost. However, the cost to maintain, update, revise the vocabulary, and repair aids must also be carefully considered. These costs, which may be quite high, recur yearly, and third-party funding sources, such as Medicaid or insurance policies, may not continue to cover them, even though they covered the initial purchase of the aid.

In considering relative costs, another important factor to consider is the cost for an assistant to aid the individual with a nonindependent technique, such as a manual communication board. Having another person available to assist the individual for even one year to allow him to complete assignments, independent work, tests, and homework using a communication board usually costs many times the purchase price of an automated communication aid. Thus, the manual communication board can often be more expensive than automated counterparts. Unfortunately, the solution to the cost problem is usually to provide the individual with a manual communication board and not provide the assistant required to allow him to use it. Use of an assistant also raises the problems discussed earlier regarding the inadvertent help that the disabled individual gains from an assistant in the completion of tests, assignments, and other activities.

Clearly, all of the requirements listed above cannot be met by a single communication technique or aid. Yet, all must be met if the individual is to have an effective system for communication. Thus, it is essential to view an individual's system in terms of a combination of complementary components, each providing a certain function that compensates for the weaknesses of another component. Developing good communication systems for individuals, therefore, requires a thorough understanding of different aids, techniques, symbol sets and systems, and strategies as well as each of their strengths and weaknesses.

## DIMENSIONS OF COMMUNICATION SYSTEM COMPONENTS

Before reviewing specific augmentative communication components, it is useful to discuss some dimensions that can be used to judge the relative advantages of each component in meeting the requirements discussed previously. A summary of the functional dimensions to be used in this chapter is presented in Table 3-2. As illustrated in this table, evaluation of the usefulness of each technique is a multidimensional task. Note also that different features or capabilities of an aid or technique may relate to several of the requirements discussed earlier. For example, the independence dimension relates to effectiveness, motivation, and cost requirements for a communication system. The three primary categories of functional dimensions include functionality/ability to meet needs, availability/useability, and accept-

## TABLE 3-2.  FUNCTIONAL DIMENSIONS OF INDIVIDUAL SYSTEM COMPONENTS.

(These may apply to the symbol portion of a technique, to the transmission mode, or to both.)

| DIMENSION | DEFINITION | IMPORTANCE/IMPACT |
|---|---|---|
| **FUNCTIONALITY/ABILITY TO MEET NEEDS** | | |
| OPENNESS | Ability to express any thought | - Reduces topic limitations<br>- Allows individual to advance on own |
| SPEED | Rate of communication | - Provides more effective system<br>- Easier for younger and retarded |
| ASSERTABILITY | Ability to interrupt; resist interruptions; and control conversation | - Provides more effective system<br>- Prevents frustration, shutdown |
| DISPLAY PERMANENCE | Permanence of the presentation or display (temporary dynamic, temporary static, displayed, printed) | - Meets writing needs<br>- Provides time to decipher<br>- Provides access to other words through cues<br>- Improves rate of communication; not necessary to wait for message receiver<br>- Provides feedback for growth, learning |
| PROJECTION | Ability to communicate from a distance | - Allows communication to/with groups<br>- Allows communication at a distance |
| CORRECTABILITY | Ability to unambiguously repair or correct utterances | - Improves clarity<br>- Allows accurate representation<br>- Facilitates learning<br>- Increases motivation |
| EXPANDABILITY | Ability of users to expand the vocabulary | - Allows user to expand topics<br>- Allows vocabulary growth |
| **AVAILABILITY/USEABILITY** | | |
| PORTABILITY | Ability to conveniently stay with the person at all times | - Can be with user in all environments |
| POSITION INDEPENDENCE | Ability to be used in any and all positions (wheelchair, couch, standing, lying down) | - Increases availability<br>- Allows use with people available only in certain environments |
| INDEPENDENCE | Ability to be used without an assistant or interpreter | - Increases effectiveness<br>- Increases motivation<br>- Lowers cost to use |
| INTELLIGIBILITY/ OBVIOUSNESS | Ability to be understood by strangers | - Increases potential communication partners, strangers<br>- Facilitates learning |
| APPROPRIATENESS | Appropriate to individual's current and future abilities (physical, cognitive, language, etc.) | - Increased effectiveness<br>- Facilitates growth |
| DURABILITY | Ruggedness, reliability | - Is more often available for use (not broken)<br>- Can go with user to more places |
| TOTAL COST | Cost of purchase, maintenance, training and assistants or aides required for use | - Decreases cost |
| **ACCEPTABILITY/COMPATIBILITY WITH ENVIRONMENT** | | |
| COSMESIS | Appearance, attractiveness | - Improves acceptability to user, others<br>- Increases communication partners (e.g., isn't removed in public) |
| MATERIALS/PRACTICE COMPATIBILITY | Compatibility of technique with materials & practices of educational or employment settings | - Facilitates use at school or job<br>- Increases acceptability to teachers, employers |
| SIMILARITY | Similarity to communication system of peers & community | - Allows more communication partners<br>- Increases number of models for the user<br>- Is more acceptable |
| TRAINING | Amount of training required of user, clinicians, others | - Improves ability to learn how to use the system when resources are limited<br>- Reduces cost overall |
| ADAPTABILITY | Ability to be customized to individual's needs, abilities, and constraints | - Facilitates adaptation to user's other aids<br>- Facilitates vocabulary customization<br>- Allows fine tuning for speed, function |
| INTERDEVICE COMPATIBILITY | Ability to use with other standard devices in the environment | - Allows access to electronic communication, learning or information systems in environment<br>- Allows control of devices in environment |
| COMPUTER COMPATIBILITY | Ability to implement the technique (or symbols) on standard computers | - Provides low cost writing system<br>- Allows computer aided teaching |

ability/compatibility with the environment. Within these categories, the items are listed roughly in order of importance. Note that requirements (Table 3-1), as discussed in this section, are in italics.


### *Functionality/Ability to Meet Needs*

The first group of dimensions relates to the ability of the particular augmentative component to meet the different communication needs of the individual.

*Openness*. This dimension refers to the ability of the system to allow the individual to express any thought. In general, aids with closed vocabulary displays, such as picture boards, would rate low on this dimension. Symbol systems that allow access to new words by combining symbols, such as Blissymbols, would rate higher. Techniques that allow full access to vocabulary, such as spelling or use of phonemes, would rate highest (assuming that the individual could spell or sound out any word desired). Openness is most important for providing the user with *unrestricted access to any topic*. Openness also facilitates independent *growth potential* with regard to vocabulary.

*Speed*. This dimension involves the rate of message transmission possible using an aid or technique. Calculations of speed should take into account the individual's accuracy or correction time. This is one of the dimensions where techniques cannot be rated on an absolute basis. The relative speed of communication on different techniques will vary for different users. The fastest technique for one individual may be the slowest technique, or an impossible technique, for another individual. Speed is one of the most important dimensions. Many persons simply will not converse with a slow communicator. Others will interact for a short period of time if the individual is brief and to the point. Thus, speed affects both *access to all communication partners* and the *effectiveness* of the communication technique. Quick, direct-selection techniques (e.g., words and phrases) would rate high and would be easier for young and retarded individuals *to learn*. Signing, for an individual with full motor control of the hands, would rate high on this dimension. Heavily time-dependent techniques, such as scanning, generally rate low on this dimension, as do techniques that require spelling out words letter by letter.

*Assertability*. This dimension refers to the ability to interrupt, to resist interruptions, and to control conversation. Certain techniques and aids, such as communication boards, are totally dependent on the attention of the message receiver, thus providing the receiver with complete control of the conversation. Techniques such as signing or automated voice output devices allow individuals to interrupt others, make themselves heard over others, and call up prestored phrases to comment or assert control.  Assertability is very important to the *effectiveness* of the communication system.  It also helps to prevent frustration and shut-down by individuals due to an inability to express themselves.  This contributes to both the *growth potential* requirement and the *motivation* requirement.

*Display permanence*.  This dimension, which refers to the temporal nature of the presentation or display, varies greatly between techniques.  Some of the categories along this continuum include:

- temporary, dynamic presentations, such as speech, signing, and gestures;

- temporary, static presentations, such as fingerspelling and pointing to pictures on a communication board;

- erasable, full-sentence presentations, such as words or symbol messages on an electronic display; and

- permanent, printed displays.

This dimension is important for addressing a wide range of the required qualities of the overall system.  If an aid provides a permanent or printed display, it would fulfill the *writing* requirement.  It can increase *access to potential communication partners* by allowing persons less familiar with the communication system time to study and decipher the individual's messages.  Use of a permanent display can also be important in allowing the individual to *express any words,* including those not on the selection display by putting up a number of "clues" on the output display that another person can study.  For particularly fast pointers, a display that will accumulate letters or message elements will allow them to communicate *at the maximum possible rate* by eliminating the need to wait for the message receiver to register each element as it is indicated.  This addresses one of the key *effectiveness* requirements.  Finally, the display that provides feedback to the individual can facilitate the *growth* and *learning potential* for the individual.

*Projection*.  This dimension refers to the ability of a technique to be used from a distance.  In addition to facilitating communication with groups, it is also important for attracting the attention of others, drawing them into communication, and encouraging conversation with individuals who are busily engaged in other activities.  Techniques with voice output rate highest, since they both project and do not require visual attention on the part of the message receiver.  Signs, gestures, and facial expressions would come next.  Systems such as pointing communication boards or manually scanned communication boards, which require close and careful attention, would rate lowest on this dimension.

*Correctability*. This dimension refers to the ability to unambiguously repair or correct an utterance. This can be done with nondisplay-based techniques, but it is easiest with visible, correctable displays. The ability to correct mistakes can affect the *effectiveness* of the individual's overall communication system by clarifying communications and providing a truer representation of the individuals's skills. It can also greatly facilitate *learning* and *motivation* in using a device. Aids with output displays would rate highest here. Next would be nondisplay techniques that allow the individual to maintain control of communication, such as signing. The lowest ratings would be for nondisplay-based techniques that are message-receiver dominated or controlled, such as manual scanning on communication boards.

*Expandability*. This dimension refers to the ability of techniques to expand easily through the addition of new vocabulary items or new ways to use existing vocabulary. The individual, as well as others in the environment, must be capable of expanding the system. Expandability is important for *growth* in the individual's system and for allowing the individual to expand or tailor the system to address new topic areas as they become of interest (*unrestricted access to novel expressions*). Preprinted communication boards, or techniques that have predefined, fixed vocabularies, would rate very low. User-programmable aids or techniques would rate high, as would techniques such as natural speech, where the user can add vocabulary spontaneously.

## *Availability/Useability*

The second group of dimensions in Table 3-2 deals with the availability of a technique in a form that is useable in the individual's current position and with the desired communication partner.

*Portability*. This dimension refers to the capability to have the communication aid available at all times. Techniques such as signing, gesturing, and use of facial expressions rate highest since they provide *unrestricted availability*. Stationary aids and computers that plug into the wall rate very low on this dimension.

*Position independence*. This dimension refers to the capability to use the technique in any positions in which the individual may find him/herself. Techniques that an individual can only use when optimally positioned would rate low along this dimension (e.g., handpointing, if the individual could only point accurately when in the special seating system in a wheelchair). Techniques that can be used in all positions (e.g., in the wheelchair, in the family easy chair, or on the couch, on a standing board, when lying on the floor, or in bed) score high on this dimension.  The rating of any technique is highly dependent upon the skills of the individual.  There are some techniques and aids, however, that rank generally better in this category, such as eye gaze or facial techniques, while others rank generally lower, such as a headstick.  Techniques that have position independence are important to enable the individual to *function in all environments* and *positions* and to have *access to all potential communication partners*.  For example, many children are never in their wheelchairs while at home and cannot use their special communication boards or other aids when seated on the couch or the floor.

*Independence*.  This dimension refers to the ability of an individual to use an aid or technique without help from an assistant or interpreter.   Aids such as communication boards require the constant attendance of an assistant, particularly for writing needs.  This restricts the *availability of the aid* to those times when an assistant is present, even though the communication board may always be in front of the individual.  In addition, the assistant often interprets the individual's communication and may anticipate (sometimes incorrectly) the individual's words or intentions.  Techniques such as signing rate high in some environments (when people know the signs) and low in others, especially in public.  Independence is important to the overall *effectiveness* of the system, particularly when addressing *writing* needs.  It is also important to *motivation* and to *affordability* when an assistant must be hired to assist in the use of the aid or technique.

*Intelligibility/obviousness*.  This dimension refers to the ability of the technique to be understood by strangers.  "Iconicity" (i.e., the degree to which something looks like what it represents) of symbol systems would affect this dimension, as would the familiarity of the symbols to the general public.  (For example, printed English is not iconic, but is familiar to and easily understood by the general adult public.)  Symbol systems that have a high iconicity would rank high.  For adults, symbols systems that involve traditional orthography would also rate high.  Direct pointing techniques rate higher in this dimension than techniques that involve coding.  Aids that print out the individual's message, or that say the message out loud in a clear, natural voice, would rate highest on this dimension.  The intelligibility or obviousness of a technique to strangers is important for *providing access to potential communication partners* for the individual.  The straightforwardness and obviousness of the techniques can also affect the *learning* of a particular technique by both the individual and those communicating with the individual.

*Appropriateness*.   This dimension refers to how appropriate a particular technique is to an individual's current and future physical, cognitive, and language abilities.  It is important that techniques be appropriate for an individual's current skill level and abilities, but they must also be capable of expanding as the individual's skill level and abilities increase. The most common mistake made here is to select an aid or technique that will be appropriate for the child at some point in the future (reflecting increased skills and abilities), rather than selecting one that is appropriate to the child's current level. Insuring the current appropriateness of techniques is essential for insuring that the system is *effective* for the individual and that it foster *the potential for growth*. For individuals with progressive or degenerative conditions, the same principle applies in reverse. Techniques must be appropriate now and have a logical path toward techniques that will be used in the future as their skills decrease.

*Durability*. This dimension refers to the ruggedness and reliability of the communication aid. Ruggedness refers to how much abuse an aid or device can sustain and remain intact in harsh environments. Reliability is the mean time between failures of a device during intended use. Ruggedness and reliability are very important to the *unrestricted availability* requirement. Aids that depend upon electronic circuitry or electromechanical devices generally rate lower, both because of reduced ruggedness and the time they may spend in repair when they fail. Wooden communication boards, signing, and gesture would rate high.

*Total cost*. No technique or aid will solve a problem if it is not *affordable*. This dimension considers the total cost for the technique or aid, not just the purchase cost. This includes costs for maintenance, training, and any assistance required for use of the technique or aid. Low-cost, low-maintenance, easily replaceable, independent communication aids score highest in this dimension, as do aids that incorporate essentially no technology, but that are highly intelligible and obvious. For conversation, a direct pointing board would score high, although it would score low for writing needs due to the need for an assistant. Signing would score high except for the high cost for training everyone outside of those already familiar with the technique. The use of under-$100 portable, electronic, battery-operated typewriters would score high along this dimension.

## Acceptability/Compatibility with Environment

The third group of dimensions in Table 3-2 deals with compatibility between the technique and the people, procedures, conventions, materials, and devices in the individual's environment.

*Cosmesis*. This dimension refers to the attractiveness or appearance of the aid overall. It directly affects the *acceptability* of the aid or technique to the individuals who use them. It also affects *access to communication partners* and the *ability to function in all environments* in which the individual can communicate. Uncosmetic techniques are often removed or forbidden to the individual when in public, thus cutting off their communication in these environments. Techniques or aids that are of interest to strangers or that enhance the perception of the user's intelligence and communicative ability would rate highest in this category. Techniques that appear childish or that decrease the impression of intelligence and attractiveness would rate lowest.

*Materials/practice compatibility.* This dimension refers to the compatibility of the technique with the materials available and the practices employed in the educational or employment setting. A communication aid would have low compatibility in a regular first- or second-grade classroom, since the individual's technique would not match any of the educational materials or practices used. A manual pointing technique also would not score high in this dimension when a large amount of worksheet and independent written work is required. A teacher who has a large number of students using a particular symbol system may find it difficult to integrate another child working with a totally different symbol system because of difficulty in converting already developed materials to the new symbol system. Compatibility can affect the usefulness of the technique in the school or job environment; it can also affect the *acceptability* of the technique to teachers or employers. In regular educational settings, traditional orthography and aids that allow the individual to produce independent work and to use worksheets would score the highest in this dimension. Conditions in other environments will change the criteria for this dimension.

*Similarity.* This dimension refers to the similarity between the techniques of augmentative communication users and those of their peers and the community. Similarity is important in maximizing *access to potential communication partners* because it makes the technique more intelligible to a larger number of persons. It also is important to the individual's *growth and learning*, in that it provides the user with very important models for communication and expression. Individuals whose system components differ from the aids, symbols, and techniques used by those around them are unable to express themselves like others in their environment. Finally, this dimension also affects the *acceptability* of system components both by the users and the community. For young children, voice output aids that are clear and easy to understand, and that have an open vocabulary, would rate highest on this dimension. For older individuals in a reading and writing environment, aids with orthographic displays would rank high. A technique that is used by everyone within a community, such as signing, or special symbol systems, would rate higher than a technique or idiosyncratic symbol system that is not used in that community.

*Training.* This dimension refers to the amount of training required of the user, clinicians, and others in the individual's environment. The user usually requires the smallest amount of training time, especially for idiosyncratic or unusual techniques that are peculiar to the individual. However, therapy personnel and other individuals often change regularly within the user's environment. Unless the technique or strategy is very intelligible and obvious, much time must be spent familiarizing each person with the techniques used by the individual. Training also will affect *access to communication partners* for the individual and the *ability to learn* the system. Training time is affected by the individual's financial resources, and thus has an effect on *affordability*. This dimension (training required), and the very high costs associated with it, is usually not considered when evaluating potential techniques. The availability of training personnel who are skilled in using the technique is also often overlooked.

*Adaptability*. This dimension refers to the capability to customize a technique to the individual's needs, abilities, and constraints. This dimension is very important, due to the unique situations that result when an individual has multiple handicaps. Aids and selection techniques must be adaptable in order to address *compatability* requirements with other devices (e.g., seating systems, etc.). Vocabulary must be adaptable in order to allow for changing skills and interests over time. The adaptability dimension is also important for fine-tuning techniques to increase the speed, function, and efficiency (*effectiveness*) of the individual's system. Aids with preprogrammed and fixed vocabularies, mounting systems, or sign systems that cannot adapt to different physical abilities would rate lowest in this dimension. More sophisticated or newer aids that allow for flexibility of input, mounting, user-programmable vocabularies, and output modes would rate high.

*Interdevice compatibility*. This dimension refers to the ability to use a communication aid or selection technique with other standard devices in the individual's environment. This may occur directly (e.g., the ability to use a headstick pointer with other keyboards, television controls, etc.), or via electrical interconnection (e.g., an individual using a communication aid to operate a computer, an environmental control, or another device through a special interface). Interdevice compatibility is important for providing *computer access* to electronic communication, learning, or information systems in the individual's environment; it is also important for control of devices in the individual's environments.

*Computer compatibility*. This dimension refers to the ability to utilize aids, techniques, or symbols with standard computers. Some symbol or sign systems lend themselves to computer display, while others do not. Those that do can potentially provide the individual with lower-cost *writing systems* using the computer screen and a dot matrix printer. They can facilitate the *learning* of the systems, or expansion of vocabulary or syntax by allowing computer-assisted instruction. They also have the advantages discussed above, under independence, especially with regard to feedback. Finally, they address the *affordability* issue by providing low-cost software implementations on standard, portable computers. Traditional orthography rates highest in this dimension, followed by symbol systems with limited shapes, such as

Blissymbols or lexigrams.  Detailed pictographs and dynamic symbols, such as signs, would score lowest in this dimension.  It should be noted, however, that with modern mass storage and animation technologies, even pictures and dynamic signing systems will soon be computer compatible.

### Using the Dimensions to Make Clinical Judgments

As you have seen, there are many dimensions that must be considered when evaluating augmentative communication components of an individual's communication system.  Each of these dimensions varies in its importance for a given individual and contributes to more than one of the requirements of the overall communication system.  There are too many dimensions and considerations to allow a person to follow a simple checklist method for prescribing aids; that is, it is generally not possible to list all of the aids in one column, score each aid across the dimensions in another column, and come up with a recommendation by adding up the points at the bottom of the page.  If the recommendation is limited to something as simple as speed (just one of the many necessary dimensions of a communication system), such a formula prescription may be possible.  When one considers, however, that many communication aids are sitting in closets unused, or are used only in speech therapy or the classroom simply because of the cosmetic considerations or incompatibility with the individual's home or classroom environment, the importance of considering all of the different factors can be clearly seen.  Or, as Albert Einstein so aptly put it:  "Everything should be made as simple as possible, but not simpler."

This still leaves the question, however, of how to deal with the myriad requirements and constraints on an individual's communication system.  They may all be important, but there are too many to keep in mind at one time.  The recommended procedure is to study the various dimensions and to understand their application and implications with regard to the various requirements of a communication system (see Table 3-1).  The dimensions can be used as a sounding board to explore the symbols, techniques, and aids in an effort to highlight the strengths and weaknesses of each.  In this manner, the differences between the various components become apparent, and a better understanding of how they can work together to provide the various functions required by an individual's overall communication system is obtained.  As the multi-component communication system is developed for an individual, the requirements listed previously can be used as a check of the overall system.  An example of this process is provided in a case study at the end of the chapter.

# STUDY QUESTIONS

1. Using the case example provided at the very end of the chapter, see if you can identify which of the components best addresses each of the requirements listed in Table 3-1.  Are all of the requirements covered?

2. Electronic systems are often considered expensive.  Why are they actually more expensive than their purchase price?  Why might a wooden communication board be more expensive overall for a child in an educational program than an electronic aid?

3. The last two sections provide a very complex and lengthy listing of considerations and requirements.  Why is it necessary to consider both the requirements and the dimensions listed above when studying the augmentative components of an individuals communication system?

4. What is the difference between the requirements and the dimensions?

5. Which dimensions seem to be least important for a severely mentally retarded child?  How could they be important?

## COMPONENTS OF A MULTI-COMPONENT COMMUNICATION SYSTEM

The components for assembling an augmentative communication system can be broken down into three categories:

1. symbols
2. transmission techniques
3. strategies for increasing speed, access to the language, or effectiveness of communication techniques

Special augmentative components generally consist of transmission techniques (such as manipulation of the hands or pointing on a board) that are used in conjunction with communication symbols or a representation system (such as gestures, American Sign Language, Blissymbols, or pictures). Various strategies are taught to help an individual use the system effectively. Such strategies include (a) cueing or combining symbols to communicate ideas outside of the vocabulary; (b) strategically using key symbols or abbreviations to increase the speed of communication; (c) using facial expressions or body motions to add emphasis; and (d) using strategies to prevent nonvocal or vocal interruption. Each of these areas is presented in the following sections.

### Symbols

Human communication involves a wide variety of communication symbols. It is customary for a discussion of symbols or symbolic representation systems to be organized according to specific dimensions or some dichotomy such as aided/unaided or static/dynamic. The reader is referred to a recent symbol taxonomy paper (Lloyd & Fuller, 1986) for a review of previously published dichotomies. Although some of the other classification schema have been used more frequently, the static/dynamic schema is used in this text to focus on the nature of the symbol rather than the production of the symbol. The definitions of static/dynamic symbols and symbol systems are as follows:

- Dynamic symbols have their meanings conveyed by change, transition, and/or movement, and therefore cannot be considered as permanent and enduring. Oral speech and most gestures and manual signs are dynamic in nature. This category generally corresponds with unaided symbols. However, synthetic productions of speech, gestures, and manual signs are examples of dynamic symbols, which are aided.

- Static symbols include both graphic symbols and objects that are permanent and enduring. They do not have to be changed or moved in order to have their meaning conveyed. Because of this, they lend themselves very well to display on communication boards, electronic devices, and other aids so that most, but not all, static symbols could be thought of as aided. The majority of the letters in manual alphabets are produced without movement and are therefore examples of static, but unaided symbols.

Table 3-3 provides a listing of all the major communication symbols and most of the infrequently used symbols. These are organized according to the static/dynamic classification schema and are generally organized along several continua:

1. from those demanding the lowest to those demanding the highest cognitive ability;

2. for the dynamic symbols, from those requiring the lowest to those requiring the highest level of motor control;

3. from nonverbal (or nonlinguistic) to verbal (or linguistic); that is, those best approximating English or other native languages of the general community;

4. from the more concrete to the more abstract;

5. from the more iconic (i.e., transparent and/or translucent) to the more opaque.

Some of the symbols listed in Table 3-3 are *symbol sets* and others are *symbol systems*. In reading this text and other publications it is helpful for the reader to understand what is meant by the terms *symbol collection*, *symbol set*, and *symbol system*. Therefore, they are defined below.

*Symbol set*. A symbol set is a defined set of symbols that is closed in nature; it could be clinician-produced or it could consist of purchased symbol books, stamps, and/or cards containing a limited number of symbols. A symbol set can be expanded, but it does not have clearly defined rules for expansion.

*Symbol system*. A symbol system refers to a set of symbols specifically designed to work together to allow for maximum communication. Symbol systems include rules or a logic for the development of symbols not already represented in the system.

## TABLE 3-3.  STATIC AND DYNAMIC COMMUNICATION SYMBOLS[a]

DYNAMIC

Gestures

    -Pointing
    -Yes/no headshakes
    -Mime
    -Generally understood
      gestures
    -Amer-Ind gestures

Natural sign languages (ASL, BSL,
  CSL, FSL, JSL, KSL, SSL, & TSL)

Gestuno

Manually coded English (Signed
  English, PGSS, SEE-I, & SEE-II)
  or manual coding for other
  spoken languages (manually
  coded Swedish)

Modified signs and esoteric (or
  idiosyncratic) signs

Synthetic manual signs and/or
  gestures

Fingerspelling or manual alphabets
  (partially dynamic)

Eye blink, gestural, and/or vocal
  alphabet codes (Morse Code)

Eye blink, gestural and/or vocal
  word and/or message codes

Oral speech

Synthetic speech

Tadoma and other dynamic
  vibrotactile codes

Speech reading and hand-cued
  speech

Auto-cued speech

Electronic speech recognition and
  display

STATIC

Objects

    -Actual objects
    -Miniature or representational
     objects

Pictures (photographs & drawings
    -simple (or basic) rebus
    -other picture sets

Sigsymbols

Pictogram Ideogram
  Communication (PIC)

Picsyms

Blissymbols

Graphic representations of manual
  signs and/or gestures (HANDS,
  pictures of signing, Sign writer,
  Sigsymbols, & Worldsign)

Modified orthography and other
  symbols

Complex (or expanded) rebus

Abstract logographs and abstract
  shapes

Traditional orthography (written &
  printed words)

Fingerspelling or manual alphabets
  (mostly static)

Graphic representations of
  fingerspelling

Braille and other static tactile
  codes

---

[a]These are "formal" or conventionalized symbols and systems; informal nonverbal
behaviors or ritualized behaviors have not been included.

**TABLE 3-4.  RELATION OF VOCAL AND NONVOCAL COMMUNICATION TO VERBAL AND NONVERBAL COMMUNICATION.**

|  | VERBAL | NONVERBAL |
|---|---|---|
| VOCAL | SPEECH (ORAL & SYNTHETIC) | CRIES MOANS SIGHS |
| NONVOCAL | WRITING ASL SIGNS BLISSYMBOLICS | GESTURES PICTURES |

These rules may be internal to the symbol system (e.g., speech in spoken English or manual signs in ASL), or may be part of the language coded by the symbol system (e.g., manual sign of Signed English or Signing Exact English).

*Symbol collection.*  This is a miscellaneous assortment of symbols; it could be a collection of symbols taken from a single source or a combination of sources.

Before discussing specific dynamic and static symbols, it would be helpful for the reader to have a clear understanding of how the symbols listed in Table 3-3 may also be considered as either verbal or nonverbal (as defined in chapter 1), and either vocal or nonvocal.  This is illustrated in Table 3-4.  For example, some nonvocal symbols are verbal (written language, American Sign Language, Blissymbolics and Lexigrams), while other symbols are nonverbal (pictures, mime, and gestures).

The dynamic and the static symbols listed in Table 3-3 are briefly discussed below.  For in-depth descriptions of these various symbol sets and symbol systems, the reader is referred to other general chapters and texts (see Fristoe & Lloyd, 1979; Jones & Cregan, 1986; Karlan & Lloyd, in press; Kiernan, Reid, & Jones, 1982; Lloyd, 1976; Musselwhite & St. Louis, 1982; Schiefelbusch, 1980; Tebbs, 1978; Vanderheiden & Grilley, 1976) or to their original sources (as cited in the brief discussions of each symbol set or system below).

**Dynamic Symbols**

Dynamic symbols tend to be production-oriented (the individual produces the symbols) instead of selection-based (where the individual simply selects the symbol from symbols that are displayed or stored).  As such, dynamic symbols can generally be transmitted more quickly (*speed*) and provide access to a larger vocabulary (*openness*) than static symbols.  Use of dynamic symbols assumes that the individual has the physical ability to produce the symbols, and the cognitive ability to encode and decode a large number of symbols.

Dynamic symbols generally do not lend themselves to static displays.  As a result, they are not easily used on communication aids.  However, the graphic representation of manual signs and gestures is currently available, providing a bridge between dynamic and static communication symbols, similar to the bridging that exists between speech and traditional orthography (and modified orthography).  In the future, graphic representations such as computer animation of manual signs will allow dynamic symbols to be "printed" on the screen.

With regard to the functional dimensions (Table 3-2), dynamic symbols are generally more *portable* and can be used more easily in different positions than static symbols.  Because of their *speed* and *openness*, they are better for *assertability*.  Their *intelligibility/obviousness* (or iconicity) ranges from arbitrary symbols, such as sign languages and speech (which are obvious only to those who know the specific system), to symbols that are designed to be iconic to uninformed message receivers (such as gestures).

The major dynamic symbol sets and symbol systems are briefly reviewed in the order in which they are presented in Table 3-3 including references when appropriate and taking into consideration the above functional dimensions (see Table 3-2).

*Gestures*

In general, while gestures can be understood by individuals with similar experiences and cultural backgrounds, they are not universally understood.  Although gestures do not have linguistic constraints in their formation and usage, they do have cultural constraints. The cultural/experiential factor has been documented. For example, the palm-back v-handshape is interpreted as "victory" in most of Europe (the same as the palm-forward v-handshape made famous during World War II), but in England, Ireland, Scotland, and Wales, it is known as a Harvey Smith and is interpreted as a sexual insult (Morris, Collett, March, & O'Shaughnessy, 1979).

Some types of gestures are generally more difficult to interpret than others. Wundt (1973) has described the four levels of gesture as mime, demonstrative, descriptive, and symbolic. *Mime* uses the whole body in direct imitation (as in acting). *Demonstrative gesturing* involves pointing or indexing, showing form and size, or displaying an object. *Descriptive gesturing* may involve drawing in the air (indicative form), shaping hands into a three-dimensional representation (plastic form), imitating movement of a person (or other creature) or thing, or using a secondary trait (connotative form). *Symbolic gesturing* involves higher-level associations with an intermediate step between the concept and the gesture. While the interpretation of all four types of gestures are experientially influenced, symbolic gestures are more culturally (and cognitively) influenced. In addition to considering levels of difficulty for typical (nonhandicapped) adults, for many augmentative communication users one must consider gestures from a developmental perspective. Some types of gestures used in augmentative communication are discussed below in a primarily developmental sequence with some reference to Wundt's (1973) levels.

*Pointing*. Although Wundt includes pointing in his second level, we consider it the most basic symbolic representation presented in Table 3-3. It is a gesture, but warrants individual discussion because of its simplistic nature and significant role in early pragmatic behavior. Its uses range from direct indexing of a referent (deixis) to pointing to one referent to represent a broader class of referent(s) not present. Pointing is very limited, primarily because a referent must be present (i.e., person, object, or place) to send the message. Pointing can often be used by individuals with very limited (but some) motor ability, and rates fairly well on dimensions such as *position independence*, *durability*, and *intelligibility*. Pointing is used as part of manual sign language and systems. For example, ASL uses pointing to body parts (e.g., ear ), pointing to other objects or things related to the object (e.g., watch), and pointing to a position (or place) to indicate pronouns (e.g., he). In addition, pointing (as well as other gestures) is frequently used when an individual does not remember the more conventional manual sign or spoken word.

*Yes/no headshakes*. Yes/no headshakes are common gestures in our culture as well as most, but not all, other cultures. Although they are easily understood in our culture, they are arbitrary and would be considered symbolic or more advanced than pointing or other demonstrative gestures. Yes/no headshakes occur relatively early in the developmental sequence. They are relatively easy to produce, but are limited in use because the communicating partner must pose questions that can be answered with *yes* or *no*, and because they can only be used for responding.   In general, yes/no headshakes rate relatively high on *intelligibility/obviousness* and *portability*, but rate poorly on *independence*, *openness*, *permanence*, and *speed*.  The major exception and real value of yes/no headshakes is when they are used in combination with other symbols. In this case, they rate high on the *speed* dimension.

*Mime*.  Mime is a special form of gesturing.  It involves the acting out or the use of motions that simulate a particular activity in order to convey a message.  Mime tends to use the whole body, while most other gestures use the hands, arms, head, and face.  Mime can be useful for individuals with good motor control and can provide projection for an individual whose communication system's transmission techniques tend to be close-quarter techniques.  It can also be used to express basic needs and to conduct simple interactions where convenience, *projection*, and 24-hour *avail-ability/useability* are important.   (Mime rates relatively poorly on *independence*, *openness*, *permanence*, and *speed*.)  It frequently takes considerable time to act out and therefore is slower than many of the other forms of gesturing.  However, mime rates relatively high on *intelligibility/obviousness* when used with relatively good guessers. Although Wundt (1973) lists mime as his first level, it requires a higher level of skill and experience than the demonstrative (and possibly the descriptive) level.

*Generally understood gestures*.  Hamre-Nietupski and colleagues have described a set of commonly used or "generally understood gestures" that can be used for communication with individuals with severe/profound mental retardation (Hamre-Nietupski et al., 1977).  Although more limited in scope than mime, they are much more quickly and easily understood because of relatively common usage within the general public (e.g., yes/no headshakes).  It is assumed that "generally understood gestures" are easily understood, but data are limited.  When used by severely impaired individuals, these gestures may have only a partial chance of being identified by strangers and some may be totally unrecognizable.  To the extent that they are recognizable to those persons familiar with the individual, these gestures can be quick, convenient, and powerful communication techniques.  In many cases they are not understood.  Fiocca (1981) found a 77 percent recognition rate by individuals working with severely handicapped persons.  Doherty, Karlan, and Lloyd (1982) found less than 40 percent of the gestures were understandable to 24 retarded adults in sheltered workshops.

*Amer-Ind gestures*.  Amer-Ind is a gestural code developed by Skelly (1979).  It is based upon the "hand talk" (or gestures) used by American Indians.  The purpose of the Indian gestures was to allow groups with totally different language systems to be able to communicate on an elementary level.  The objective of Amer-Ind is to communicate ideas by using gestures that Skelly presumed to be easily recognized.  As with mime and "generally understood gestures," these symbols are designed to rate high along the dimension of *intelligibility*, but their transparency is not as high as some early reports indicate. Amer-Ind was originally reported as 80 to 90 percent transparent (Skelly, 1979; Skelly, Schinsky, Smith, Donaldson, & Griffin, 1975; Skelly, Schinsky, Smith, & Fust, 1974), but more recent research indicates that it is approximately 50 percent transparent for nonretarded young adults, and even less so for retarded individuals (Daniloff, Lloyd, & Fristoe, 1982; Doherty, Daniloff, & Lloyd, 1985; Imhoff & McMillen, 1984; Kirschner, Algozzine, & Abbot, 1977). The Amer-Ind gestural code permits agglutination (i.e., the combining of symbols to represent new concepts). Thus, it is intended to represent a large number of referents (i.e., to have *openness*). However, the ability to comment very specifically or to carry out detailed discussion is limited.

Although Amer-Ind has some practical and conceptual limitations, it is probably the best known gesture system used with severely handicapped individuals. In addition to Skelly's book (1979), the reader is referred to other recent papers for general educational/clinical considerations (e.g., Daniloff & Schafer, 1981; Lloyd & Daniloff, 1983; Musselwhite & St. Louis, 1982, pp. 126-131). For example, Doherty et al. (1982) made a direct comparison of "generally understood gestures" and Amer-Ind presented in an elaborated form (e.g., with parakinesic cues) and in an unelaborated form. "Generally understood gestures" were more easily guessed than the Amer-Ind and elaborated forms did not enhance gestural transparency, and in some cases actually reduced the transparency of Amer-Ind.

Both generally understood gestures and Amer-Ind use all four of Wundt's levels. The use of other gestures with severely handicapped individuals has been reported (Barten, 1979; Berger, 1972a,b; Bricker, 1972; Ricks & Wing, 1975; Rutter, 1965; Topper, 1974, 1975; Webster, McPherson, Sloman, Evans, & Kaucher, 1973). Sometimes, these gestures and expressions will be specific to an individual or to an environment, and may be referred to as "esoteric or idiosyncratic signs or gestures." Within a specific environment, they can be a very effective means of communication that ranks high along the dimensions of *availability*, *portability*, *projection*, and *speed*. Their weakness is generally in the areas of *intelligibility/obviousness* once they leave a familiar environment. These gestures are generally limited in their ability to be used to communicate new ideas (*openness*).

## Natural Sign Languages

Natural sign languages are not directly related to the native spoken language of the country of origin. For example, American Sign Language (ASL) is not a mechanism for signing English, although there are systems to manually sign an approximation of English (discussed below). American Sign Language has its own vocabulary, syntax, and grammar, which are totally different from English. Sign languages are not directly related to various spoken languages and they are not universal.   Different sign languages have developed in different countries.   For example, in addition to ASL, there is a British Sign Language (BSL), a Chinese Sign Language (CSL), a French Sign Language (FSL), a Japanese Sign Language (JSL), a Korean Sign Language (KSL), a Swedish Sign Language (SSL), a Taiwanese Sign Language (TSL), and so on; none is related to the spoken languages from those countries.   It appears that different sign languages may have approximately 10 to 15 percent of sign formations produced in an identical way.   In some cases an identical production has a different meaning.   For example, the sign WHAT in BSL is made in the same way WHERE is made in ASL.   The natural sign languages rank very high for *assertability*, *availability*, *independence*, *openness*, *portability*, *projection*, and *speed*.   They do require manual dexterity, although signs can be made with limited manual dexterity as well.   Limitations in manual dexterity generally affect the rate and openness of the system as the individual's recognizable vocabulary decreases.   Sign language systems are generally not *intelligible* or *obvious* to individuals not trained in or familiar with the system.   Further information about ASL and BSL are provided in Deuchar, 1984; Friedman, 1977; Klima & Bellugi, 1979; and Wilbur, 1976 and 1979.

## Gestuno

Gestuno is an "international sign language" (or compromise language) developed by the Unification of Signs Commission of the World Federation of the Deaf (WFD) for use as an auxiliary language at WFD meetings (Rubino, Hayhurst, Guejlman, Madison, & Plum, 1975).   This publication had 1,470 signs selected from American Sign Language and British Sign Language plus a number of European, Latin, and Scandinavian sign languages.   The WFD commission chose what they thought were the more iconic, naturally spontaneous, and most common forms of signs from the different sign languages and attempted to avoid alphabetical or initialized signs. Gestuno is not in common use by native deaf signers, but it has provided an important resource for lexical expansion in some sign languages.   As a total system, Gestuno would seem to have limited use as an augmentative communication technique for individuals with severe communication problems.   However, it is a valuable resource for signs and gestures.   Although there are no published data to support the assumption, Gestuno seems more iconic than natural sign languages (e.g., ASL, BSL, CSL).   In other words, it seems to have more *intelligibility/obviousness* than natural sign languages.

## Manually Coded English

A number of manual systems have been developed in an attempt to code English word distinctions, syntax, and grammar to varying degrees.   Signing in an

English word order has been referred to as "artificial," "contrived," "devised," "educational," and "pedagogical" in the attempt to distinguish these symbol systems from natural sign languages such as ASL. We prefer the generic terms *manually coded English* (MCE) or *pedagogical signs* because the objective of these systems is to provide a signing communication technique that allows for an easier transition to written English or to speech.

These systems share some of the the same basic advantages and disadvantages as sign languages. Communication in spoken English and in ASL can occur at approximately the same rate, but MCE is slightly slower. This is in part because of the need to produce more signs in MCE than in ASL to communicate the same thoughts, and because of the need to translate from one code (e.g., English) to another (e.g., MCE). The rationale is that MCE may make it easier for an individual to learn a written communication system, because it has essentially the same syntax and grammar as English. However, some linguists point out that it would be easier to learn ASL and then learn written English as part of learning a second language. The major advantage of MCE over a natural sign language is that MCE provides more consistency between simultaneously signed and spoken symbols.

MCE or pedagogical systems that fall into this general category are the Paget-Gorman Signed System (PGSS) (previously referred to as the New Sign Language and Systematic Sign Language) (Bishop, 1982; Feinmann, 1982; Paget, 1951; Paget & Gorman, 1968; Paget, Gorman, & Paget, 1976); Seeing Essential English or SEE-I or SEE-1 (Anthony, 1966, 1971, 1974); Linguistics of Visual English or LOVE, LoVE, or LVE (Wampler, 1971); Signing Exact English or SEE-II or SEE-2 (Gustason, Pfetzing, & Zawolkow, 1972, 1980); Manual English (Washington State School for the Deaf, 1972); Signed English (Bornstein, 1973, 1974; Bornstein & Saulnier, 1984; Bornstein, Hamilton, Saulnier, & Roy, 1975; Bornstein, Saulnier, & Hamilton, 1976, 1983). The basic characteristics of these six pedagogical sign systems and pidgin signed English are summarized in Table 3-5. SEE-2 and Signed English have emerged as the two most commonly used pedagogical systems in the United States for a number of reasons. Probably the most critical factor is the availability of materials. Both systems do a reasonably good job of approximating spoken English structure, but as with any attempt to translate from one language to another, something is lost. The modification of signs to code onto English words results in some loss of the natural properties of the signs.

The relationship between ASL, pidgin signed English, spoken English, MCE (pedagogical systems) and signs supporting English (Sutcliffe, 1983) is illustrated in Figure 3-1. ASL and spoken English should not be considered to be on a continuum any more than spoken English, spoken French, and/or spoken Spanish can be considered to be on a continuum. When the users of two different languages attempt

**TABLE 3-5. BASIC CHARACTERISTICS OF PEDAGOGICAL SIGN SYSTEMS AND PIDGIN-SIGNED ENGLISH[a]**

| SYSTEM | AUTHOR(S) | ASL/BSL SIGNS | FINGERSPELLING | BASIC MORPHOLOGICAL PRINCIPLE(S) |
|---|---|---|---|---|
| Paget-Gorman Sign System (PGSS) | Paget (1951, 1971); Paget & Gorman (1968); and Paget, Paget, & Gorman (1972, 1976) | No | Only for proper names | One meaning—one sign |
| Seeing Essential English (SEE-1) | Anthony (1967, 1971, 1974) | For the most part ASL | Some | Two-out-of-three: Sound, meaning, and spelling |
| Signing Exact English | Gustason, Pfetzing, & Zawolkow (1972, 1980) | Same as SEE-1 | Same as SEE-1 | Same as SEE-1 |
| Linguistics of Visual English | Wampler (1971, 1972) | Same as SEE-1 | Same as SEE-1 | Same as SEE-1 |
| Manual English | Washington State School for the Deaf (1972) | Yes, ASL | More than SEE-1 | Variable; one meaning—one sign; some same as SEE-1 |
| Signed English | Bornstein et al. (1973, 1975, 1983) | Primarily ASL | Yes, variable amounts | To string together ASL signs with 14 markers and fingerspelling |
| Pidgin Signed English Also known as: signed English, Siglish, and Ameslish | Riekehof (1963); Fant (1964, 1972); Watson (1973); Bragg (1973); O'Rourke (1973) | Yes, ASL | Yes | Pidginization of ASL signs and English markers and word order |

[a]Modified from Fristoe & Lloyd (1979, p. 405) and Wilbur (1976, p. 453).

**FIGURE 3-1. RELATIONSHIP OF ASL, PIDGIN-SIGNED ENGLISH, MCE (OR PEDAGOGICAL SYSTEMS), AND SIGNS SUPPORTING ENGLISH.**

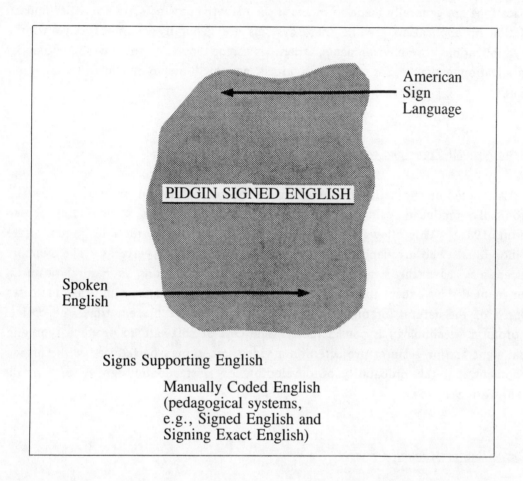

to communicate, they frequently develop a pidgin. In the case of ASL and spoken English, it is referred to as "pidgin signed English." MCE is not spoken English, ASL, or pidgin signed English, but it is closer to pidgin signed English as it uses signs in an approximation of English. It may be theoretically desirable to have an exact one-to-one correspondence of sign to spoken word. However, in actual practice, most clinicians/teachers sign only part of the spoken words (usually the "key words"), while they speak in grammatically correct sentences. The practice of signing only key words while speaking full sentences has been referred to as "signs supporting English" (Sutcliff, 1981, Sutcliffe, 1983). In addition to checking original sources, there are several reviews of pedagogical sign systems (Bornstein, 1973, 1982; Karlan & Lloyd (in press); Musselwhite & St. Louis, 1982, pp. 104-110; Wilbur, 1976, 1979, pp. 203-228).

## *Modified Signs and Esoteric (or Idiosyncratic) Signs*

Just as there are idiosyncratic or nonstandard gestures that can be part of an individual's system, there may also be modified signs or modified sign systems.  These modifications are generally made to increase the effectiveness of signs for a particular population or application.  While these systems are generally more effective within these applications or environments, there is some loss in the overall potential communication audience for these individuals as noted above in the discussion of gestures.

## *Synthetic Manual Signs and/or Gestures*

Animated or synthetic representations of manual signs and/or "gestures" can be electronically produced using robotic or animated hands on a computer screen (Johnson, 1981).  This allows those unfamiliar with manual systems to communicate with individuals who are dependent upon manual signs and/or gestures.  The symbols produced may have the same general strengths and limitations as natural gestures and/or manual signs except that they may not have the *independence* and in some cases the *speed* of the natural (or unaided) symbols.  Also, at the present time, the cost of such prototype technology is considerable.  The cost of software to produce synthetic manual signs and/or gestures projected on a video screen may be reduced with further development, but the probability of developing low-cost robotic sign systems in the near future is very low.

## *Fingerspelling or Manual Alphabet*

Fingerspelling is sometimes referred to as an alpha-dactyl code because it uses fingers to encode the letters of the alphabet.  (Several other alphabet encoding techniques will be discussed in later sections.)  Theoretically, the manual alphabet is a dynamic system rather than a static system.  In most manual alphabets, letters are formed by different shapes of the hand and fingers, with a few letters represented by movement.  In other words, some letters are dynamic, but most are static.  Therefore, in Table 3-2, manual alphabets are listed as mostly static and partially dynamic.  In the one-handed American Manual Alphabet (see Figure 3-2), only two letters (J and Z) are represented by movement.  The manual alphabets of other countries may have more or less movement (three additional samples are shown in Figure 3-2).  For example, in the one-handed Swedish alphabet, J and Z do not require movement, but four other letters do (Å, Ä, Ö, and Y).  In the two-handed British manual alphabet, only two letters J and H require movement.  The one-handed Lorm Manual Alphabet

## FIGURE 3-2. ONE- AND TWO-HANDED MANUAL ALPHABETS

### British Manual Alphabet

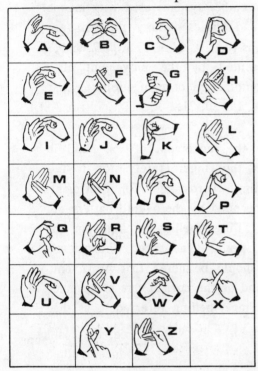

### Swedish Manual Alphabet

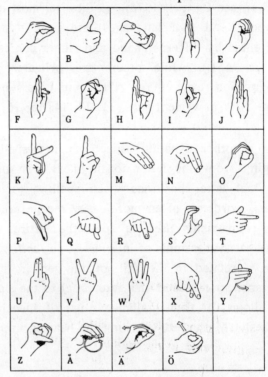

### American Manual Alphabet

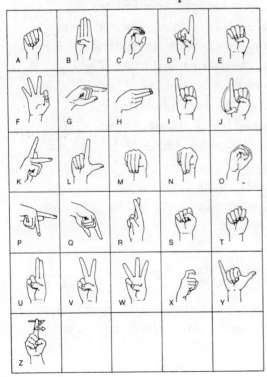

### Lorm Manual Alphabet

(one of the systems used in our country by deaf-blind individuals) requires movement for all letters.  For samples of other manual alphabets, including the international manual alphabet (adopted by the World Federation of the Deaf in Stockhom, Sweden in 1963), see Carmel (1975).  Likewise, most of the number systems used with manual alphabets (and sign languages) are both dynamic and static.  Many numbers are represented by different hand and finger configurations (e.g., 1, 2, 3, 4, 5, 6, 7, 8, 9, & 100 for ASL), while others are primarily represented by the movement of a configuration (e.g., 10 for ASL), and others by a combination of configurations that change with movement (e.g., 11, 12, 14, 15, 16, 17, 18, 19, 20, 21, . . . , 30, . . . for ASL).

Another dynamic aspect of fingerspelling is the movement of the hand in changing from one letter to the next.  In practice, the fingers rarely stop in the individual letter positions when spelling (or encoding) words, and for proficient readers, words are often more easily recognizable or decoded by the overall pattern of finger movements used to spell the entire word.  Fingerspelling is high on the functional dimensions of *openness*, *portability*, and *speed*.  The speed dimension is naturally related to the skill of the sender, but it should be noted that proficient fingerspellers can send at a rate equal to the slower end of the normal rate of speech. This allows for the simultaneous use of speech and fingerspelling referred to as the "Rochester Method" of teaching the hearing impaired.

## *Eye Blink, Gestural, and/or Vocal Alphabet Codes*

There are a number of ways that eye blinks, gestures, and vocalizations can be used separately or in combination to represent alphabets.  They can be used to encode or decode letters.  The best known and most efficient of these methods is to use contrasting features (e.g., dot/dash, short/long), as in the International Morse Code (see Figure 3-3).  Morse Code adapts any two consistent contrasting features with considerable efficiency.  Vanderheiden and Grilley (1976) have illustrated this with right and left movements for the dots (.) and dashes (-) of Morse Code.  (This is illustrated later in the chapter in Figure 3-22.)  The dots versus dashes of Morse Code may also be considered short versus long for eye blinks, gestures (e.g., waving) or vocalizations.  Such codes are high on the functional dimensions of *openness* and *portability*, but are generally not as fast as other alphabet coding (e.g., as fingerspelling).  They are poor on *intelligibility/obviousness*.

## *Eye Blink, Gestural, and/or Vocal Word and/or Message Codes*

There are various ways to encode words and/or messages with eye blinks, gestures, and/or vocalizations (of different quality, sound, and/or duration).  These

**FIGURE 3-3. INTERNATIONAL MORSE CODE**

| | | | | |
|---|---|---|---|---|
| A | .- | V | ...- |
| B | -... | W | .-- |
| C | -.-. | X | -..- |
| D | -.. | Y | -.-- |
| E | . | Z | --.. |
| F | ..-. | 1 | .---- |
| G | --. | 2 | ..--- |
| H | .... | 3 | ...-- |
| I | .. | 4 | ....- |
| J | .--- | 5 | ..... |
| K | -.- | 6 | -.... |
| L | .-.. | 7 | --... |
| M | -- | 8 | ---.. |
| N | -. | 9 | ----. |
| O | --- | 0 | ----- |
| P | .--. | Period | .-.-.- |
| Q | --.- | Comma | --..-- |
| R | .-. | ? | ..--.. |
| S | ... | Error | ........ |
| T | - | Wait | .-... |
| U | ..- | End | .-.-. |

are usually idiosyncratic codes and therefore are limited in the functional dimension of *independence* and *intelligibility/obviousness*. However, they may be fast (i.e., high on the *speed* dimension) and therefore often save time when used in combination with static symbols and assistive devices. While idiosyncratic codes may be useful, more standard gestures allow more people to understand the communication. In general, the eyeblink, gestural, and/or vocal word and/or message codes are high on the *portability* dimension, but relatively low on the *openness* dimension.

*Oral Speech*

Where speech is possible, it is, of course, extremely effective for communication. Unimpaired speech is very high on the *independence*, *openness*, *portability*, and *speed* dimensions. It is one of the most powerful symbol systems, which is why it is used so extensively. Its major limitations are in the area of *permanence*, which is why it is augmented by written traditional orthography in the communication systems of most people. Theoretically, speech would rank quite low in the area of *obviousness* or *intelligibility*, since it is very specific to the group of individuals who understand a particular language; that is, an individual who does not understand English would have extreme difficulty in understanding someone who was speaking in English--much more difficulty, in fact, than in understanding the same individual using common gestures, mime, or Amer-Ind.  On the practical level, however, individuals who speak English have a very large group of potential message receivers.

For individuals with disabilities, the usefulness of speech usually first degrades along the dimension of *intelligibility* or *understandability* by the general public.  Even after the speech is totally unintelligible to the general public, it is often still functional with persons familiar with the disabled individual.  The next area to degrade is generally the *openness* of the system.  Persons familiar with disabled individuals are generally capable of understanding their speech, but often cannot do so if they do not have some preconceived notion of the topic of communication or discussion and the specific words that will probably be used.  For these individuals, speech may be very effective for expressing basic needs and common communications with those familiar with them.  For discussion of other topics or new and different terms or words, and for communicating with those less familiar with them, some other augmentative form of communication must be provided.  A very common occurrence in this situation is parents who "understand everything a child says," even when trained clinicians can understand little or no speech after working with the child for some time.  Often, the parent is completely correct.  The parent and child work out what amounts to a vocal code for common needs and comments.  This is combined with the fact that the child does not try to communicate things outside of this limited repertoire, since he knows that he will not be understood.  The result is that the parent does indeed understand everything that the child says, even though the child's speech is not functional with other communication partners except for a limited number of topics or sentences.  Augmentative components should be provided to allow the child to communicate on a broader range of topics.  Another dimension that is often affected is the *speed* of communication.  However, because even impaired speech is generally so much faster than other augmentative modes (particularly the selection-based modes), speech, when possible, is usually the communication method of choice.

## *Synthetic Speech*

There are two basic techniques for creating voice output from communication aids.  The first and oldest technique is digitized speech.  This is essentially speech recorded in digital format.  The second approach is true synthetic speech.  True synthetic speech is never spoken by a human being, but is generated using mathematical and phonological rules that model the human speech production system.  Both digitized speech and synthesized speech are often incorrectly referred to as "synthesized speech."  There are some fundamental differences clinically, however, which makes their distinction important.

Digitized speech is digitally recorded. The sound quality can be very good (e.g., on compact discs) or poor ("Speak and Spell") depending on the amount of data stored. High quality digital recording, however, uses up very large amounts of memory. For example, digitally recorded speech (as used in prerecorded telephone messages) requires 6,000 bytes of memory for each second of speech. Compact discs require 90,000 bytes of memory for each second of stored music/speech. The memory constraints can be reduced by limiting the amount of information stored, but this reduces the quality of the speech, giving it an artificial sound (e.g., "Speak and Spell"). As a result, people have thought of poor quality digitized speech as being artificial or synthetic speech. Digitized speech recording and playback techniques are therefore often confused with true synthetically generated speech.

With true synthetic speech aids, words are generated from scratch using vocal tract models. The vocabulary of synthetic aids is not limited to words that have been recorded and stored. Instead, limitations are based upon the rules that are stored as part of the model. Synthetic speech generally includes text-to-speech translation rules. As such, they can take any spelled word and pronounce it vocally. The intelligibility of the word is dependent upon the accuracy and extensiveness of the set of pronunciation rules in the synthesizer. Proper names and foreign words are often "mispronounced" because they are not part of the synthesizers special pronunciation dictionary.

There is one other category of voice output communication aids (VOCAs) that somewhat blurs the picture. Some developers have come up with a mechanism for taking English speech and breaking it down into a set of between 64-700 sounds that can be linked together to produce a fairly good pronunciation of English words. In some cases, the sounds are synthesized; in other cases, they are doctored clips of digitally recorded or compressed human speech. If these aids or techniques are combined with text-to-speech rules, the following statements about the two categories, digitally recorded speech and synthesized speech, would both apply.

1. *Digitally recorded speech is potentially the clearest speech.* When one remembers that the laser disk is digitally recorded, the high quality potential of digitally recorded speech is clear. This high quality, however, is achieved at the cost of a very high electronic storage capability. The clarity of digitally recorded speech is a direct function of the amount of memory used to store the speech and the quality of the speech reconstruction algorithms. Systems using digitally recorded speech can have high or low quality. In all cases, however, the vocabulary of the system will be limited strictly to those words that have been prestored as spoken words in the system.

2. *Synthesized speech aids do not have direct limitations on their vocabulary.* Any word that can be spelled by the user can be pronounced by the aid. As a result, synthetic speech aids rate very high in the *openness* category. To access this openness,

however, the user must be able to "spell" out the words using either the standard alphabet or a phoneme alphabet.  Otherwise, the individual will be limited to those words whose spelling has been prestored in the system.  The quality of synthetic speech will always be lower than the very best digitally recorded speech.  However, recent advances in synthetic speech technology indicate that synthetic speech will rival human speech in quality in the not too distant future.  The cost for implementing synthetic speech is also dropping rapidly with advancing technologies in this area.

### *Tadoma and Other Vibrotactile Codes*

Vibrotactile techniques allow reception of speech by deaf individuals.  A number of electronic vibrotactile hearing aids have been proposed and researched (Sanders, 1976).  At the present time, however, these have demonstrated only limited success for speech recognition.  A manual technique that has proven successful is the Tadoma method (Alcorn, 1932; Grover, 1955; Hanson, 1930; Norton et al., 1977; Van Adestine, 1932; Vivian, 1966).  With this technique, an individual places his hand on the speaker's jaw and lips in such a way that he can feel the breath from the speaker's nose, the movement of the speaker's lips and jaws, and the vibration from the speaker's throat simultaneously.  Speech recognition has been demonstrated using this technique, even with completely deaf and blind individuals.  Although this technique cannot be easily used by individuals who have physical disabilities, it can be used by individuals whose communication problems are primarily a result of sensory disabilities.  In addition, it does demonstrate that speech can be presented in a completely tactile form and be understandable, even though automated systems have not yet been developed for individuals who are more severely physically handicapped.  These techniques are important, since there is a significant number of individuals who require augmentative communication techniques who are also deaf or severely hearing impaired.  While most of the symbols or codes discussed to this point are for sending and receiving, vibrotactile codes are receptive only.  Such codes may be considered high on *independence*, *openness*, *portability*, and *speed*.

### *Speechreading and Hand-Cued Speech*

Because of the power, speed, and openness of speech, techniques have been developed to aid the message receiver as well as the speaker to facilitate the use of speech where it would not normally be effective.  One example of this is speechreading (or lipreading), where the individual is taught to "read" what the person is saying by carefully watching the lips and other cues of the speaker.  Unfortunately, it is very difficult to understand everything that is said, since only a limited amount of information is available from the lips alone.  Features such as voicing, nasality, and fricatives are all controlled by articulators that cannot be seen.  To help increase the amount of information available to the speechreader, a number of cueing systems have been developed over the centuries (e.g., Bell's speech glove, Lyon's Phonetic Finger Alphabet, and Periere's dactylology) (Evans, 1982). The best-known current systems for the hand cueing of speech are Forchhammer's Danish Mouth-Hand System (Forchhammer, 1903; Holm, 1972) and Cornett's Cued Speech (1967, 1975). Both systems use the same phonetic-based principles. The Danish Mouth-Hand System cues consonants, while Cued Speech cues both consonants and vowels. In hand cueing, the speaker makes cues with his hands near his mouth to indicate what the unseen portions of his mouth and throat are doing at any point in time. The speechreader is thus able to see more of what is going on, greatly increasing the ability to understand the individual's speech. This technique requires that all speakers know how to cue their speech for the hearing-impaired or deaf individual. As a result, the deaf individual's communication partners are limited to those persons who know how to cue their speech (i.e., it is low in *obviousness*).

## Auto-Cued Speech

To help alleviate some of the problems of hand-cued speech, work is underway to develop an automatic cuer. This miniaturized microprocessor device is worn by the deaf individual. It automatically analyzes the speech of those talking to the deaf individual, providing automatic cues by way of special optics on the deaf individual's glasses. The visual cues are typically flashing light patterns that appear to float in space to either side of the mouth of the person whom they are watching. As with hand-cued speech, the patterns only provide part of the information needed to understand the speaker (i.e., the symbol is actually a combination of light patterns and lip movements plus other cues used in lip reading).

## Electronic Speech Recognition and Display

Although auto-cued speech could provide the deaf individual with the ability to lip-read with a high degree of accuracy, the technique still requires the deaf individual to master lipreading (speechreading). This is difficult for many, especially people with acquired deafness. Advances in electronic speech recognition, however, will eventually result in a portable, wearable system that can recognize most speech and translate it into printed text. With special optics, this text could be projected onto the deaf person's glasses so that the words would appear to float in space about 3 feet in front of the user, thus providing "subtitles" of whatever was being said and picked up by the system. This is currently, however, beyond the state of the art.

**Static Symbols**

Static symbols differ from dynamic symbols in that movement and change are not factors in conveying their meaning.  The most common static symbols are graphic representations.  Graphic symbols permit individuals who are not able to produce symbols to select them using some pointing technique.  They can be used to produce hard copy or written copy of the individual's message and may be printed on electronic displays or paper.  They can provide feedback on output to the user, allow message receivers to study an individual's output in order to decipher poorly constructed or confusing messages, and can be used to provide preprinted or computer-based instructional materials.  The ability to do this varies with different symbols, ranging from very difficult (with detailed pictographic techniques, to fairly simple with limited line symbols such as Blissymbols or, of course, traditional orthography).

In general, static symbols can be used more easily than dynamic symbols by individuals with more severe physical handicaps.  They are also, however, generally slower.  Most (but not all) require some type of a communication aid or assistive device.  When an aid is used, the symbols may also be limited by the functional dimensions (see Table 3-2) associated with it, such as *durability*, *independence*, *portability*, *speed*, and sometimes *cosmesis*.  Symbols requiring an aid are frequently referred to as "aided symbols" (Bloomberg & Lloyd, 1986; Fristoe & Lloyd, 1979; Goossens' & Lloyd, 1981; Lloyd, 1980a,b, 1984; Lloyd & Fuller, in press; Lloyd & Karlan, 1984; Romski, Sevcik, & Joyner, 1984).  As with dynamic symbols, static symbols cover a wide range of the *intelligibility/obviousness* and *openness* dimensions.  Static symbols also rank high in the *permanence* dimension.

There are many ways that static representation systems can be presented or transmitted, including:

- manual production of the symbols (e.g., fingerspelling),

- drawing of the symbols,

- direct pointing to previously drawn symbols,

- having another person point to the symbols and stopping the person when he gets to the desired item, and

- sending a code that is used to look up the symbol on a chart or in one's memory.

The major static symbol sets and symbol systems are briefly reviewed in the order in which they are listed in Table 3-3.

## *Objects*

Actual (or full size) objects and miniature objects may be used for symbolic or representational purposes. Within certain limitations noted below, objects may rate fairly high on the intelligibility dimension, but are relatively low on *openness*, *portability*, *projection*, and *speed*.

*Actual objects*. Individuals can communicate by "pointing" to the actual objects they are interested in communicating about. As discussed earlier, this pointing could take place through a wide variety of techniques, ranging from actually pointing to having someone or something point for the individual. Sometimes the object will stand for itself; for example, the individual might point to a doll, a toy, the television, a computer, or a dish of food on the table. At other times, an object may represent something other than itself; pointing to the door may indicate that the individual wants to go outside, or pointing to a bed may indicate that the child is tired. Difficulties can arise when the individual wants to communicate about the object that is used to represent something else. For example, a child whose toy rolls under a bed may point to the bed, whereupon he is taken from his chair and to the bed for a nap. Because of the ambiguity of this approach, it is good to check all answers with a yes/no question to the individual. Pointing to objects can be a very useful strategy for cueing message receivers to topics or ideas.

*Miniature or representational objects*. Miniature three-dimensional objects can also be used as "symbols" to represent real objects (or what the real objects represent). Care must be taken, however, that the miniature objects (symbols) actually represent the real objects (referent) to the disabled individual. Although a small chair or toilet is easily generalized to its large version by an adult familiar with the many forms that an object can take, it may not be obvious to the child. Small representations may be very different from the large representations both in appearance and function. For example, a small toilet with a water closet on the back may not look anything like the toilet that is built into the wall at an institution. Further, using a toilet to represent a bodily need to defecate may have no meaning at all to a child who has never used a toilet for that purpose. Objects also have the obvious disadvantage in that they cannot be used to easily represent many very early communicative concepts, such as *more*, *sick*, *pain*, *want*, and so on. It is also extremely difficult to find objects that match all of the concepts desired for an individual's communication system.

*Pictures*

A wide variety of pictographs can be used for symbolic representation.  A pictograph is a picture that is used to represent a thing or a concept and may range from photographs and hand-drawn symbols to prepackaged sets of symbols.  With all of these, it is important to make sure that the pictures (symbols) are clearly representational *for the individual with the handicap,* and not just for the adults working with the handicapped individual.  Even photographs may look very different from the real objects to young or retarded individuals.  Individualized photographs and hand-drawn symbols generally enable the individual's vocabulary to be expanded in any direction or to include any concept within the creative abilities of the people working with the disabled individual.  Prepackaged pictures (or symbol sets) are easier to use, but tend to limit the topics or specific symbol choices to those that happen to be provided in the set.  Some symbol sets (and symbol systems) support the use of preprinted and hand-drawn symbols and individualized photographs, thus providing the advantages of both.  In general, communication boards using preprinted symbols should always include custom drawn symbols to expand and individualize the displays to meet the specific needs of the user.

Figure 3-4 provides examples of pictographs for a sample of relatively common referents from the two most frequently used picture dictionaries: *Picture Communication Symbols* (Johnson, 1981, 1985) and the *Oakland Picture Dictionary* (Kirstein & Bernstein, 1981).  Figure 3-4 also provides examples of pictographs from five other symbol sets and symbol systems (to be discussed below) that use some pictographs in combination with other graphic symbols.

Although there are some differences between the pictures, their similarity is more striking than their differences.  The major differences between prepackaged symbol sets and symbol systems relate to representation of objects and actions that are not easily illustrated by pictures.  Different approaches to this problem are presented below in the discussion of Blissymbols, Picsyms, and Sigsymbols.

*Simple (or basic) rebus*.  Rebus is a common name given to pictographs.  Rebus is actually based upon the Latin for "thing," and rebus is defined as "a representation of words or syllables by pictures of objects or by symbols whose names resemble the intended words or syllables in sound; also, a riddle made up wholly or in part of such pictures or symbols. . . ." (Gove, 1976, p. 1983).  There are two levels of rebus--the *simple* (or *basic*) *rebus* and the *complex* (or *expanded*) *rebus*.  Rebus may be used for pictographs such as those shown in Figure 3-5 (*simple* or *basic rebuses*), or for much more linguistically, cognitively, and experientially demanding symbols (*complex* or *expanded rebus*) as discussed in a later section.

**FIGURE 3-4. EXAMPLES OF PICTOGRAPHS (BLISSYMBOLS USE IDEOGRAPHS FOR *CANDY* AND *COOKIE*).**

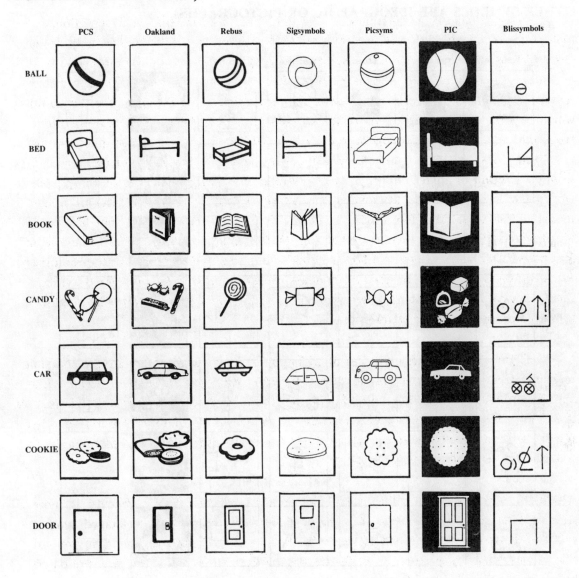

Although there is a wide variety of rebuses (see Clark & Woodcock, 1976), the most common source of pictographs labeled rebus in this country is the AGS (American Guidance Service) Rebuses (or the Peabody Rebus Reading Program Symbols) developed by Woodcock and his colleagues (Clark, Davies, & Woodcock, 1974; Clark & Woodcock, 1976; Woodcock, 1965; Woodcock, Clark, & Davies, 1968). This rebus system was not developed for communication or to be a communication symbol set. It was developed to provide a mechanism for teaching young unimpaired children to learn to read. Further, it is based upon an assumption of phonetic skills in the children, all of whom could speak. Because the system included a large number of

**FIGURE 3-5.  ADDITIONAL PICTOGRAPHIC REPRESENTATIONS (SIGSYMBOLS FOR** *COLD, DIRTY, FALL, MAKE,* **AND** *WANT* **ARE SIGN LINKED. ALL OF THE OTHER SYMBOLS ARE IDEOGRAPHIC OR PICTOGRAPHS)**

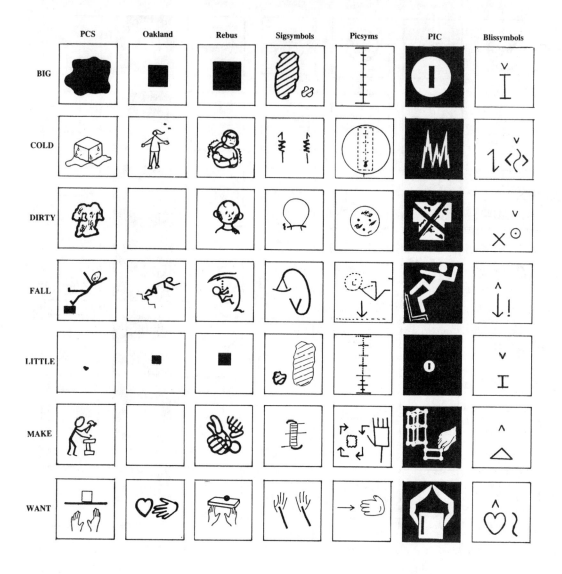

preprinted, simple, small pictographs, they were seen by individuals who were putting together communication boards as a source of small pre-made pictures.  Because of this application of the symbols, and the fact that the complex rebus symbols were unsuitable for this application, educators in the United Kingdom have developed other pictograph sets in recent years that include more simple pictographs (to avoid complex rebuses that were previously used) and to add additional symbols to the set to make them more appropriate for disabled users (e.g., Chapman, 1982; Chapman & Lees, in press; Devereux & van Oosterom, 1984; Jones, 1972, 1976, 1979; Lees & Chapman, in press; van Oosterom & Devereux, 1982, 1984)).  Figure 3-5 shows examples of the simple rebuses (pictographs) from the AGS Standard Rebus Glossary (Clark, Davies, & Woodcock, 1974).

   *Other picture sets*.   A number of other sets of pictures have been produced to assist speech-language pathologists and others in assembling communication boards and other picture-based communication aids.   These include the *Oakland Picture Dictionary* (Kirstein & Bernstein, 1981); *Picture Communication Symbols* (PCS) (Johnson, 1981); *Sigsymbol Dictionary* pictures (Cregan, 1982; Cregan & Lloyd, 1984a); *Communicaid* (Gethen, 1981) and other picture communication charts; Compics (Bloomberg, 1985); various picture aids for travelers (Drolet, 1982; Earl, 1972); and children's picture dictionaries (e.g., Parnwell, 1977).   Examples of pictographs from various symbol sets and symbol systems are shown in Figure 3-4.   Many referents are too abstract to be represented by pictographs; for other referents, the pictograph may be too context specific.   Figure 3-5 provides a few examples of referents that are difficult to represent by pictographs and illustrates how the same seven symbol sets and symbol systems in Figure 3-4 would depict these more difficult concepts.   In the following sections, Sigsymbols, Picsyms, Pictogram Ideogram Communication (PIC) symbols, and Blissymbols are presented as approaches for representing the more difficult concepts. It should be noted that the different pictures for the same referent in Figure 3-4 are frequently similar, while the symbols in Figure 3-5 are typically quite different.

   All pictographic symbol sets rate low on the functional dimension of *openness*, since they do not provide direct access to any words or concepts beyond those pictured on the board.   The *intelligibility/obviousness* dimension of pictures is reasonably good, but varies from user to user.   While many pictographs may rate relatively high for individuals with relatively good cognitive abilities and some experience with the referents, they rate relatively low for many individuals with intellectual impairments and/or limited experience.   Although pictographs are more *intelligible* and *obvious* than most other graphic representation systems, they are less *obvious* than might first be thought.   The meanings of the pictures are generally not obvious to others unfamiliar with the communication board.   As a result, the English (or other native language) word or phrase represented by the picture or symbol should be printed above each symbol, so that the symbols can be easily understood by at least those in the individual's environment who can read.   Removing the words from above the symbols generally makes the communication boards unintelligible to many message receivers. A primary reason for pictographs is to facilitate the *learning* of symbols by children, rather than their obviousness to others.   However, once individuals with normal cognitive ability see that a specific picture represents a specific referent, it is easy to remember the relationship illustrated in Figure 3-5.   In other cases, the pictures are *intelligible* to nonhandicapped individuals as might be seen in Figure 3-4.   In other words, some pictures are *intelligible* (or *obvious*) to some people, but all pictures are not *intelligible* to all people.

The Sigsymbols, Pictogram Ideogram Communication symbols, Picsyms, and Blissymbols discussed in the following four subsections include pictographs as well as other types of symbols (ideographs, sign-linked, and/or arbitrary).

## Sigsymbols

Sigsymbols consist of pictographs, ideographs, and sign-linked symbols (Cregan, 1980, 1982, 1984; Cregan & Lloyd, 1984a,b).   Therefore, they may be classified, in part, under the heading *pictures*, and, in part, under the heading *graphic representations of signs and/or gestures*.  They are discussed at this point for two reasons:  (a) there are many pictographs in Sigsymbols, and (b) they are one of several bridges between pictographs and more arbitrary (or abstract) symbol systems.  Sigsymbols are designed to be easily drawn by the nonartist.   They can provide a stable visual cue for nonreaders to reinforce language learning and support its expression.  Developed in a classroom setting for use with the severely mentally handicapped, they can also be used as a tool in teaching populations with expressive language difficulties (e.g., deaf, autistic, or aphasic individuals).  Sigsymbols are related to manual signs and to graphic symbols (e.g., pictographs and ideographs).   Therefore, Cregan (1980) coined the term Sigsymbols as a contraction of *sig* from *manual sign*, and *symbol* from *graphic symbol*. Sig may also be used as a further contraction of Sigsymbol.  Sigs are appropriate for individuals using sign because signing is relevant to a number of Sigsymbols.  Some Sigs are pictographic and some are ideographic.  Sometimes pictographs and ideographs are inappropriate because they are too specific to a certain context (e.g., *bad*, *build*) or impractical, being relatively abstract (e.g., *now*, *and*).  In such cases, the design of Sigs is based on established manual signs (e.g., signs from BSL or ASL).  Cregan's original Sigsymbols are based upon BSL signs, but the same principles can be used with symbols relating to signs from any sign language or pedagogical system.  Examples of an American version of Sigsymbols with the sign-linked symbols based upon American signs (Cregan & Lloyd, 1984a), such as Signed English (Bornstein et al., 1983) are provided in Figures 3-4 and 3-5.  Predrawn symbols in the dictionaries facilitate the advanced preparation of material for instructional purposes and communication boards, but the simplicity of Sigsymbols allows clinicians, teachers, and others to quickly draw them during communication interactions when the appropriate symbols are not readily available.  Sigsymbols that are pictographic and ideographic rate the same as previously discussed graphic systems on the *intelligibility/obviousness* dimension.  However, because of the bridging to more abstract concepts through sign-linked symbols, Sigsymbols rate higher on *openness*.  Sigsymbols also are faster to draw than some of the more detailed pictographs previously discussed.

## *Pictogram Ideogram Communication*

The Pictogram Ideogram Communication (PIC) materials (Maharaj, 1980) includes pictographs as well as ideographs, and was specifically designed for disabled individuals. PIC symbols differ from most other symbol sets in that, in an effort to increase their visual saliency, they are depicted as white symbols on black background. Although the saliency advantage of white on black drawings seems logical, the limited data available are equivocal. Meador, Rumbaugh, Tribble, and Thompson (1984) found that illuminated white-on-black lexigrams and an advantage over randomly assigned colors on black lexigrams, but Campbell and Lloyd (1986a) did not find that nonilluminated white on black line drawings had an advantage over black-on-white pictographs. Examples of the PIC symbols are provided in Figures 3-4 and 3-5. PIC is limited in the *openness* dimension for several reasons. First, any symbol set that is dependent upon a specific number of pictograms and ideograms without a method of agglutination (or combining) to represent additional referents is by definition limited in the *openness* dimension. This would be true of all the graphic symbols discussed above to the extent that one is limited to pictographic and ideographic symbols. The exception is that some of the pictographic sets are supplemented by alphabet letters or words (e.g., PIC), or by sign-linked symbols (i.e., Sigsymbols). To some extent pictographic and/or ideographic symbols can be supplemented by clinician/educator drawn symbols of a similar design or style. However, PIC is difficult to draw because of its white on black feature. Therefore, PIC is essentially limited to the 400 symbols purchased. The author states that "PIC . . . was designed as symbols having little analytical requirements and a high representational component" (Maharaj, 1980, p. 5). This would suggest good *intelligibility/obviousness*; however, PIC is similar to all of the symbols discussed above on this dimension, in that some symbols are easily guessed by most people and others are difficult to guess (i.e., experience and cognitive ability are critical factors). In comparing several different symbol sets and systems for a sample of 41 initial lexical items, Bloomberg (1984) found PIC less easily guessed by nonhandicapped adults than more pictographic symbols (e.g., PCS).

## *Picsyms*

Picsyms are a combination of predrawn symbols and user-drawn symbols. Picsyms include extensive materials and instruction on how individuals who cannot ordinarily draw a square can draw recognizable and useable pictographic symbols (Carlson, 1981, 1982, 1984; Carlson & James, 1980). It also includes predrawn symbols that were copied by a nonartist. The objective of the system is to facilitate the construction of communication boards by providing some predrawn symbols and suggestions for drawing additional symbols to expand and customize the individual's communication system. Therefore, Picsyms rate higher on *openness* than most of the symbols discussed above. The exception is again the use of letters and sign-linked symbols, which require knowledge of those symbols in order to be utilized. The *intelligibility* of Picsyms was significantly less than the pictographs in Bloomberg's (1984) study. The Picsyms were statistically less intelligible than PIC for nouns and verbs, but equally intelligible for modifiers. Both Picsyms and PIC were more intelligible than Blissymbols. This illustrates an inverse relationship between the *intelligibility/obviousness* and *openness* in that Blissymbols rate higher on *openness* than Picsyms, PIC, or pictographs. Picsyms are higher on openness than PIC or pictographs. The openness of Picsyms (and Blissymbols and Sigsymbols) is a major clinical/educational advantage for individuals who are not limited to a small lexicon. Picsyms also have a potential clinical/educational advantage over the previously discussed graphic symbols in that they are available in a computerized form (Frumkin, Geiger, Wilansky, & Cohen, 1984). Examples of Picsyms symbols are provided in Figures 3-4 and 3-5.

## *Blissymbols*

Blissymbols consist of pictographic, ideographic, and arbitrary symbols as shown in Figure 3-6. They were originally developed by Charles Bliss (1965) as an international second language. His intention was to provide a graphic medium that could be used by persons with different spoken languages, following the centuries-old model in China. Although Blissymbolics did not catch on as an international written language, McNaughton and others at the Ontario Crippled Children's Center (OCCC) developed Blissymbols for use with nonspeaking individuals in the early 1970s. Blissymbols offer a bridge between limited pictographic symbols and totally arbitrary written words. They are designed to communicate the maximum breadth of information with a limited number of shapes and a number of strategies for combining the shapes. Blissymbols are composed of meaning-based units. Some of these depict the outline shape of the concept represented (pictographic), others utilize shapes relating to an idea associated with the referent (ideographic), and some are arbitrary. Whether the Blissymbol consists of one unit or several, it is intended that the root meaning of the symbol be explained in a way that relates to the cognitive level of the learner (e.g., more advanced users would be taught the symbols based upon the meaning-based shapes of the symbols, but very young or retarded individuals would be taught to just associate meaning with the whole symbol). The original 1,400 Blissymbols published by the Blissymbolics Communication Institute (BCI) represent general concepts rather than specific instances. New Blissymbols are being added annually to the vocabulary; because they maintain the logical sequencing of meaning-based units, these symbols provide rather abstract representations of concepts (see *cookie, candy,* Figure 3-4). In combining the shapes, it is critical to maintain their relative positions and proportions because such relationships also convey meaning.

**FIGURE 3-6.  BLISSYMBOLICS.**

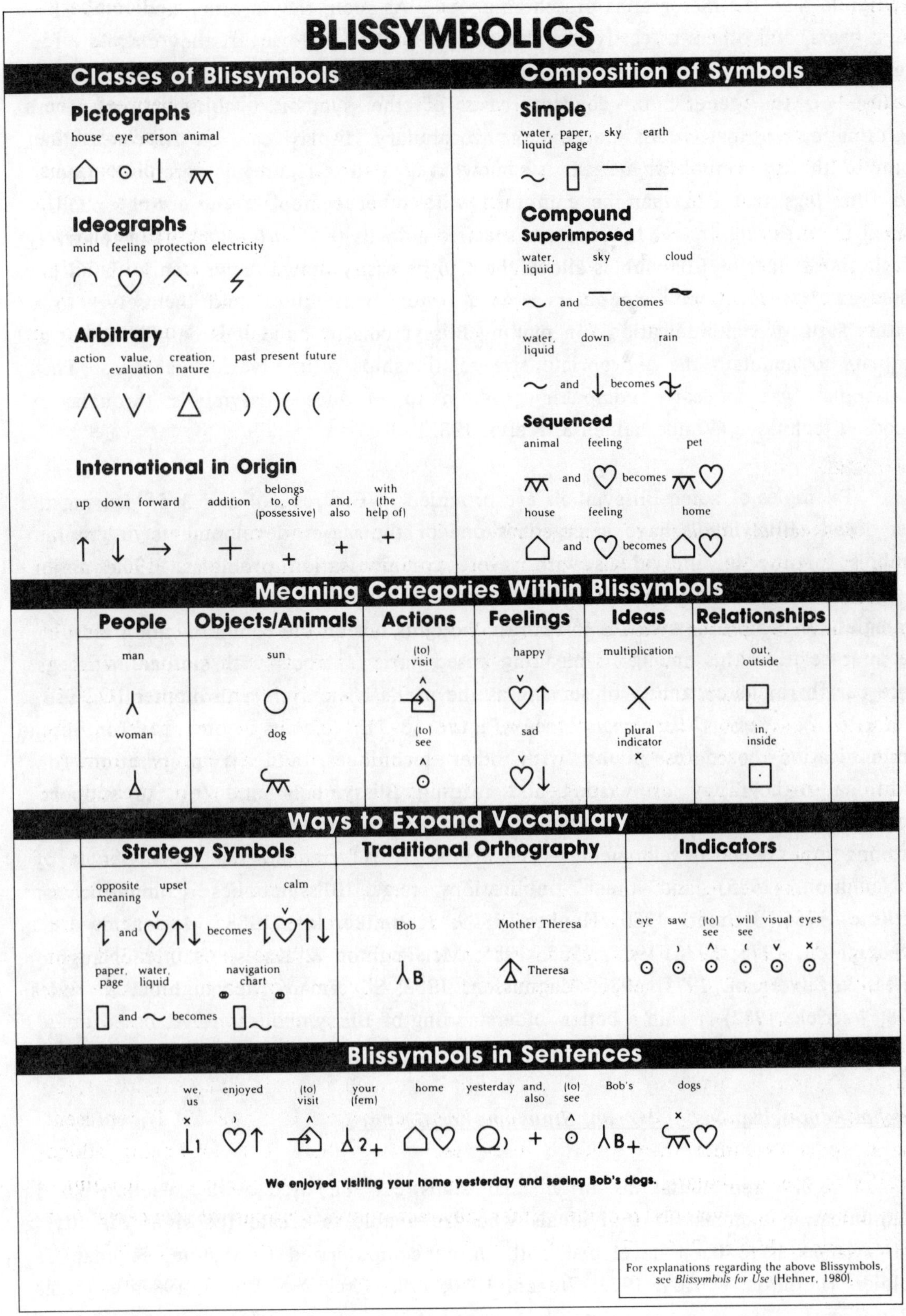

# BLISSYMBOLICS

## Classes of Blissymbols

### Pictographs
house  eye  person  animal

### Ideographs
mind  feeling  protection  electricity

### Arbitrary
action  value,  creation.  past present future
evaluation  nature

### International in Origin
up  down  forward  addition  belongs  and,  with
                              to, of  also  (the
                              (possessive)      help of)

## Composition of Symbols

### Simple
water, paper,  sky   earth
liquid   page

### Compound
#### Superimposed
water,     sky        cloud
liquid

~  and  ‾  becomes  ⌐

water,     down       rain
liquid

~  and  ↓  becomes

#### Sequenced
animal     feeling         pet

house    feeling    home

## Meaning Categories Within Blissymbols

| People | Objects/Animals | Actions | Feelings | Ideas | Relationships |
|---|---|---|---|---|---|
| man | sun | (to) visit | happy | multiplication | out, outside |
| woman | dog | (to) see | sad | plural indicator | in, inside |

## Ways to Expand Vocabulary

| Strategy Symbols | Traditional Orthography | Indicators |
|---|---|---|
| opposite meaning  upset  calm | Bob  Mother Theresa | eye  saw  (to) see  will see  visual  eyes |
| paper, page  water, liquid  navigation chart | Theresa | |

## Blissymbols in Sentences

we,   enjoyed   (to)    your     home   yesterday   and,   (to)   Bob's        dogs
us              visit   (fem)                        also   see

**We enjoyed visiting your home yesterday and seeing Bob's dogs.**

For explanations regarding the above Blissymbols,
see *Blissymbols for Use* (Hehner, 1980).

Blissymbols are conceptually based and typically less pictographic and intelligible than the pictographs presented above. As such, they are not understood by users, peers, and others as easily as pictographic symbols. However, they do allow for communication on a much broader range of topics and have an advantage in *openness*, because of the generic or concept basis of the symbols. Blissymbols permit agglutination so that words not on the vocabulary display can be formed. For example, the Blissymbol for *animal* is somewhat of a stick-figure pictograph of a body and four legs that can then be combined with other symbols representing specific animal features (e.g., *teeth*) to represent specific animals (e.g., *alligator*). The relatively simple line shapes of Blissymbols allows them to be easily drawn or written by hand or displayed or printed with computers. As a result, Blissymbols lend themselves to a written form of communication. In making Blissymbols by hand it is helpful to use a template to maintain the appropriate size relationships of the various shapes. The "Blissapple" was an early computer program to produce Blissymbols through an encoding technique (Vanderheiden & Kelso, 1982).

Examples of some Blissymbols are provided in Figures 3-4 and 3-5. During the past decade Blissymbols have emerged as one of the major developments in graphic symbols for use by individuals with severe communication problems. The major strengths of Blissymbolics lie in (a) the system's openness through its principles and strategies for combining symbols to express thoughts not on the communication aid; (b) the inter-relationships among its meaning-based parts (symbols with similar meanings share parts); (c) its capability of serving as the user's basic system through initial use with *Picture Your Blissymbols* (see Figure 3-7); (d) its potential for broad communication board use along with other techniques, and its preparation for traditional orthography by writing and reading Blissymbols; and (e) the support provided by the Blissymbolics Communication Institute through training, publications, and ongoing system development. The reader is referred to the recent book by McNaughton (1985) and other publications (e.g., Blissymbolics Communication Institute, 1985; Hehner, 1980; Hughes, 1979; Kalimikerakis, 1983; McDonald, 1980; McNaughton, 1975, 1976, 1981, 1982, 1985; McNaughton & Kates, 1980; McNaughton, Kates, & Silverman, 1975, 1976; Magnusson, 1982; Silverman, McNaughton, & Kates, 1978; Warrick, 1982) to gain a better understanding of Blissymbolics.

## *Graphic Representations of Manual Signs and/or Gestures*

Graphic representations of manual signs can be used with selection-based communication systems for individuals who are unable to create the signs directly. Such systems have been developed both in noncomputerized (Bornstein, Kannapell, Saulnier, Hamilton, & Roy, 1973; Cregan, 1980, 1982; Cregan & Lloyd, 1984a,b; Evans, 1982; Orcutt, 1984; Savage, Evans, & Savage, 1981; Sutton, 1981) and computerized

**FIGURE 3-7. PICTURE YOUR BLISS.**

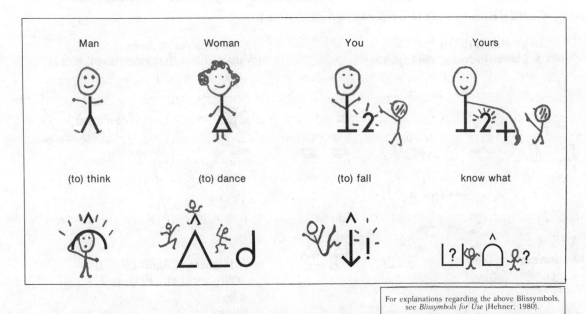

For explanations regarding the above Blissymbols, see *Blissymbols for Use* (Hehner, 1980).

(Blissymbolics used herein derived from the symbols described in the work, Semantography, original copyright see K. Bliss, 1949.) (Exclusive license, 1982-- Blissymbolic Communication Institute, 350 Rumsey Road, Toronto, Ontario, Canada M4G 1R8)

forms (Llewellyn-Jones, 1983, 1984; Watts & Llewellyn-Jones, 1984a, 1984b). Examples of graphic symbols for manual sign are shown in Figure 3-8. The graphic representations shown are designed primarily for use by individuals who know (or are learning) manual signs. Two of the systems (Sigsymbols and World Sign) represent some referents with graphics other than sign-linked symbols. As discussed above, Sigsymbols (Cregan, 1980, 1982; Cregan & Lloyd, 1984a,b; Lloyd & Cregan, 1984) include pictographs and ideographs (see Figures 3-4 and 3-5) in addition to sign-linked symbols. World Sign (Orcutt, 1984) symbols include gesture-linked symbols, pictographs, and ideographs in addition to sign-linked symbols. The intelligibility primarily varies from system to system, but in all cases full use is dependent upon knowledge of the signs, the graphic representations of signs, or gestures that the graphics represent. In general, their *intelligibility* would be high for signers, but low for nonsigners.

The graphics allow one to present printed words paired with graphic symbols for manual signs and/or gestures. This facilitates communication between an individual who knows manual signs (or gestures) and another who does not know manual signs (or the specific gestures), but who knows how to read. The HANDS computer program (Llewellyn-Jones, 1983, 1984; Watts & Llewellyn-Jones, 1984a, b) provides three options for presenting the sign-linked symbols with and

## FIGURE 3-8. GRAPHIC REPRESENTATION OF SIGNS AND/OR GESTURES (*CONTINUED ON NEXT PAGE*).

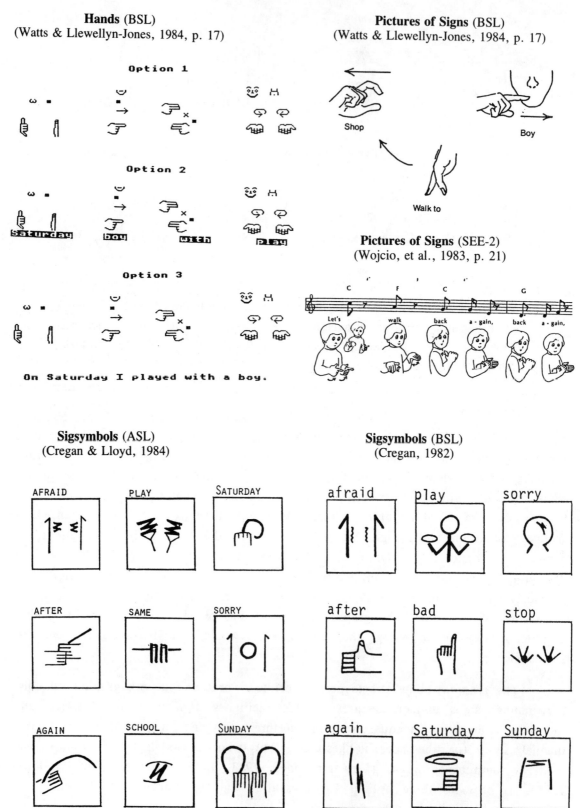

**Hands** (BSL)
(Watts & Llewellyn-Jones, 1984, p. 17)

**Pictures of Signs** (BSL)
(Watts & Llewellyn-Jones, 1984, p. 17)

**Pictures of Signs** (SEE-2)
(Wojcio, et al., 1983, p. 21)

**Sigsymbols** (ASL)
(Cregan & Lloyd, 1984)

**Sigsymbols** (BSL)
(Cregan, 1982)

**FIGURE 3-8 (*CONTINUED*).**

**Sign Writing** (ASL)
(Sutton, 1981, p. 14)

Dear friend,
Now you can read
and write what you
sign. Here is your first
letter in Sign Writing.
Please write me a letter
back (again) in Sign Writing.
Thank you.
Love , Valerie
Copyright © 1981 By Valerie J. Sutton
ALL RIGHTS RESERVED
Pan American And Universal Copyrights Secured

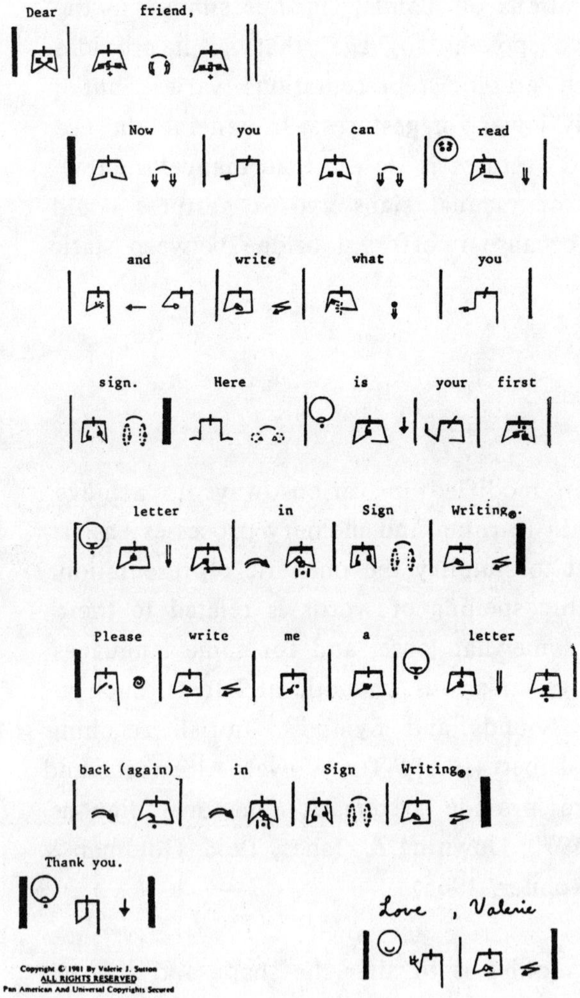

**Worldsign**
(Orcutt, 1985, p. 24)

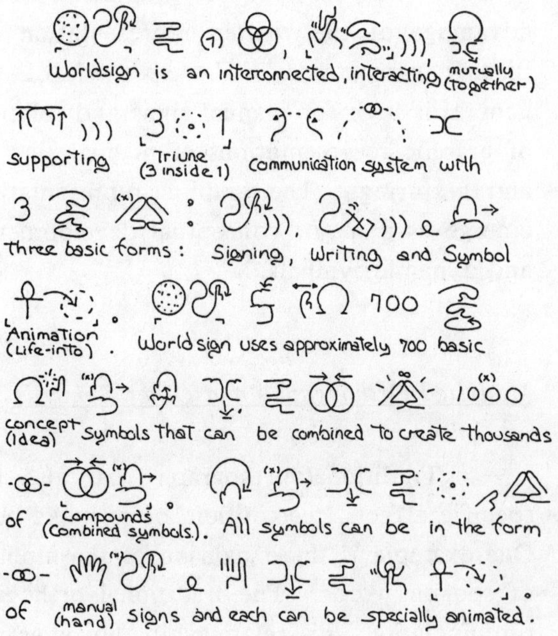

Worldsign is an interconnected, interacting, mutually (together)
supporting Triune (3 inside 1) communication system with
three basic forms: Signing, Writing and Symbol
Animation (Life-into). Worldsign uses approximately 700 basic
concept (idea) symbols that can be combined to create thousands
of compounds (combined symbols). All symbols can be in the form
of manual (hand) signs and each can be specially animated.

without printed words.  This is illustrated in Figure 3-8.  In option #1, the four sign-linked symbols are presented in the order in which they would be signed in BSL without an English gloss.  In option #2, the four sign-linked symbols each have an English gloss.  In option #3, the four sign-linked symbols are presented with English words providing the gloss for the sentence.  The HANDS program is currently being modified for use with ASL (M. Llewelyn-Jones, personal communication, July, 1986).  A major advantage of the graphic representations of manual signs is similar to the advantage of the written representation of a spoken language, that is, it provides display *permanence*.  The *openness* of such graphic representations varies, but in general is high for manual signs and relatively lower for gestures.  In general, the use of graphic representations of manual sign and gestures is slower than manual signing and gesturing.  The graphic representation of manual signs and/or gestures could emerge as a major conceptual development because it offers a bridge between static and dynamic symbols.

## *Modified Orthography and Other Symbols*

Traditional orthography has also been modified in various ways to achieve specific effects, recognition, or to make certain learning and memory processes easier.  One example is the expansion of the alphabet to simplify the phonetic representation of spoken words.  The traditional orthographic spelling of words is related to their pronunciation; this relationship, however, is somewhat loose, and for some languages (e.g., English) follows an irregular set of rules.  Various phonetic alphabets, such as Fonetic English Alphabet, Goldman-Lynch Sounds and Symbols, Initial Teaching Alphabet (i.t.a.), International Phonetic Alphabet (IPA), Ten-Vowel Alphabet, and UNIFON have therefore been developed to provide systematic and unambiguous spellings for English words (Downing, 1963, 1970; Downing & Jones, 1966; Goldman & Lynch, 1971; Malone, 1962; Mathews, 1966; Rohner, 1966).

Another approach to modified orthographies is to alter the shape and size of and/or embellish letters with drawings, alphabet letters, and/or words (e.g., Devereux & van Oosterom, 1984; Fuchs & Fuchs, 1984; Jeffree, 1981; Marko, 1967; Miller, 1967, 1968; Miller & Miller, 1968, 1971; Wendon, 1979).  For further discussion of modified orthographies, see Clark and Woodcock (1976).

Other graphic symbols may also be modified by adding drawings or sketches in an attempt to increase intelligibility.  Clinicans/teachers have used this technique for years.  Recently, an extensive set of Blissymbol embellishments, known as *Picture Your Blissymbols* (Blissymbolics Communication Institute, 1984; McNaughton & Warrick, 1984) was published in an attempt to offer concrete and pictographic support to the beginning Blissymbol user, without reducing the logical composition of Blissymbols.  By adding colored illustrations to the Blissymbols, students can be introduced directly to a system offering long-term, broad usage. *Picture Your Blissymbols* can be introduced in the form published by BCI or with embellishments added by the clinician/teacher to provide personally meaningful information to the learner. As the student progresses, the illustrations can be removed and the strategies of Blissymbolics (e.g., special symbols for *opposite meaning*, *combine symbol*, *part of*) and of traditional orthography (initial consonant, proper names) can be introduced.

Increasing the iconicity of alphabet letters, words, or other symbols may enhance initial learning and/or retention for some individuals. However, as indicated in the discussion of pictures, one must be cautious about the assumptions made about pictures and other emblishments added to symbols. They may not be perceived the same way by the client/student as by the developer. For some, such modifications may be of considerable assistance, but for others may interfere with effective learning (e.g., in the case of stimulus overselectivity and figure-ground problems).

## *Complex (or Expanded) Rebus*

As mentioned in the earlier discussion of simple (or basic) rebus, the complex (or expanded) rebus includes pictographs and more complex symbols. This section will consider rebus as a representation of words or syllables by pictures of objects whose names resemble the intended words or syllables in sound. In other words, rebuses are pictures whose names sound like words or syllables. For example, the picture of a *stinging insect* next to a picture of a *leaf* would be a rebus for the word *belief*. Expanded (or complex) rebus also includes combining such pictures with alphabet letters, which requires considerable phonetic skill plus processing the letter sound with picture associated sounds. For example, the letter *C* next to a *bald man* would be a rebus for the word *cold* (likewise, B + *bald man* = *bold*, F + *bald man* = *fold*, T + *bald man* = *told*, etc.). In other words, this use of the picture of a *bald man* stands for the sound *old* rather than representing the concept of old or other concepts we might associate with the picture (e.g., *bald* or *man*). However, the picture of a small boy representing the word or concept *boy* is a pictograph. Examples of the complex or expanded rebuses are presented in Figure 3-9. Programs for teaching reading to nonhandicapped children using the rebus concept have been developed. The best known set of rebus materials in the United States were developed by Woodcock (1965) and his colleagues at Peabody College. The programs started off using pictograms, which were then combined with letters to form the more complex rebuses; thus, the program contained many direct pictographs as well as complex (or expanded) rebuses. Because of the use of rebuses, the authors called the system the Rebus Reading Series (Woodcock, 1965) and later the Peabody Rebus Reading Program (Woodcock, Clark, & Davies, 1968), which contains simple pictographs as well as complex rebus symbols. This program (and materials) is also referred to as the "Peabody Rebus" as a

## FIGURE 3-9.  COMPLEX REBUSES.

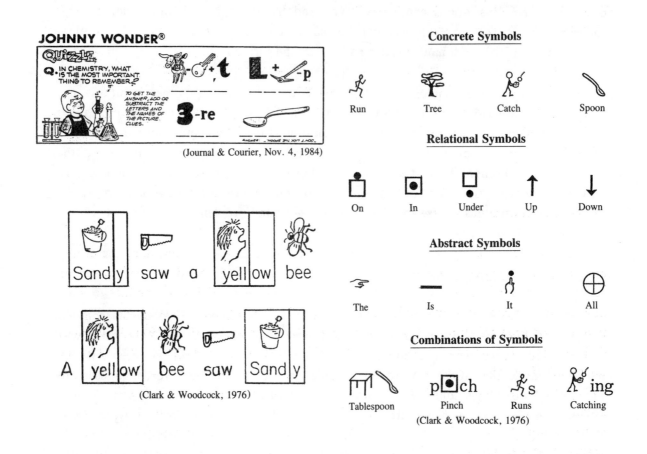

(Journal & Courier, Nov. 4, 1984)

(Clark & Woodcock, 1976)

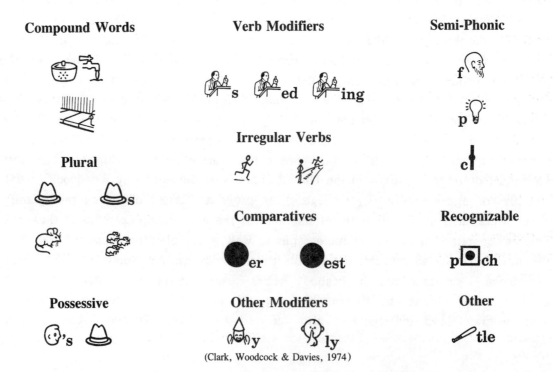

(Clark, Woodcock & Davies, 1974)

shorthand, the "Woodcock Rebus" after its author, and the "AGS Rebus" after the publisher (American Guidance Service). The *intelligibility* of rebuses using letters and/or rhyming is limited to the level of language and cognitive devleopment of the user. While simple rebuses (or pictographs) may be used with many severely speech-impaired clients, the complex rebuses are much more limited.

The *intelligibility/openness* of complex rebuses is much poorer than pictographs (or simple rebuses). The *portability*, *projection*, and *speed* also rate relatively low. They would rate higher on *openness* than pictographs, PIC, and Picsyms, but not as high as completely open symbols such as Blissymbols, traditional orthography, manual signs, or speech.

## Abstract Logographs and Abstract Shapes

Abstract logographs and shapes are similar in basic assumptions and, therefore, are discussed together. Of the number of abstract symbol forms developed in recent years, the two best known have stemmed from research originally conducted with nonhuman primates to study their ability to acquire and use abstract language. These two are the Premack-type symbols used by Premack (Premack, 1970, 1971a,b; Premack & Premack, 1974) and later by Carrier (Carrier, 1976; Carrier & Peak, 1975) and the lexigrams used by Rumbaugh (Rumbaugh, 1977; Rumbaugh, Gill, & von Glaserfeld, 1973) as part of the Yerkish system. The symbols were purposely made as abstract as possible in order to combat criticisms that had been leveled at earlier research by Gardner and Gardner (1969) which used manual signs with chimpanzees. Critics argued that because some of the signs often resembled the concepts that they were communicating, they did not truly represent language. The Premack symbols and lexigrams are designed so there is absolutely no relationship between the symbols and their referents. The finding that nonhuman primates used these symbols led to research showing that retarded individuals could learn these symbols (Carrier, 1976; Romski, White, Millen, & Rumbaugh, 1984). In fact, Romski, Sevcik, and Rumbaugh (1985) reported that individuals who had learned lexigrams were able to retain and use lexigrams for communication 18 months after daily teaching sessions had ceased. While no evidence has yet been found that the symbols themselves are superior to any other available symbols in terms of learnability, lexigrams are easier to discriminate that traditional orthographic letters (Romski, Sevcik, Pate, & Rumbaugh, 1985). In fact, one study showed that although a pictographic system (e.g., simple rebus) was learned much faster than abstract symbols (traditional orthography), there was no significant difference in time for acquisition of the traditional orthography and lexigrams (Kuntz, Carrier, & Hollis, 1978).

Language intervention research based on the application of this nonhuman primate model continues, focused on the symbol learning process and the communicative use of symbols in naturalistic settings (Romski, 1986; Romski, Sevcik, & Joyner, 1984; Romski, Sevcik, & Pate, 1986). Because of the amount of research conducted with lexigrams, the nine basic design elements as well as a sample of 10 lexigrams are shown in Figure 3-10. They are an excellent example of contrived, arbitrary graphic symbols for the exploration of abstract symbol use.

By definition, abstract logographs and shapes rate at the bottom of the *intelligibility/obviousness* dimension. They also rate relatively poorly on the *portability*, *projection*, and *speed* dimensions. Premack symbols and lexigrams would rate relatively high on *openness*, but not as open as Blissymbols, manual signs, traditional orthography, or speech. The major limitation is that one is limited by the numer of symbols one can form with two-dimensional shapes or nine basic elements. The remaining static symbols are codes. These symbols do not have a direct relationship with the referent, but have an indirect relationship through encoding and decoding.

## *Traditional Orthography*

Traditional orthography means spelling in accord with the regular printed letters of the English alphabet or orthography. The term *orthography* may also be used, but traditional orthography is in common usage in reading as opposed to "modified orthography," as discussed above. The use of printed words, phrases, and letters to construct messages is an extremely powerful communication technique if one has the ability to spell and read. Orthography is not easily learned, especially by nonspeaking children or those with no knowledge of phonetics. Printed words bear no relationship to the concepts they represent; thus, orthography is a totally abstract system. In the alphabets of some languages, there is a one-to-one correspondence of letters to the phonemes of the language. However, in English, the letters have only a rough phonetic relationship to the spoken language. Further, if someone does not understand phonetics or cannot synthesize and analyze phonemes to interpret words, as some handicapped individuals cannot, this sound-shape relationship is of no value to them. For these individuals words must be learned as very complex visual shapes, each representing a different concept.

As an advanced form of communication, traditional orthography is very powerful and has a number of distinct advantages in addition to being understood by the public at large. It is one of the highest ranking symbol systems on the *openness* dimension. It is also easily supported when used with simple and complex electronic devices providing for correctable displays, printed output, and conversion to speech. In addition, just 26 letters can be assembled to form any of the words in the language (the same as fingerspelling). The individual's access to the language is limited only by his ability to spell, and not by the vocabulary that can be displayed on his system. The letters of the alphabet can also be represented in other forms (e.g., manual

**FIGURE 3-10. EXAMPLES OF LEXIGRAMS.**
(Romski, Sevcik, & Pate, in press)

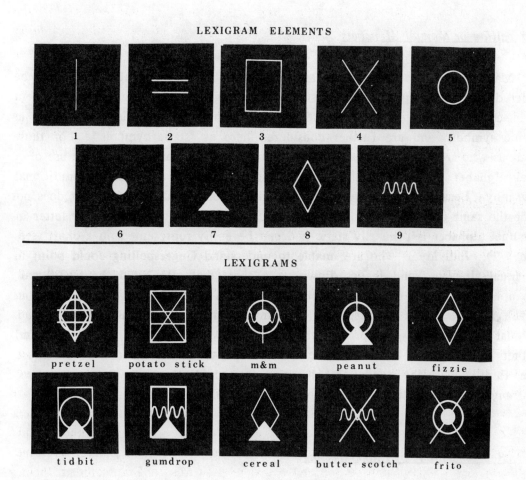

LEXIGRAM ELEMENTS

1  2  3  4  5

6  7  8  9

LEXIGRAMS

pretzel  potato stick  m&m  peanut  fizzie

tidbit  gumdrop  cereal  butter scotch  frito

alphabet, Braille and vibrotactile representations, and  Morse Code) that have a one-to-one correspondence to the letters of the alphabet.  Some of the modified orthographies as discussed above have a one-to-one correspondence of letters to sound by using more than 26 letters.  Examples of the one-to-one encoding and decoding are provided in the following sections.

### *Fingerspelling or Manual Alphabets*

Manual alphabets (also known as finger alphabets or hand alphabets) may be considered dynamic or static symbol systems depending upon the amount of movement used in coding the letters.   Therefore, manual alphabets were discussed above as "dynamic symbols" and are further considered here as "static symbols."  For those individuals who are unable to speak but who have some manual dexterity, the use of a manual alphabet or fingerspelling can provide the same *openness* as traditional orthography.  Because it is not recognized by the general public, however, it does not provide the same access to untrained communication partners.  Almost every letter in the manual alphabet is primarily static and can be easily represented on a chart (see Figure 3-2).  Individuals who are unable to understand fingerspelling could point to the manual alphabet hand shapes drawn on a chart that also listed the traditional orthographic equivalents (or use an "alphabet board" as a back-up).  Although such an approach is slower than fingerspelling, a combination of the manual alphabet and traditional orthography would provide the individual with *projection, convenience*, and the other advantages of a manual system that they would be able to use with those persons familiar with the manual alphabet, and yet provide the ability to *communicate with strangers* using the traditional orthographic equivalents to the manual alphabet.

### *Graphic Representations of Fingerspelling*

As with the graphic representation of manual signs, the graphic representation of fingerspelling provides display *permanence* and the pairing of the fingerspelling and the letters of the alphabet.  As with fingerspelling, these graphic symbols rate high on *openness*.  However, the use of graphic symbols would tend to be slower than fingerspelling.  Their intelligibility is related to the user's knowledge of fingerspelling.

### *Braille and Other Static Tactile Codes*

Like manual alphabets, Braille and tactile codes allow blind individuals to access and use traditional orthography.  With tactile codes, the letters are generally represented on a one-to-one basis with the codes.  With Braille, three "grades" have been developed. Grade 1 is a one-to-one relationship between the Braille cell configurations and the letters of the alphabet. The Braille cell consists of six positions that may or may not have raised dots arranged in a specific configuration. Grade 2 and Grade 3 use additional codes and contractions to reduce the number of cells necessary to spell out a word or sentence. Microprocessor-based devices are now available that can automatically translate fully spelled out text into Grade 2 or 3 Braille, and translate Grade 2 or 3 Braille back into fully spelled out text to facilitate communication and translation of materials for both sighted and blind users.

## STUDY QUESTIONS

1. Both iconicity and openness/expandibility are positive features of symbols, but they have an inverse relationship. Which symbols offer the best compromise of these two features?

2. List all symbols in Table 3-1 in the format of Table 3-4 to indicate which are verbal and which are nonverbal.

3. Which symbols have a direct relationship with their referents and which symbols have an indirect relationship with their referents through encoding and/or decoding?

4. Considering developmental levels (where appropriate) and future potential, select three to five symbols that might be selected for initial use for: (a) a 7- to 9-year-old child with severe intellectual impairment; (b) a 5- to 6-year-old child with severe physical impairment, but normal intellectual capabilities; (c) an adult with global aphasia; (d) an adult with a tracheostomy who is severely dysarthric secondary to a severe head injury; (e) a college freshman with intermittent aphonia secondary to a high spinal cord injury; and (f) an ambulatory, unintelligible 3-year-old child with speech motor problems.

## Transmission Techniques

Transmission techniques are procedures that are used to transmit message elements (symbols) to the message receiver. Pointing, speaking, and signing are transmission techniques that can be used with pictures, English words (auditory), and ASL symbol systems, respectively. In general, there is more than one transmission technique that can be used with any given symbol system, and vice versa. For example, spoken English symbols may be sent to the message receiver through speech, a talking typewriter device, or via a pointing board and an "interpreter."

There is a wide variety of transmission techniques available to meet the specific needs, abilities, and constraints of children and adults having different types and degrees of disability. All of the techniques, however, can be classified as either production- or selection-based, or a combination of the two.

### Production-Based Techniques

With production-based techniques, the individual actually produces the symbols used for communication. Individuals can use extremely large vocabularies, since all vocabulary items they remember are accessible to them. However, production-based techniques generally require considerable motor control. Some examples of production-based techniques are speech production, body movements (yes/no headshakes, facial gesture, body gesture, etc.), and manual production (e.g., manual gestures, signs, etc.).

Most production-based transmission techniques are the same as those used by unimpaired individuals (as part of their communication system)--use of the oral-vocal mechanism for speech, use of the hands and arms for gesture, use of the head for yes and no, use of the face for facial gestures and expression, and use of the general body for bodily gestures and emphasis. Most other production-based techniques are merely extensions or modifications of these techniques. For example, use of the hands for gesturing can be extended to using them for signing. The hands may also be used for cued speech. Individuals who are unable to use their larynx to phonate due to neurological or physical damage to the larynx may be taught esophogeal speech, in which the individual forces air into the esophagus and then releases it in a very controlled extended "burp" that is used, instead of the vocal folds, to produce "phonation" for speech. Production-based techniques can also involve the use of aids. Artificial larynges that use a mechanical vibrator instead of the vocal folds may be used to help an individual to produce speech. Special prostheses are now available for allowing tracheal esophogeal speech for tracheotomized patients. Voice amplifiers are also included in this category of aided, production-based techniques. On a more sophisticated level, sound synthesizers are now available that could be incorporated into a device that would potentially allow individuals to use their hands and arms to produce speech directly using special aids that directly simulate the vocal tract in real time. (Mastering such an aid would require extensive practice, due to the very complex nature of speech, and would only yield speech approximations.) Research is also being conducted on techniques for sending manual signs over telephone lines using special data compression techniques and low-resolution displays. Thus, production-based transmission techniques may be aided or unaided. At the present time, however, the most widely used production systems are unaided.

**Selection-Based Techniques**

Selection-based techniques refer to those techniques that do not involve the creation of symbols. Instead, the user selects or indicates desired symbols from a pre-formed set of symbols. One advantage of selection-based techniques is that they require much less physical control than production-based techniques. In general, however, they also limit the individual's access to the language, since vocabulary is limited to those items in the selection set. The rate of communication is also usually slower. Examples of selection-based techniques include direct selection (pointing to objects, pictures, words), scanning (where items are presented one at a time to the user), and direct encoding (where the individual uses a code to indicate the desired vocabulary items).

Selection-based techniques, like production-based techniques, can be either aided or unaided. For example, an individual may use direct pointing to a communication board (aided) or to actual objects or people in the environment (unaided). Scanning, where items are presented one at a time to the individual, may be done using either a communication board (aided), or a kind of "twenty questions" (unaided). Encoding techniques may be implemented on a device that accepts Morse Code sent to it from a switch operation, or by simply having the individual use eye motions or simple vocalizations to communicate with people using a predetermined code.

The major problem with these techniques is that unless an alphabet or its equivalent is included on the display, the individual's access to language is restricted. Further, practical constraints generally make the vocabulary display much smaller than the expressive vocabulary of an individual. For example, a large, 500-symbol communication board is only a fraction of the vocabulary of a 4- or 5-year-old, which usually exceeds 2,500 words.

**Selection-Assembly Techniques**

A third category of transmission techniques, called *selection-assembly techniques*, involves the combination of some of the advantages of both selection-based and production-based techniques.  As such, it overcomes some of the problems of each.  Specifically, it overcomes the closed vocabulary problem of selection-based techniques, yet can still be used with individuals having severe physical handicaps.

As discussed above, the greatest problem with selection-based techniques is that the individual's vocabulary is limited to those words that are present in the selection set.  Selection-assembly techniques overcome this difficulty by providing a comprehensive alphabet (e.g., letters) as a part of the selection set.  With the alphabet, the user can construct (or produce) all of the symbols (e.g., printed words) in the language.  For example, the use of an alphabet on a pointing board would permit individuals who can only select items to assemble the letters to produce word symbols.  In this manner, any word that the individual can spell is accessible.

Traditional orthography is the most common comprehensive "alphabet."  It is, however, not the only alphabet.  A phoneme set could also be used and would also provide an individual using a voice output communication aid with the ability to assemble or produce any word tht the individual could sound out and enter as a phoneme approximation.  The Blissymbol system is also made up of a set of 50 different basic symbol shapes that, when assembled and positioned, form the full set of Blissymbols.

Selection-assembly techniques combine the advantages of both selection and production, but retain some of the disadvantages of both as well.  The primary disadvantages relate to speed and cognitive load.  First, it is often slower to communicate using alphabets, since a greater number of selections must be made to construct messages.  The second disadvantage, and an important constraint with young or retarded individuals, is that use of the alphabets requires specific skills.  For example, to use traditional orthography, the individual must be able to spell.  To use a phoneme alphabet, the individual must know how to sound out words and assemble phonemes to recreate those sounds.  To use the Blissymbol elements, the individual must know how to combine meaning elements together to express desired messages.  Advances in technology and in our therapy and communication skill development programs, however, provide children with effective ways to use special alphabet systems at earlier ages.  One possibility is that as low-cost, phoneme-based communication aids become more available, severely speech-impaired children, provided with such aids at very early ages, may learn to "sound out" and imitate words that they hear in a manner similar to that of normal children who often play with sounds and recreate or make up new words.  This would probably be most easily achieved if the actual phoneme assembly process, as well as the final speech output, were modeled by adults. It is also possible that the availability and use of phonemic-based speech output aids may directly facilitate the development of phonemic skills in children.

## Overview of Selection-Based and Selection-Assembly Techniques

Whether the individual is selecting whole symbols (selection-based) or elements of an alphabet (selection-assembly based), the basic selection process remains the same. The individual must be provided with some mechanism for selecting desired message elements.

In fact, most aids that use alphabets also use whole symbols as well. To accommodate the extremely wide variety of types and degrees of disabilities, an equally wide variety of selection-based techniques is available. All of the techniques, however, are based upon one of two approaches: direct selection and scanning. Encoding techniques have been developed that can be used with either direct selection (direct encoding) or with scanning (scan encoding) to increase the speed of communication or the size of the selection vocabulary available to the individual (Vanderheiden & Grilley, 1976; Vanderheiden, in press,a).

### *Direct Selection*

With direct-selection techniques, the individual, by pointing or some other mechanism, directly indicates the desired item from the selection set. This pointing may be achieved using the finger, thumb, fist, elbow, eyes, knee, or any other part of the body. Often, some type of pointing aid is used to facilitate this process. Handpointers, for example, can provide individuals who cannot open their fists with a "finger" with which to point to smaller symbols, allowing them a larger vocabulary. Headsticks and mouthsticks can also be used (see Figure 3-11).

More recently, lightbeam pointers, which require little effort on part of the individual, have been used very successfully (Hodgetts, Beard, & Hobson, 1980; Levy & Waksvik, 1977; Vanderheiden, 1982). Lightbeam pointers allow the individual to use headpointing, but involve much less head movement than headsticks and essentially no trunk movement. Lightbeam pointers can also be attached to hands, arms, and feet for individuals who have control of these extremities, but who lack the control or range to be able to otherwise point directly to a large vocabulary (see Figure 3-12).

**FIGURE 3-11.  DIRECT SELECTION USING A HEADSTICK**

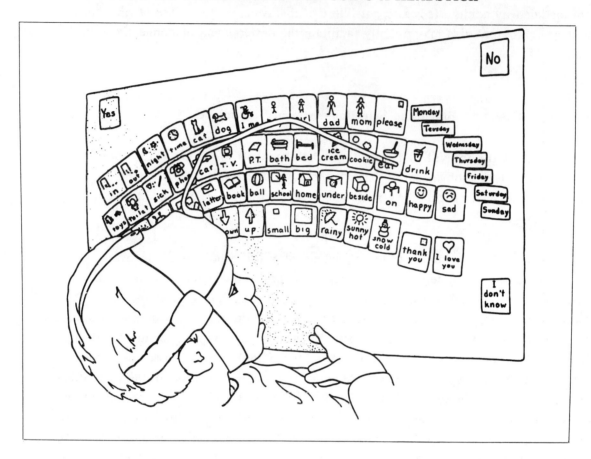

**FIGURE 3-12.  DIRECT SELECTION USING A LIGHTBEAM POINTER**

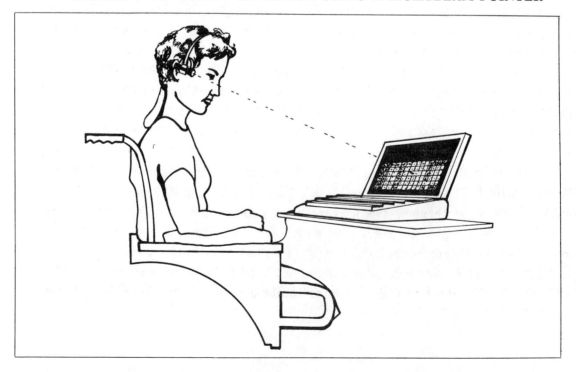

**FIGURE 3-13.  TWO-MOVEMENT ENCODING FOR EYE GAZE SELECTION**

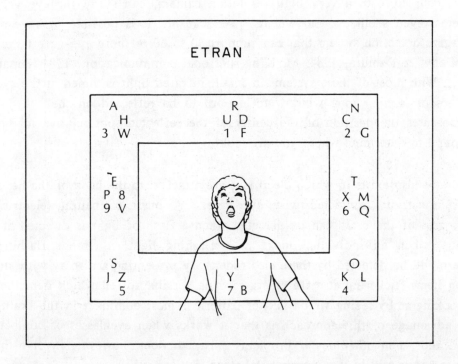

The eyes can also be used for direction selection, which can be a particularly powerful technique.  Because of their physical and neural relationship to the brain, they are often the last system to be impaired.  Eye movements are also low energy movements and are largely independent of postural and other body movement systems. Use of the eyes does, however, have two disadvantages.  First, the eyes are used for looking.  As a result, eye gaze systems may result in listener confusion when the system user simply looks around.  Second, it is difficult for others to determine precisely where an individual is looking.  As a result, eye gaze is generally only useful for a small number of widely spaced items.  Some type of encoding is usually required if the individual is to be provided with a selection vocabulary of useful size (Figure 3-13).  One simple technique has been developed that does use direct eye gaze.  It is based on the principle that it is easy to tell when someone is looking directly at you. The alphabet or word choices are placed on a large, clear piece of plastic that is held between the message sender and receiver.  The sender locks his gaze directly on the desired item on the plastic chart.  The message receiver then moves the plastic chart until the message sender's eyes are looking directly into the eyes of the message receiver.  When the chart has been successfully maneuvered so that the sender's eyes are looking directly at the message receiver, the selected item (the item the sender is staring at) will be directly in line with the gaze of both the receiver and the sender. This technique, although very effective, is physically fatiguing for the message receiver, who must constantly hold and move the chart.  Direct eye gaze can also incorporate the use of electronic monitoring devices.  While it is difficult for a human being to determine exactly where someone's eye is looking, a high-speed microprocessor, coupled with a very high resolution camera, can study the eye very closely and detect even small eye movements. As a result, it is possible to have an electronic eye-gaze detection system that can support 30 to 60 or more eye-gaze targets (Friedman, Kiliany, & Dzmura, 1984; M. King, personal communication, 1984; Rinard & Rugg, 1978). With most of these systems, a small, infrared light is aimed at the eye, which causes a spot (similar to a window reflection) to be reflected on the eye. A camera then measures the position of the center of the reflected spot relative to the center of the pupil to determine where you are looking.

A technique also exists in which electrodes are attached to the back of the head to monitor brain activity associated with eye gaze. A burst of neural (electric) activity in this area of the brain can be detected when a flash of light is directed at the eye. Thus, when an individual looks at a flashing light, a similar flashing electrical pattern will be detected by these electrodes. By presenting a display with all of the selection items flickering at different rates, it is possible to tell which item the individual is looking at by seeing which flicker pattern is most dominant in the brain activity. The advantage of this approach is that it works when eyeglasses or contact lenses are used and when other ocular problems exist. It does, however, involve the use of electrodes and is still in the experimental stage (Sutter, 1983).

Use of electronics also facilitates other direct-selection techniques. In addition to using aids to physically point, it is possible to create a selection panel that has an indicator, usually a light, under direct user control. One group developed a technique that uses two muscle bioelectric signals to control the up-down and left-right movement of the indicator (Copeland, 1974) (Figure 3-14). For example, tensing muscles on one arm would cause the indicator to move up; tensing the muscle on the other arm would cause the indicator to move to the right. By controlling the tension in the two muscles, the indicator can be quickly and directly moved to any point on the selection panel, even though the individual does not have the strength to physically move either arm. This technique can be used with any two continuous signal sources. The technique can also be used to amplify very small or weak head movements (or movements of a finger or any other part of the body) in order to move the indicator around on the large selection panel.

The Target System (Nelson, Park, Farley, & Cote-Baldwin, 1981) involves the use of a small joystick mounted for use with the mouth. Two versions have been developed. One (shown in Figure 3-15) uses a small metal pin that extends from the end of the pointer and makes contact with the target when the user puffs on the pointer. The second version uses a mouth-operated joystick to position a moving lightspot cursor on a computer-based selection panel and a puff switch to activate or

**FIGURE 3-14. GENERAL MAN-MACHINE INTERFACE (GMMI).** (This is a direct-selection aid using range-of-motion expansion, shown here with the muscle potential [EMG] input connected to the user's forearms. One controls up and down positions; the other controls left and right positions.)

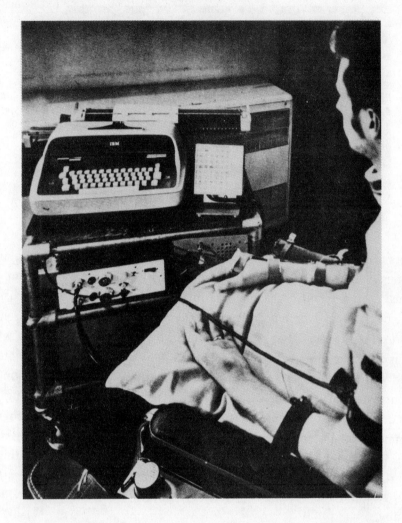

confirm the selection. For those unable to puff, simply holding the spot on a letter for a short time would confirm the desired selection. Researchers in Michigan developed a related technique, where the movements of a person's foot on a special footpad allowed direct selection of items from an array of 256 selections on a selection grid ("The Jim Brooks System," 1980).

Another direct-selection technique is speech recognition. With this technique, the individual selects the words they want by saying them aloud. This technique is relevant for those individuals who can speak but cannot write. In the near future, voice recognition will be an extremely powerful technique for individuals with clear speech, and perhaps also for individuals with mild to moderate speech impairments. At the present time, however, low-cost speech recognizers are limited to a vocabulary of between 40 and 400 items and, more importantly, are not able to reliably recognize

**FIGURE 3-15.  THE TARGET SYSTEM.**  (This system uses a mouth-operated pointer with a puff-operated contact at the end, which pops out to touch the desired selection.)

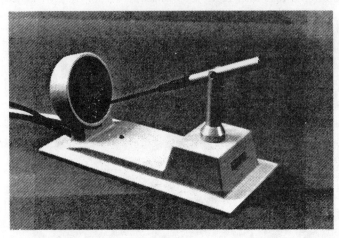

the different letters of the alphabet.  The letters B, D, E, and G, for example, all tend to sound very much alike and cannot be easily distinguished by current voice recognition systems.  As a result, it is not possible to directly spell out words.  One technique that can be used to overcome this is to use words in place of letters, such as *Able, Baker, Charlie, David*, etc.  It is very difficult, however, to think about what one is saying when it is necessary to spell in this fashion.  It is also important to note that even for those individuals who can speak and who use these voice recognition units reliably, it is often faster to use other direct-selection techniques (headpointing to an array of letters and words, for example).  It is also difficult to use voice recognition systems in environments where speaking aloud is either not permissible or is disruptive (e.g., taking notes in a meeting, the library, or in class; taking exams; writing in a noisy environment).  Since speech recognition technology is advancing steadily, however, its utility as input for vocal but physically handicapped individuals will also be increasing steadily.

Direct-selection techniques are the most straightforward and cognitively simple techniques.  They are, therefore, more obvious both to users and message receivers.  They are motivating to the user, since the individual is a continually active participant in the process.  This is in contrast to scanning, where the individual is mostly passive.  As such, direct-selection techniques are generally easier to use with very young or retarded individuals, whose attention is difficult to maintain.  They are also generally faster than other approaches.  Direct-selection techniques, however, do require some type of graded motor control.  Clinical experience has shown that for many individuals, even those who may have severe motor impairments, this graded motor control can be developed and results in an increase of 200 to 1,000 percent in overall communication rate over scanning approaches.

Some individuals, however, are not able to develop direct-selection pointing skills. Others will develop direct-selection skills later, but need a communication system to use in the meantime. For these individuals, scanning techniques have been developed.


## *Scanning Selection*

The scanning category includes all techniques that involve presenting choices to the individual one at a time and having the individual select the desired item, or group of items, by signaling at the proper time.

*Linear or circular scanning*. The simplest type of scanning is "twenty questions." The communication partner presents choices to the handicapped individual one at a time until the desired item is reached. This is one of the most commonly used communication techniques, especially when aids (communication boards, etc.) are not immediately available. This unstructured type of scanning has two major problems. First, the range of communication is limited to whatever thoughts occur to the communication partner. Although obvious or commonly occurring messages may come to mind, it is unlikely that the communication partner would be able to guess that the disabled person "would like to go to the zoo tomorrow," that "these pants are uncomfortable," that "something is bugging me," or that the individual wishes that "people would just leave me alone." The second problem with this technique is that it uses linear scanning; that is, the items are presented one at a time. This is the slowest of all possible scanning techniques.

In addition to the twenty questions technique, linear scanning is also used with a number of simple communication and training aids. Rotating pointers, or aids that employ use of a light, are examples of linear scanning devices (Figure 3-16). These devices can be useful for providing a child with up to 15 choices and can be useful for assessment/testing activities or with very young children. Once the number of choices exceeds approximately 16 items, this one-dimensional or linear scanning approach becomes very time-intensive; the individual is constantly waiting while the device points to the wrong choices before it finally reaches the desired one. Further, the device must move quite slowly, so that when it does reach the correct choice, the individual has the time to respond and activate the switch. For example, an individual who, when using a linear scanning technique with an alphabet, can respond accurately and consistently in less than a second would take from two to five minutes to spell out a single word. For these reasons, linear scanning is generally not used as a communication technique, but is limited to training, assessment, or for individuals whose vocabulary still contains less than 15 items.

**FIGURE 3-16.  CIRCULAR/LINEAR SCANNING**

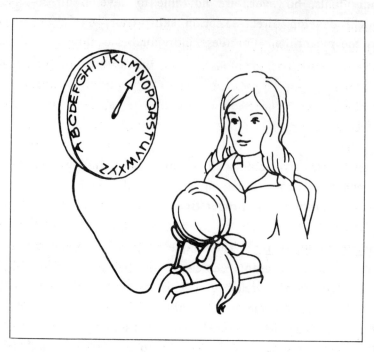

**FIGURE 3-17.  ROW COLUMN SCANNING**

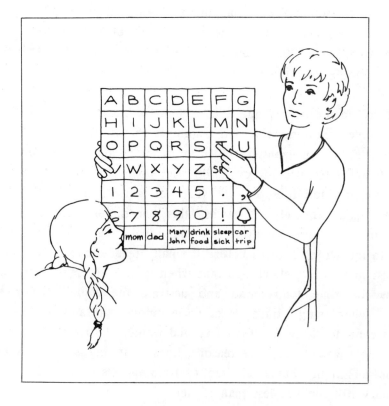

*Multi-dimensional scanning*. To increase the rate of communication, various multi-dimensional or group-item scanning techniques have been developed. The most common group-item scanning technique is the row-column technique. With this technique, the user is asked to indicate when the correct row (i.e., that row containing the desired item) is being presented. After the individual indicates the correct row, the items in that row are presented, one at a time, until the individual selects the correct item (Figure 3-17). Group-item scanning techniques can take other forms as well. Cards may be held up, each containing a number of choices, until the individual signals the card containing the desired item. The items on that card would then be scanned one at a time. In another case, topic areas may be presented to the individual until the desired topic area is selected; individual choices within that topic area may then be presented. The objective of these techniques is to get past the wrong choices quickly and zero in on the desired choice. For large vocabularies, the selection process can be made even faster by using a group-group-item approach. For example, pages of choices can be presented until the individual indicates the desired one, at which time the rows of choices on that page and, finally, the individual items in the selected row are presented. Theoretically, each time another dimension is added to the scanning process, the process becomes more efficient. However, each dimension requires more signals from the user to get to the selected item. Whether these techniques are actually more efficient depends on many factors: the complexity of the system, the visual skills of the user, the ease and speed of making the signal, the speed with which the individual can recover and be ready to signal again, and the way in which the entire process is implemented. In general, scanning techniques are so slow that two-dimensional scanning (e.g., row-column) is required for anything above 10 to 20 items, and three-dimensional scanning (area-row-column or page-row-column) is advised for vocabularies that contain more than 200 items. When used properly, row-column techniques are not much more complicated than linear scanning itself and can be understood and used by very young children. To make the process as visually and cognitively simple as possible, aids should be designed to light up the entire row of choices when the rows are being presented (rather than just lighting up a marker at the end of the row). In this way the user can tell when the desired row is lit even if they do not take their eyes off the desired choice on that row. When hand pointing is used, the individual should also point to the entire row rather than just pointing to the end.

*Frequency of use strategy*. A strategy that can be used with scanning techniques to increase the rate of communication involves placing the most frequently used items close to the beginning of the scanning process. In a row-column panel, these would be the squares in the upper left-hand corner.

Figure 3-18 shows a scanning panel with the number of seconds required to select each square on the panel given (one step per second). As illustrated, the most frequently used items are in the upper left-hand corner and the less frequently used items are in the lower right-hand corner. Placing the most frequently used letters (E,T,A,O,N,I,S,H,R) in the upper left-hand positions can decrease the selection time to two-thirds of what it would take if the letters were in alphabetical order. A similar strategy can be used with the most frequently used words.

### Directed Scanning

The directed-scanning category includes all techniques where both the type or direction of movement and the timing of the movement influence the item selected. Examples would be a four- or eight-position joystick or an armslot control that drives a spot of light around on a selection panel (see Figure 3-19). With this technique, the individual controls selection by either pushing the joystick in the correct direction or hitting the appropriate switch on the armslot control. The device then scans in that direction until the individual releases the switch, thus, selecting the desired item.

### Encoding

The term encoding is used with any technique where the individual gives multiple signals which, taken together, specify the desired item from the individual's selection vocabulary. An individual who selects 1, 3, and 5 to indicate that he wants the 135th item on the list is using an encoding technique. Either direct-selection or scanning can be used to make the individual selections that make up the code. An individual pointing to 1, 3, and 5 to indicate that he would like the 135th word on a chart would be using a direct-encoding technique; an individual who used scanning to select 1, then 3, and then 5 would be using a scan-encoding technique. An individual who used two switches to send dot-dash-dash to select the letter A would be using a two-switch, direct-encoding technique.

Encoding techniques are generally used either to increase the number of items that can be selected or to decrease the amount of time required to select a given item. Direct-encoding techniques are usually used to increase the number of selections that can be made. For example, an individual who can only operate two switches could use encoding and Morse Code to select the entire alphabet. An individual who can only point to 10 items could use a two-number encoding scheme to indicate any one of 100 items, or a three-number encoding scheme to indicate any one of 1,000 items (Figure 3-20) (Vanderheiden, 1985). Scan-encoding techniques are generally used to decrease the

**FIGURE 3-18. SCANNING PANEL.** (This panel shows letters arranged according to frequency of occurrence. The number of steps needed to access each letter is shown in the corner of the square.)

| SP $_2$ | T $_3$ | N $_4$ | R $_5$ | F $_6$ | B $_7$ | . $_8$ | $_9$ |
|---|---|---|---|---|---|---|---|
| E $_3$ | O $_4$ | H $_5$ | U $_6$ | G $_7$ | Q $_8$ | $_9$ | $_{10}$ |
| A $_4$ | S $_5$ | C $_6$ | Y $_7$ | J $_8$ | $_9$ | $_{10}$ | $_{11}$ |
| I $_5$ | D $_6$ | W $_7$ | X $_8$ | $_9$ | $_{10}$ | $_{11}$ | $_{12}$ |
| L $_6$ | P $_7$ | K $_8$ | $_9$ | $_{10}$ | $_{11}$ | $_{12}$ | $_{13}$ |
| M $_7$ | V $_8$ | $_9$ | $_{10}$ | $_{11}$ | $_{12}$ | $_{13}$ | $_{14}$ |
| Z $_8$ | $_9$ | $_{10}$ | $_{11}$ | $_{12}$ | $_{13}$ | $_{14}$ | $_{15}$ |

**FIGURE 3-19. DIRECTED SCANNING PANEL.** (This panel is depicted with a four-position joystick on a four-direction push-button array.)

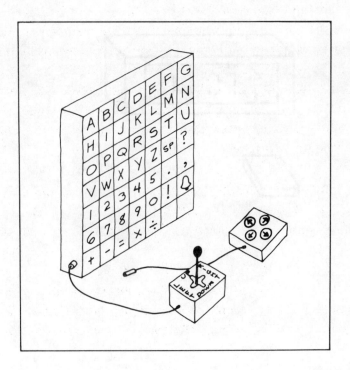

**FIGURE 3-20. THREE-DIGIT SCAN ENCODING.** (This can be used to access any of 1,000 items. Each digit, in turn, rolls from 0 through 9 until the user hits the switch to freeze the digit at that number. When all digits have been frozen, the selection is made based upon the three-digit number selected.)

| | |
|---|---|
| 001 Space | 100 Want |
| 002 A | 101 Can |
| 003 B | 102 Could |
| 004 C | . |
| 005 D | . |
| 006 E | . |
| 007 F | |
| 008 G | |
| 009 H | |
| 010 I | |
| 011 J | |
| . | |
| . | |
| . | |

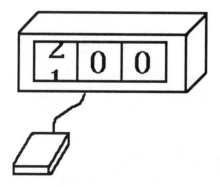

time required to select an item. Selecting item number 256 on scan-encoded aid would only take 13 step times (i.e., the time it takes to move from one item to the next in a scanning sequence) versus 256 step times on a linear scanner or 32 on a row-column scanning aid.

All encoding techniques can be implemented in three different ways:

1. memory-based,
2. chart-based, and
3. display-based.

*Memory-based encoding techniques*. These techniques require that both the sender and the receiver know each item in the selection vocabulary as well as the code for each item. They can be totally unaided; eye movements, vocalizations, or physical movements can be used to transmit the code to the message receiver. Memory-based techniques tend to be limited in their utility and selection vocabulary size, mostly because of the limitations of the message receiver rather than the message sender. This can be offset with the introduction of an electronic aid or computer that automatically interprets the codes as they are sent and displays the various message elements on an electronic display or printer. Such a technique would still be categorized as memory-based, since both the user and the aid must recall the codes and words from memories. However, the receiver need not know the code or even the technique, since the message appears plainly on the output display. Fairly quick access to a large selection vocabulary can be made in this fashion.

*Chart-based encoding*. These encoding techniques are identical to the memory-based techniques except that the words and their codes are listed on a chart. As a result, neither the message-sender nor the receiver needs to remember the code in order to use it. The chart for the message-sender typically has the words arranged alphabetically or in some other logical sequence with the code next to each word (the code would not be in any order). The chart for the message receiver typically has words listed in logical order by code. For example, the message-sender's vocabulary might be arranged alphabetically, with the code number next to each item, while the message-receiver's chart would have the vocabulary items listed in order by the code number to facilitate looking the words up by the code.

Very young children who do not know how to count or even identify numbers can use number encoding techniques; they simply look up the picture or word that they would like communicate and then point out the sequence of shapes (numbers) listed next to the picture or word. As long as the individuals can match and sequence, they can use chart-based encoding techniques of this type. Retarded individuals have

**FIGURE 3-21.  AN ETRAN NUMBER BASE EYE GAZE CHART**

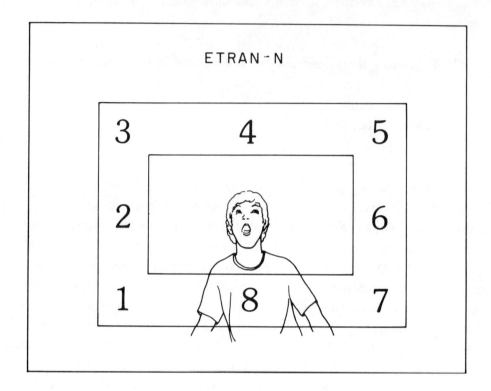

also used memory-based encoding techniques with smaller vocabularies.  The message receiver, however, usually still needs a chart.  One very common use of chart-based encoding techniques is the use of an Etran number-based eye-gaze chart (see Figure 3-21).

*Display-based encoding*.  These techniques involve the use of the same motions or signals by the user as the memory- or chart-based encoding techniques.  However, with display-based techniques, the user is simply responding to a display, rather than sending a code that is memorized or selected from a chart (Vanderheiden, 1985).  For example, Figure 3-22a shows an individual using two switches to send Morse Code. The individual remembers or looks on a chart to find the code for each letter and then activates the left or right switch to send the dots or dashes necessary to transmit the desired letters.  To send the word *tan*, for example, the individual would send dash, dot-dash, dash-dot, for T, A, N.  To do this, he would hit left, right-left, left-right.  The individual in Figure 3-22b is using a display-based encoding technique. With this technique, the individual looks at an inverted binary tree diagram.  Each time he hits the left switch, the cursor light moves down and to the left one step.  To

**FIGURE 3-22. MORSE CODE.** A, Chart-Based; B, Display-Based.

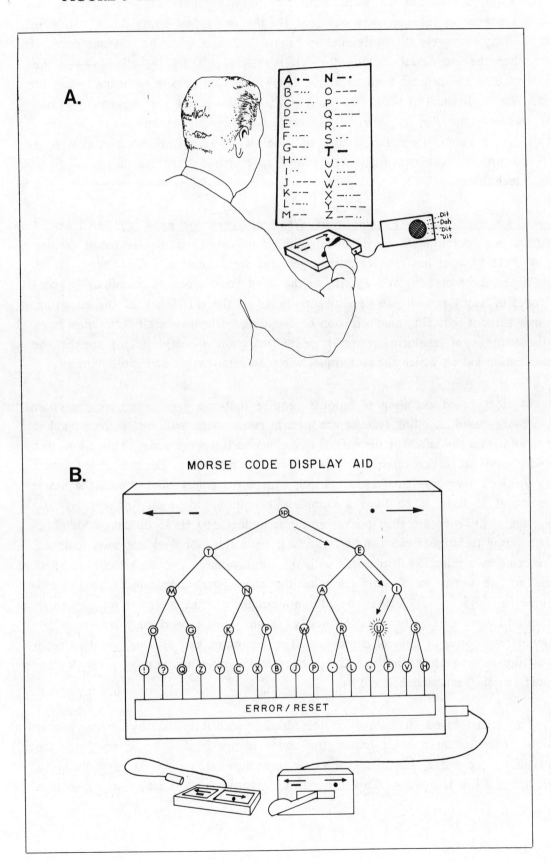

select the letter S, for example, the individual hits the right switch three times.  For this individual to spell out the word "tan," he hits left, right-left, left-right.  This signal is identical to the one that was sent by the individual using Morse Code in Figure 3-22a.  However, the individual in Figure 3-22b is using no obvious code.  In fact, neither the individual making the letter selections from the display nor the person watching the process need to know that Morse Code exists in order to use the system.  The individual is simply sending signals that control the movement of the cursor light on the display.  With display-based encoding techniques, no code is evident.  As a result, they are usually not identified as encoding techniques (e.g., direct-encoding or scan-encoding), but rather as multiple-signal scanning or direct-selection techniques.

*Advantages and disadvantages of different forms of encoding*.  All encoding techniques can be implemented in memorized, chart-based, or display-based formats.  Each of these formats has relative advantages and disadvantages.  The display-based format is the most obvious and eliminates the need for anyone to memorize or deal with codes of any type.  It provides essentially all of the efficiency of the encoding technique without requiring memorization or decoding.  Display-based techniques have the disadvantage of requiring some type of selection display.  This makes the communication aid on which the technique is implemented larger and more expensive.

Memory-based encoding techniques require that the user memorize the codes.  Most memory-based encoding systems are used in conjunction with an electronic aid in order to eliminate the need for the message-receiver to learn the code.  This allows the disabled individual to communicate with a wider audience.  Because there is no display or chart, memory-based encoding aids can be extremely small.  With the newer computers, it is possible to have a complete encoding aid, including display and printer, that will fit into a shirt pocket and cost under $500 (1985 dollars).  Memory-based encoding techniques can also be quite fast, since the user does not need to spend time reacting to a selection display (as with the display-based encoding techniques) or looking up the words on a chart (as with the chart-based implementations).  This technique can also be very effective with individuals who have visual impairments, are blind, or have difficulty fixating their gaze on a chart or display due to head movement restrictions or control problems.  The technique can also be operated from any position as long as the individual can operate the interface (e.g., a joystick, sip-and-puff switch, head switches, etc.).

The chart-based technique is essentially identical to the memory-based technique, except that a chart listing the codes is provided.  It differs from the memory-based technique only in that the user must also carry about or have displayed a chart listing all of the codes.  This is somewhat inconvenient.  Large charts may also block the forward vision of an individual, which may be somewhat of a problem in the classroom or for individuals who operate their wheelchairs. Charts that can be mounted flat on the laptray, however, do not pose as serious a problem in this area. A chart-based technique does not require memorization of codes, as they can be read from the chart as needed. Almost all individuals who use a chart-based technique can eventually remember the codes for the most frequently used items. Individuals working toward a memory-based technique usually start with a chart-based technique on a temporary basis or to remember the less frequently used items.

*Display-based techniques commonly known by other names*. Many display-based encoding techniques are not widely recognized as such. For example, a row-column scanning technique is, in fact, a display-based encoding technique. Multiple signals are used by the individual to make a selection; in this case, the selection of the row and then the selection of the item. The parallelism between this and other encoding techniques can be seen in Figure 3-23. In Figure 3-23a, a two-digit rolling number scan encoding technique is illustrated. With this technique, the individual would select the letter G by waiting for three step times on the first rolling number, hitting the switch, waiting for two step times on the second rolling number, and hitting the switch again, to send the code 32, representing the letter G on the chart. In Figure 3-23b, a row-column scanning device is illustrated. With this system, the individual waits three step times until the third row is indicated and hits the switch to select that row; waits two step times until the second square, the letter G, is indicated and hits the switch to select it. In both cases, the individual waits three step times, hits the switch, waits two step times, and hits the switch again.

Careful examination will show that any technique that involves more than one motion to select an item is a variation on an encoding technique. If it does not look at all like an encoding technique, then it probably is a display-based encoding technique. This realization has several direct clinical implications. First, it demonstrates that the efficiency of any encoding technique can be made available to individuals who are not able to remember codes easily. Second, it is possible to create variations on any technique to allow its use by individuals having specific difficulties. For example, one might wish to use a row-column scanning technique with a visually impaired individual. Due to poor vision or lack of head control, however, the individual is not able to keep his eyes on the display. By having the system make a clicking noise each time it steps, the individual can still use the device by remembering the number of clicks down and the number of clicks across as a code to select the given item. If the individual has some sight, a scanning display may be used to supplement the clicking. If the individual is totally blind, the visual display can either be used to indicate the selected items to the message receiver (if pictures, etc., are being used), or as a mechanism for allowing the teacher to "see" what mistakes the individual is making

**FIGURE 3-23.  OTHER ENCODING TECHNIQUES.**  A, Chart-Based; B, Display-Based.

**A.**

```
A-13     I-22     R-41
B        J        S-23
C        K        T-21
D        L        U
E-12     M        V
F        N-31     W
G-32     O-13     X
H        P        Y
I        Q        Z
                  Space 11
```

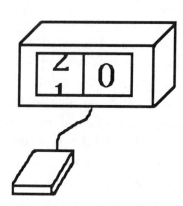

**B.**

| SP | E | A | O |   |   |   |   |
|----|---|---|---|---|---|---|---|
| T  | I | S |   |   |   |   |   |
| N  | H |   |   |   |   |   |   |
| R  |   |   |   |   |   |   |   |
|    |   |   |   |   |   |   |   |
|    |   |   |   |   |   |   |   |
|    |   |   |   |   |   |   |   |
|    |   |   |   |   |   |   |   |

while learning the code. In addition, the clinician's knowledge about the design and arrangment of vocabularies on a scanning display can be used to design the auditory scan-encoding system for a visually impaired individual.

*Variable depth encoding systems (direct selection)*. Most of the direct-selection techniques discussed above use the same length codes to select items in the selection vocabulary. For example, the three-number encoding technique of Figure 3-20 requires the individual to select three numbers for each item in the selection vocabulary. If all items in the selection vocabulary were used with equal frequency, this would be the optimum encoding strategy (Vanderheiden, in press, b). Normal English usage, however, is very skewed. Some letters of the alphabet are used far more frequently than others. The 10 most frequently used words are used three times more often than the next 10 most frequently used words, and 10 to 400 times more frequently than most of the other words in the vocabulary (Gains, 1939, pp. 218-219). The individual's communication system would, therefore, be more efficient if these very frequently used letters and words involved the use of shorter codes. Techniques that have shorter selection times for some items, and longer selection times for others, are termed *variable-depth techniques* (Vanderheiden, in press, a). All scanning techniques are variable-depth techniques. In addition, those encoding techniques that have variable-length codes are generally faster and more efficient than fixed-length encoding schemes. Morse Code is an example of a variable-depth encoding technique; examination of the code reveals that the most frequently used letters have the shortest codes. E and T are a single dot and dash, respectively; A, I, N, and M are two tones long; and so on.

Level or shift squares operate like the shift key on a typewriter (i.e., completely changing the meaning of the number keys). The use of level or shift squares is an examples of a variable-depth display-based encoding technique. For example, Figure 3-24 shows two different implementations of an encoding technique. Figure 3-24a illustrates a special keyboard that can be used directly to type letters and frequently used words. Each selection takes one pointing motion. An additional 260 words can be selected using a two-character code that consists of a code number and a letter of the alphabet and requires two pointing motions. Figure 3-24b shows the same encoding technique, except in this illustration each square contains not only the direct-selection item, but also the words that can be selected. Note that with both techniques, the word *banana* is selected by pointing to the 2 square (key) and then the square containing the letter G. Whereas Figure 3-24a looks like an encoding technique, Figure 3-24b does not, which is again a characteristic of chart-based encoding techniques. Each of these implementations has its own advantages. Figure 3-24b is a more straightforward and obvious approach, if there is room in the squares to print the additional words. Figure 3-24a is more effective on smaller keyboards, where

**FIGURE 3-24. VARIABLE-DEPTH ENCODING TECHNIQUES.** A, Two-Movement Encoding and Use of a Shift Level Square; B, Illustrated Encoding.

**A.**

| 1A — want | 2H — |
|-----------|------|
| 1B — like | 2I — |
| 1C — because | 2G — banana |
| 1D — hello | - |
| 1E — - | - |
| 1F — - | - |
| IG — - | - |
| - | 9X — go home |
| - | 9Y — turn me |
| - | 9Z — get lost |

| A | B | C | D | E | F | G | H | I |
|---|---|---|---|---|---|---|---|---|
| J | K | L | M | N | O | P | Q | R |
| S | T | U | V | W | X | Y | Z | SP |
| 1 | 2 | 3 | 4 | 5 | 6 | 7 | 8 | 9 |
|   |   |   |   |   |   |   |   | 0 |

**B.**

| A<br>1 want<br>2 was | B<br>1 like<br>2 stop | C<br>1 because | D | E | F | G<br>1<br>2 banana | H<br>1 | I |
|---|---|---|---|---|---|---|---|---|
| J | K | L | M | N | O | P | Q | R |
| S | T | U | V | W | X | Y | Z | SPACE |
| WORD 1 | WORD 2 | WORD 3 | WORD 4 | WORD 5 | WORD 6 | WORD 7 | WORD 8 | WORD 9 |
|   |   |   |   |   |   |   |   |   |

there is no room to print the additional words on the keys. It also is more effective for including phrases and sentences in the selection vocabulary that do not fit well on any size square or key. Both techniques are, however, variable-depth techniques, in that they allow very quick, one-motion access to the most frequently used items (the alphabet and frequent words), and use a longer, two-motion sequence for less frequently used words.

*Abbreviation expansion*. A technique that can be used in conjunction with all techniques that include an alphabet in their selection vocabulary is called abbreviation expansion. Words, phrases, or entire sentences can be coded and recalled by the user using a short abbreviation. This technique can be used with unaided techniques, simple communication boards, or electronic communication devices. When used with nonelectronic implementations (e.g., a communication board), the message-receiver must know and recall the meaning of the abbreviations. In these applications, only commonly used or obvious abbreviations (such as removing some of the vowels) should be used. With electronic aids, however, any code can be used, including idiosyncratic codes established by the user. Once the aid is programmed with the abbreviations and expansions, it will always remember them perfectly and can instantly convert the abbreviation into the expansion any time it is used. One generic abbreviation expansion technique called QuicKey (formerly Speedkey) (Vanderheiden, 1984) allows any other abbreviation expansion technique to be generated as a subset, and can provide increases in rate to 200 percent of spelling rate for normal conversation and logical abbreviations. It would be 300 percent or more efficient for text on a familiar topic. Although common sense abbreviations, such as "abbv" for the word "abbreviation," can be used, shorter and more cryptic letter combinations, such as "e2" for enough, can also be used in order to have an additional number of shorter codes for higher efficiency. (A two-key abbreviation is 50 percent faster than a three-key abbreviation.) Using unusual codes is no different, and much simpler, than learning a foreign spelling for a word when you do not know the language. Cryptic codes are only useful, however, for very frequently used words, where the time to learn the codes would be justified by the frequency of use. Most abbreviations, especially seldom used ones, should, therefore, be easy to remember or reconstruct.

*Predictive techniques*. Researchers have also explored the use of prediction techniques to increase the rate of communication (Beukelman et al., 1984; Foulds et al., 1975; Heckathorne et al., 1983; W. Woltosz, personal communication, 1983). These techniques have ranged from scanning techniques that involved the rearrangement of the letters in the scanning array to word prediction techniques. In the letter prediction schemes, the last letters selected are examined and, based upon digram (two-letter) or trigram (three-letter) frequency information (i.e., letters that appear together most frequently in English), the letters that are most likely to follow are placed on the individual's scanning panel. With this technique, the individual's scanning panel changes after each selected letter. Gains in theoretical efficiency are offset somewhat by the perceptual delays introduced, since the individual must now observe and react to the changing display.

Word prediction techniques operate in somewhat the same manner. Here, the first letters typed are used to predict the entire word, or the last word typed is used to predict the next word (W. Woltosz, personal communication, 1983). Aids using the beginning letter to predict the word can be confusing to some users, since they keep putting words onto the screen that are similar in spelling to the desired word. These techniques work best when the predicted words show up directly on the selection panel, so that the individual does not have to look back and forth between two places when assembling the message.

Study of prediction techniques is still very much in its infancy at this point. It appears that the techniques work less well for very fast users and that they increase the cognitive load on the user. Prediction techniques appear to have their greatest application with slow users and slow techniques. Use of prediction techniques would be devastating to a touch typist (e.g., where the letters on the keyboard shift after each keystroke to move the next most likely letters closest to the fingertips if letter prediction were used, or where they would have to stop after each keystroke to see if the computer had guessed their word if word prediction were being used). An individual using a scanning aid with very slow step times, however, would have much more time to observe the display and might find the technique quite useful, unless perceptual problems prevent rapid understanding of the rearranged letters. The actual efficiency of prediction techniques seems to be less than their theoretical efficiency and is dependent upon both the specific implementation of the technique and the skills of the user. Please note that aid prediction schemes, where the predictions are always the same (e.g., *th* always causes the aid to predict *then*) are not prediction techniques, but are usually "cued abbreviation expansion techniques." The abbreviation expansion discussion would apply to them.

*Spelling*. At this point, it can be seen that spelling can itself be viewed as an encoding technique that allows an individual to use a small number of selections (the letters of the alphabet) to access a very large number of symbols (printed or synthetically spoken words). Like most encoding techniques, spelling requires that the message-receiver understand the code (understand the spelling), or that some device be available to translate the code (spelling) into a form that is recognizable to the message receiver (e.g., into synthesized speech). Like all encoding techniques, spelling allows the individual to access a very large vocabulary using a smaller number of selection items. If the individual could direct select the entire vocabulary (as in speech), then using this or any encoding technique would be slower and would not be used (i.e., an individual would not vocally spell out words if the words can be spoken directly). However, if one is using a scanning technique, it would be much faster to use scanning to select the individual letters than it would be to try to scan an array large enough to contain the entire vocabulary of an individual (unless a different multi-dimensional, display-based technique, such as page-section-row-column scanning, were used).

*Semantic encoding--Minspeak*. One problem with memory-based encoding techniques is that the larger they get, the more difficult it is to recall codes for all of the words, phrases, sentences, and so on. The Minspeak semantic encoding approach was developed to address to problem. With this approach, a code consisting of polysemic (multiple-meaning) symbols (little pictographs) is used to recall prestored phrases and sentences (see Figure 3-25). For example, if the code for "What time do we eat?" is entered into an electronic communication aid with a question mark (?), a picture of an apple, and a picture of clock, it will be very easy to recall or reconstruct the "What time do we eat?" In fact, recognition memory, rather than recall memory, will be used in this process. Further, it is not necessary to remember the exact form of your sentence (i.e., was it What time do we eat?, When do we eat?, etc.), as you would if you were using a letter-based encoding system and used the first letter of each word to encode the sentence. Minspeak can also be used to store words; the procedure, however, gets more complicated and involves grammatical knowlege (see Figure 3-26). This would be more complex than levels or abbreviations for a small set of words, but becomes less complex or cognitively taxing for large vocabularies (over 800 words or so).

Minspeak's principal advantage lies in its ability to facilitate the memory recall of a large number of codes. As with any encoding system, all words, phrases, and sentences to be communicated with it must be prestored. This would include sentences that are either multifunctional, commonly used, or predictable prior to a particular interaction so that they can be prestored. Minspeak, when well applied, can be very powerful for a wide range of potential users. However, applying Minspeak well can be a demanding and time-consuming task for the clinician. Using Minspeak to encode sentences and phrases is only moderately difficult. Using it to encode single words for novel sentence construction demands a more thorough knowledge of syntax on the part of the clinician and, to a lesser degree, on the part of the user. Because of the increased demands of the Minspeak for novel sentence construction, alterations in the device have been made. These changes allow not only the advantage of Minspeak, but permit access to novel sentence creation and writing.

Minspeak is not a transmission technique *per se*, but rather a strategy for

# FIGURE 3-25. EXAMPLE OF TYPICAL MINSPEAK KEYBOARD WITH SAMPLE OF WORD MODE SENTENCE

**TOUCH TALKER ™ WITH MINSPEAK ™**

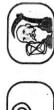

## What time are we going home

FIGURE 3-26. EXAMPLE OF MINSPEAK IN WORD MODE

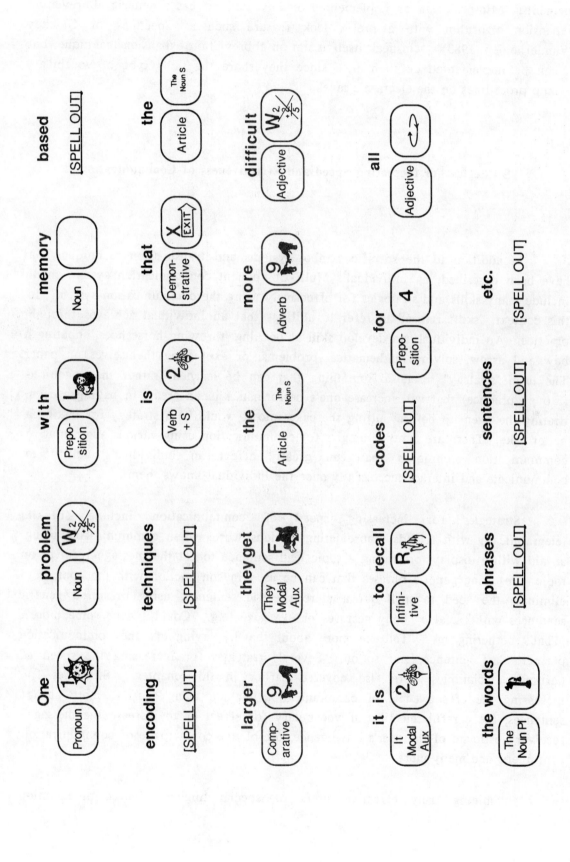

remembering large numbers of codes through the use of pictographs as the coding elements. Minspeak can be implemented on any aid that has a generic abbreviation expansion algorithm with a prefix lock feature such as Speedkey or Quickey (Vanderheiden, 1983). Minspeak itself is not an abbreviation expansion technique, but it can be implemented on such aids, since they share the same type of vocabulary lookup procedures on the electronic level.

## Strategies For Increasing Speed and Effectiveness of Communication

In addition to the specific symbol systems and transmission techniques that have been described, an individual's Multi-Component communication system should include many skills and strategies for effectively using the communication system. In this context, "skill" is used to refer to abilities that an individual achieves through practice. An individual can develop skill at bowling, throwing horseshoes, shooting a bow and arrow, solving mathematical problems, or expressing themselves on paper. The term "strategy" refers to something that can be learned (rather than acquired through practice) that will increase one's performance in an area. In baking a cake, heating the oven up before putting the cake into it would be a strategy for baking a better cake. There are many strategies for communication using various augmentative communication techniques that can greatly affect an individual's ability to communicate and interact successfully once the individual knows them.

Strategies for increasing speed of communication include speaking telegraphically with friends, abbreviating obvious words when communicating using an aid with a display, prestoring a topic lead sentence to get the message-receiver on topic, prestoring generic phrases that can be used in conjunction with the context to eliminate the need to spell out a more specific sentence, using prestored generic sentences with facial or body gestures or eye gaze (e.g., "Could I have some more?," "That's bothering me," "Tell me more about that"), playing off the communication partner's last sentence, and so on. Several strategies for increasing the speed of particular techniques were also covered earlier in this chapter. Strategies for increasing the effectiveness of communication include using shorter, more abrupt sentences; the careful selection of vocabulary for effect or to increase the message-receiver's estimate of the user's intelligence; use of eye contact; use of communication continuers; and many more.

Examining truly effective users of special augmentative communication components reveals that their success is not due to the specific techniques or technologies used, but rather to the strategies they use for communication. It is the provision of information and training on strategies for communication, however, that is most often missing or weakest in the augmentative communication service delivery process. These and other communication strategies are covered in more detail later in this book. Their importance as a part of the overall Multi-Component communication system for the individual cannot be overstated.

## SUMMARY

Developing an overall Multi-Component communication system for an individual, therefore, consists of selecting different symbols, techniques (with or without communication aids), and strategies. From the list of requirements for the communication system (see Table 3-1), it is clear that there are no symbols or techniques that meet all requirements. It is not possible, for example, to provide severely physically handicapped individuals with a mechanism for writing that will be with them at all times. Again, it is important to remember that the communication system for able-bodied individuals consists of many different symbols or techniques, including speech, writing, facial gesture, eye gaze, and so on. To help illustrate this principle, the following case study will examine a communication system for an individual.

### *Case Example*

This individual is a 7-year-old boy. He is of normal intelligence, but has severe athetoid cerebral palsy. He is in the first grade, where he spends part of his time mainstreamed and part of his time in special education and therapy programs. While at school, he uses a power wheelchair; however, there is no mechanism for transporting it home. Further, there is not sufficient space in his parents' house to allow him to stay in his wheelchair at home. As a result, he spends most of his time either in the easy chair or on the couch or floor. His family is quite active, and he and his brothers and sisters (older and younger) go on many outings. Although he is unable to use his arms, he is able to use a lightbeam mounted on his head to point fairly accurately and rapidly to squares of approximately 1" x 1." His speech is sufficient for a few words that are understandable by his parents and some but not all of his siblings.  The grandparents, who also spend a lot time with him, recognize a couple of his words.

The communication system for this boy is designed around a communication board, but involves speech, eye gaze, and gesture extensively, especially in the home. Wherever it is effective, speech is his first choice, since it is quick and convenient and allows him to communicate even if others are not paying close attention.  Often, he will use his speech even when it is not intelligible in order to attract attention and to initiate more intelligible communication.  He has been taught to use his eyes extensively and can often communicate basic needs through vocalization in combination with an eye gaze toward an object, person, or place.  For those familiar with him, he has worked out an idiosyncratic communication technique, whereby he can communicate many common thoughts by gazing at objects in his environment.  For example, to ask "When do we go?" he looks at his watch and then at the door.  He has also picked up a number of very gross signs or gestures that he makes with his arms. Again, these are only functional with a very small group of people, but they are quick and effective and can be easily seen from across a room.

He has several communication boards.  One is made out of a piece of paper covered with clear contact paper and small enough for him to keep tucked into the waistband of his pants.  It remains with him at all times, even as he moves or is carried about the house.  Sealed in plastic, he can even take it into the bathroom and the swimming pool, so that he is never without the ability to communicate.  A second manual board, which is mounted to a piece of wood, is his primary communication board at home.  Most of the time, he uses it with the lightpointer mounted on his head. He is able to use the lightpointer when he is in a stable position (including on the floor, if one of his brothers or sisters holds him while he is using it).  The wooden board allows words and phrases to be changed more easily and, as a result, is more functional and includes the words and topics that are of most interest to him.  Since he is just learning to spell, he does not yet have open access to the entire range of words and topics about which he would like to communicate.  To facilitate his communication, therefore, the board has been developed with a topic strategy.  There are a number of squares on the board, each of which deals with a different general topic (e.g., playing, politics, television, eating, etc.).  When he begins to communicate, he first indicates the general area or topic that he would like to communicate.  He can then use the other symbols and pictures on his board in different ways.  He also has a square on his board saying "This word is not on my board, but I'll give you clues," thus enabling him to use a cluing strategy for accessing words not on his board.  For example, he recently used "red truck hot" to indicate a fire engine.  Similarly, he used "politics person big" to indicate the President.  In addition to using the lightbeam pointer to indicate words and phrases on his communication board, he also uses it for general pointing.  With this he is able to play games, exactly controlling the movement of his pieces on the board. He is also able to direct his feeding activities so that he can eat the items on his plate in the order and at the time he wishes.

When doing homework and work at school, he has an electronic aid that allows him to use the lightbeam pointer to point to items on a selection panel. As he points to them, they are spoken and/or printed out for him. This ability to print out his messages allows him to complete his work, take tests, and participate in classroom activities where other children use pencil and paper. The printout on his aid also allows him to use the strategy of messaging for longer communications when the message receiver is not willing or able to wait for him to spell out his message. The flexible display on his aid allows him to correct mistakes he makes so that his schoolwork is truly representative of his current cognitive skills. A portable printer built into this aid allows him to take his "pencil and paper" with him from class to class and back and forth to school. A small printer that can handle full-size sheets of paper is also used to allow him to be able to complete standard 8 1/2" x 11" worksheets and use other materials that his nonhandicapped peers are using. This was an important consideration in determining his ability to participate in the regular educational classroom. At school, he is not able to rely as heavily on some of his faster but more idiosyncratic communication techniques. Some of his close friends, however, are familiar with some of his techniques; he carefully chooses the mode of communication that will be the fastest with his different communication partners.

A voice output capability on his aid allows him to respond in class. The teacher sometimes leads up to a question, giving him a little additional time to respond. He has also been taught strategies for assembling answers using prestored sentence fragments or answering questions with only a few words, even though they do not make a complete sentence. He practices making intelligible responses in class, giving sufficient information to the teacher and the class so they understand his meaning.

Recently, his school system incorporated some computer-based drill and practice programs into its curriculum. Also, the third and fourth grades began to do experiments in their science and mathematics courses using computers. Since he is very interested in pursuing these areas, there was concern that he might not be able to operate the computers used at the school and would, therefore, not be able to participate in those classes. A special adaptation is now available, however, that lets him hook up his lightbeam pointer aid to the computer in such a way that it can function as the standard keyboard on the computers. As a result, he is now able to use all of the programs that will be part of his curriculum later this year and next; he can, therefore, continue to participate in the regular education program.

# STUDY QUESTIONS

1. When comparing the rate of communication between an individual using a manual pointing communication board and an automated pointing communication, it can be shown that, if the boards were identical and were being used in the identical way, the automated board would be faster. Why? Can you think of strategies that the user of the manual communication board might use to increase the rate of communication?

2. Describe a communication system that might exist for an ambulatory retarded child with no functional speech but very little motor impairment.

3. One component of a communication system for a physically handicapped individual might be a pointing communication board with letters and words on it. Analyze this communication board and discuss its ability to meet the various requirements for a communication system.

4. What strategies might the user of the communication board be taught to help overcome the weaknesses cited in your answer to Study Question 3?

5. List the functional dimensions for communication techniques down the left hand side of a page. Now create two columns to the right, titled "Stronger" and "Weaker." Fill in as many different techniques and symbol systems as you can for each of the strength ratings in each of the functional dimensions. For example, under "projection" you might list speech, signing and gesture in the "Stronger" column, and manual communication board in the "Weaker" column.

# REFERENCES

Alcorn, S. (1932). The Tadoma method. Volta Review, 34, 195-198.

Anthony, D. (1966). Signing Essential English. Unpublished paper, Eastern Michigan University.

Anthony, D. (Ed.). (1971). Seeing Essential English. Anaheim, CA: Educational Services Division, Anaheim Union High School District.

Anthony, D. (1974). The Seeing Essential English manual. Greeley, CO: The University Northern Colorado Bookstore.

Barten, S. (1979). Development of gesture. In N.R. Smith & M.B. Franklin (Eds.), Symbolic functioning in children (pp. 139-151). Hillsdale, NJ: Lawrence Erlbaum Associates.

Berger, S. (1972a). A clinical program for developing multimodal language responses with atypical deaf children. In J.E. McLean, D.E. Yoder, & R.L. Schiefelbusch (Eds.), Language intervention with the retarded: Developing strategies (pp. 212-235). Baltimore: University Park Press.

Berger, S. (1972b). Systematic development of communication modes: Establishment of a multiple-response repertoire for non-communicating deaf children. Report of the proceedings of the 45th meeting of the convention of American instructors of the deaf (pp 118-122). Little Rock, Arkansas, Arkansas School for the Deaf. Washington, DC: U.S. Government Printing Office.

Beukelman, D., Yorkston, K., Poblete, M., & Naranjo, C. (1984). Frequency of word occurrence in communication samples produced by adult communication aid users. Journal of Speech and Hearing Disorders, 49(4), 360-367.

Bishop, D. (1982). Comprehension of spoken, written and signed sentences in childhood language disorders. Journal of Child Psychology and Psychiatry, 23, 1-20.

Bliss, C. (1965). Semantography. Sydney, Australia: Semantography Publications.

Blissymbolics Communication Institute (1984). <u>Picture your Blissymbols instructional manual</u>. Toronto: BCI.

Blissymbolics Communication Institute (1985). <u>Blissymbolics independent study program</u>. Toronto: BCI.

Bloomberg, K. (1984). <u>The comparative translucency of initial lexical items represented by five graphic symbol systems.</u> Unpublished master's thesis, Purdue University, West Lafayette, IN.

Bloomberg K. (1985). <u>Compics: Computer pictographs for communication</u>. Presentation on behalf of the Victorian symbol Standardization Committee at the Australian Group on Severe Communication Impairment Study Day, Melbourne, Australia.

Bloomberg, K., & Lloyd, L. (1986). Graph/aided symbols and systems: A resource list. <u>Communication Outlook</u>, <u>7</u>(4), 24-30.

Bornstein, H. (1973). A description of some current sign systems designed to represent English. <u>American Annals of the Deaf</u>, <u>118</u>, 454-463.

Bornstein, H. (1974). Signed English: A manual approach to English language development. <u>Journal of Speech and Hearing Disorders</u>, <u>39</u>, 330-343.

Bornstein, H. (1982). Toward a theory of use for Signed English: From birth through adulthood. <u>American Annals of the Deaf</u>, <u>127</u>, 26-31.

Bornstein, H., Hamilton, L., Saulnier, K., & Roy, H. (1975). <u>The Signed English Dictionary for preschool and elementary levels</u>. Washington, DC: Gallaudet College Press.

Bornstein, H., Kannapell, B., Saulnier, K., Hamilton, L., & Roy, H. (1973). <u>Basic preschool Signed English Dictionary</u>. Washington, DC: Gallaudet College Press.

Bornstein, H., & Saulnier, K. (1984). <u>The Signed English starter</u>. Washington, DC: Gallaudet College Press.

Bornstein, H., Saulnier, K., & Hamilton, L. (1976). <u>A guide to the selection and use of the teaching aids of the Signed English System</u>. Washington, DC: Gallaudet College Press.

Bornstein, H., Saulnier, K., & Hamilton, L. (1983). Comprehensive Signed English dictionary. Washington, DC: Gallaudet College Press.

Bragg, B. (1973). Ameslish: Our national heritage. American Annals of the Deaf, 118, 672-674.

Bricker, D. (1972). Imitative sign training as a facilitator of word-object association with low functioning children. American Journal of Mental Deficiency, 76, 509-516.

Campbell, A., & Lloyd, L. (1986a). Graphic symbols and symbol systems: What research and clinical practice tell us. Paper presented at the Conference of the American Association on Mental Deficiency, Denver.

Carlson, F. (1981). A format for selecting vocabulary for the nonspeaking child. Language, Speech, and Hearing Services in Schools, 12, 240-245.

Carlson, F. (1982). Alternate methods of communication. Danville, IL: Interstate Printers and Publishers, Inc.

Carlson, F. (1984). Picsyms categorical dictionary. Lawrence, KS: Baggeboda Press.

Carlson F., & James, C. (1980). Picsyms systems and symbol system. Unpublished paper, Meyer Children's Rehabilitation Institute of the University of Nebraska Medical Center.

Carmel, S. (Ed.). (1975). International hand alphabet charts. Rockville, MD: Studio Printing, Inc.

Carrier, J., Jr. (1976). Application of a nonspeech language system with the severely language handicapped. In L. Lloyd (Ed.), Communication assessment and intervention strategies (pp. 523-547). Baltimore: University Park Press.

Carrier, J., Jr., & Peak, T. (1975). Non-slip: Non-speech language initiation program. Lawrence, KS: H & H Enterprises.

Chapanis, A., Ochsman, R., Parrish, R., & Weeks, G. (1972). Studies in interactive communication modes on the behavior of teams during cooperative problem solving. Human Factors, 14, 487-509.

Chapman, B. (1982). Computer assisted teaching of communications to handicapped users project. In Research unit handbook (p. 22). University of Bristol: School of Education.

Chapman, B., & Lees, G. (in press). Computer assisted communication for language development. British Journal of Educational Technology.

Clark, C., Davies, C., & Woodcock, R. (1974). Standard rebus glossary. Circle Pines, MN: American Guidance Service.

Clark, C., & Woodcock, R. (1976). Graphic systems of communication. In L. Lloyd (Ed.), Communication assessment and intervention strategies (pp. 549-605). Baltimore: University Park Press.

Copeland, K. (1974). Aids for the severely handicapped. London: Sector Publishing, Inc.

Cornett, R. (1967). Cued speech. American Annals of the Deaf, 112, 3-13.

Cornett, R. (1975). Cued speech and oralism. Audiology and Hearing Education, 1, 26, 28-29, 32-34.

Creech, R., & Viggiano, J. (1981). Consumers speak out on the life of the non-speaker. Asha, 23(8), 550-552.

Cregan, A. (1980). Sigsymbols: A nonvocal aid to communication and language development. Long study submitted in partial fulfillment of the Advanced Diploma in Education of Children with Special Needs. Cambridge, England: Cambridge Institute of Education.

Cregan, A. (1982). Sigsymbol dictionary. (Printed at Cambridge by LDA) (Printed by LDA, but available from A. Cregan, 76 Wood Close, Hatfield, Herts AL10 8TX England)

Cregan, A. (1984, January). Sigsymbols: A graphic aid to communication and language development. A paper presented at the Curriculum Conference, Cambridge Institute of Education.

Cregan, A., & Lloyd, L. (1984a). Sigsymbol dictionary: American edition. (Experimental edition may be obtained from L. Lloyd, 1717 Sheridan Road, West Lafayette, IN 47906)

Cregan, A., & Lloyd, L. (1984b). Sigsymbols: Graphic symbols conceptually linked with manual signs. Abstract of Proceedings of the Third International Conference on Augmentative and Alternative Communication, International Society for Augmentative and Alternative Communication, (p. 44). Cambridge, MA: MIT.

Daniloff, J., Lloyd, L., & Fristoe, M. (1983). Amer-Ind transparency. Journal of Speech and Hearing Disorders, 48, 103-110.

Daniloff, J., & Shafer, A. (1981). A gestural communication program for severely-profoundly handicapped children. Language, Speech, and Hearing Services in Schools, 12, 258-268.

Deuchar, M. (1984). British sign language. Oxford: Routledge and Kagan.

Devereux, K., & van Oosterom, J. (1984). Learning with rebuses. Stratford-upon-Avon: National Council for Special Education (Developing Horizons in Special Education Series, No. 8). (Also available from EARD, Blackhill, Ely, Cambridgeshire, England)

Doherty, J., Daniloff, J., & Lloyd, L. (1985). The effect of categorical presentation on Amer-Ind transparency. Augmentative and Alternative Communication, 1, 10-16.

Doherty, J., Karlan, G., & Lloyd, L. (1982). Establishing the transparency of two gestural systems by mentally retarded adults [Abstract]. Asha, 24, 834.

Downing, J. (1963). The Downing readers. London: Initial Teaching Publication. (Teacher's manuals included)

Downing, J. (1970). Cautionary comments on some American i.t.a. reports. Educational Research, 13, 70-72.

Downing, J., & Jones, B. (1966). Some problems of evaluating i.t.a.: A second experiment. Educational Research, 8, 100-114.

Drolet, C. (1982). Unipix: Universal language of pictures. Los Angeles: Imaginart Press.

Earl, C. (1972). Don't say a word! The picture language book. London: Charles Knight & Co. Ltd.

Evans, L. (1982). Total communication: Structure and strategy. Washington, DC: Gallaudet College Press.

Fant, L., Jr. (1964). Say it with hands. Washington, DC: American Annals of the Deaf.

Fant, L., Jr. (1972). Ameslan: An introduction to American Sign Language. Silver Spring, MD: National Association for Deaf.

Feinmann, J. (1982). The visual-motor complexity, transparency, and translucency of the Paget-Gorman Sign System and British Sign Language. Unpublished master's thesis, University of Manchester.

Fiocca, G. (1981). Generally understood gestures: An approach to communication for persons with severe language impairments. Unpublished master's thesis, University of Illinois.

Forchhammer, G. (1903). On Nodvendigheden of Sikra Meddelelesmidler Dovstumme under Ervisingen. Copenhagen: J. Frimodts, Fortag. (Text of English translation, The Need of a Sure Means of Communication in the Instruction of the Deaf, Royal National Institute for the Deaf Library, London)

Foulds, R., Baletsa, G., & Crochetiere, W. (1975). The effectiveness of language redundancy in nonverbal communication. Proceedings of the Conference on Systems and Devices for the Disabled (pp. 82-86). Philadelphia: Krusin Center for Research and Engineering at the Massachusetts Rehabilitation Hospital, Temple University Health Sciences Center.

Friedman, L. (Ed.) (1977). On the other hand: New perspectives in American Sign Language. New York: Academic Press.

Friedman, M., Kiliany, G., & Dzmura, M. (1984). An eye gaze controlled keyboard. Proceedings of the Second International Conference on Rehabilitation Engineering (pp. 446-447). Ottawa, Canada: RESNA.

Fristoe, M., & Lloyd, L. (1979). Nonspeech communication. In N. Ellis (Ed.), Handbook of mental deficiency: Psychological theory and research (2nd ed.) (pp. 401-430). New York: Lawrence Erlbaum Associates.

Frumkin, J., Geiger, C., Wilansky, L., & Cohen, C. (1984). Magic symbols. Syracuse, NY: Schneier Communication Unit, Cerebral Palsy Center.

Fuchs, L., & Fuchs, D. (1984). Teaching beginning reading skills: A unique approach. Teaching Exceptional Children, 17(1), 48-53.

Gains, H. (1937). Elementary cryptoanalysis. Boston: American Photographic Publishing Co.

Gardener, R., & Gardener, B. (1969). Teaching sign language to a chimpanzee. Science, 165, 664-672.

Gethen, M. (1981). Communicaid. (Available from author, 173 Old Bath Road, Cheltenham, Gloucestershire GL53 7DW, England)

Goldman, R., & Lynch, M. (1971). Goldman-Lynch sounds and symbols developmental kit. Circle Pines, MI: American Guidance Service.

Goossens', C., & Lloyd, L. (1981). Clinical experience and research: Implications for teaching nonspeech communication (Abstract). Asha, 23, 697.

Gove, P. (Ed.). (1976). Webster's third international dictionary of the English language (unabridged). Springfield, MA: G&C Merriam Co..

Grover, M. (1955). The Tadoma method. Volta Review, 57, 17-19.

Gustason, G., Pfetzing, D., & Zawolkow, E. (1972, 1980). Signing Exact English. Rossmoor, CA: Modern Signs Press.

Hamre-Nietupski, S., Fullerton, P., Holtz, K., Ryan-Flottum, M., Stoll, A., & Brown, L. (1977). Curricular strategies for teaching selected nonverbal communication skills to nonverbal and verbal severely handicapped students. In L. Brown, J. Nietupski, S. Lyon, S. Hamre-Nietupski, T. Crowner, & L. Gruenewald (Eds.), Curricular strategies for teaching nonverbal communication, functional object use, problem solving, and mealtime skills to severely handicapped students (Volume III, Part I). Madison: University of Wisconsin-Madison and Madison Metropolitan School District.

Hansen, A. (1930). The first case in the world: Miss Petra Heiberg's report. Volta Review, 32, 223.

Heckathorne, C., Leibowitz, L., & Strysik, J. (1983). Microdec II--Anticipatory computer input aid. Proceedings of the Sixth Annual Conference on Rehabilitation Engineering. RESNA.

Hehner, B. (1980). <u>Blissymbols for use</u>. Toronto, Ontario: Blissymbolics Communication Institute.

Hodgetts, M., Beard, J., & Hobson, D. (1980). Electronic device control using the retro-reflective concept. <u>Proceedings of the International Conference on Rehabilitation Engineering</u> (pp. 242-243). Toronto: RESNA.

Holm, A. (1972). The Danish mouth-hand system. <u>Teacher Deaf</u>, <u>70</u>, 486-490.

Hughes, J. (1979). Sequencing of visual and auditory stimuli in teaching words and Blissymbols to the mentally retarded. <u>Australian Journal of Mental Retardation</u>, <u>5</u>, 298-302.

Imhoff, T., & McMillen, M. (1984). The transparency of Amer-Ind and S.E.E. to untrained peers [Abstract]. <u>Asha</u>, <u>26</u>(10), 149.

Jeffree, D. (1981). A bridge between pictures and print. <u>Special Education Forward Trends</u>, <u>8</u>(1), 28-31.

Jim Brooks system: A foot-operated portable communication. (1980). <u>Communication Outlook</u>, <u>2</u>(2), 11.

Johnson, R. (1981). <u>The picture communication symbols</u>. Salana Beach, CA: Mayer-Johnson.

Johnson, R. (1985). <u>The picture communication symbols: Book II</u>. Salana Beach, CA: Mayer-Johnson.

Jones, K. (1972). Rebus Materials in Pre-School Playgroups. <u>Teachers' Research Groups Journal</u>. Bristol, England: Research Unit, School of Education, University of Bristol.

Jones, K. (1976). The development of pre-reading procedures based upon the reading of rebus materials. In A. Cashdan (Ed.), <u>The content of reading</u>. London: Ward Look Educational.

Jones, K. (1979). A rebus system of non-fade visual language. <u>Child Care, Health and Development</u>, <u>5</u>, 1-7.

Jones, K., & Cregan, A. (1986). <u>Sign and symbol communication for mentally handicapped people</u>. Beckenham, England: Croom Helm.

Kalimikerakis, C. (1983). <u>Training mentally handicapped children to use Blissymbolics</u>. Unpublished master's thesis, University of London Institute of Education.

Karlan, G., & Lloyd, L. (in press). <u>Communication intervention for the moderately and severely handicapped</u>. Austin, Texas: Pro-Ed.

Kiernan, C., Reid, B., & Jones, L. (1982). <u>Signs and symbols: A review of literature and survey of the use of non-vocal communication</u>. London: Heinemann Educational Books.

Kirschner, A., Algozzine, B., & Abbott, T. (1977). Manual communication systems: A comparison and its implications. <u>Education and Training of the Mentally Retarded, 14</u>, 5-10.

Kirstein, I. (Compiler), & Bernstein, C. (Illustrator). (1981). <u>Oakland schools picture dictionary</u>. Pontiac, MI: Oakland Schools Communication Enhancement Center.

Klima, E., & Bellugi, U. (1979). <u>The signs of language</u>. Cambridge, MA: Harvard University Press.

Kuntz., J., Carrier, J., & Hollis, J. (1978) A nonvocal system for teaching retarded children to read and write. In C. Meyers (Ed.), <u>Quality of life in severely and profoundly mentally retarded people: Research foundations for improvement</u> (pp. 145-191). Washington, DC: American Association on Mental Deficiency.

Lees, P. & Chapman, B. (in press). CATCHUP - A computer mediated reading and language development scheme for children with language difficulties. <u>Support for Learning</u> (successor to Remedial Reading).

Levy, R., & Waksvik, K. (1977). Simple equipment for the handicapped. <u>Proceedings of the Fourth Annual Conference on Systems and Devices for the Disabled</u> (pp. 14-18). Seattle: University of Washington School of Medicine.

Llewellyn-Jones, M. (1984). <u>Computer program-HANDS</u>. Unpublished progress report, Derrymount School, Nottingham, England.

Llewellyn-Jones, M. (1983). <u>Signed reading project -- Computer programme.</u> Unpublished report, Arnold Derrymount School, Nottingham, England.

Lloyd, L. (Ed.) (1976). <u>Communication assessment and intervention strategies</u>. Baltimore: University Park Press.

Lloyd, L. (1980a). Nonspeech communication: Discussant's comments. In B. Urban (Ed.), <u>Proceedings of the 18th Congress of the International Association of Logopedics and Phoniatrics. (Vol. II)</u> (pp. 43-48). Washington, DC: American Speech-Language-Hearing Association.

Lloyd, L. (1980b). Unaided non-speech communication for severely handicapped individuals: An extensive bibliography. <u>Education and Training of the Mentally Retarded, 15</u>, 15-34.

Lloyd, L. (1984). Comments on terminology. <u>Communicating Together, 2</u>(1), 19-21. (Reprinted in <u>Augmentative and Alternative Communication</u>, 1985, <u>1</u>, 95-97.)

Lloyd, L. & Cregan, A. (1984). Sigsymbols: Simplified graphic symbols conceptually linked with manual signs. <u>Asha, 26</u>(10), 90. (Abstract of a videotape presentation at the November, 1984 ASHA Convention, San Francisco, CA)

Lloyd, L. & Daniloff, J. (1983). Issues in using Amer-Ind code with retarded persons. In T. Gallagher & C. Prutting (Volume Eds.), <u>Pragmatic Assessment and Intervention Issues</u> (pp.171-194). San Diego, CA: College-Hill Press.

Lloyd, L., & Fuller, D. (in press). Augmentative and alternative communication symbol taxonomies. <u>Augmentative and Alternative Communication, 2</u>.

Lloyd, L., & Karlan, G. (1984). Nonspeech communication symbols and systems: Where have we been and where are we going? <u>Journal of Mental Deficiency Research, 28</u>, 3-20.

Magnusson, M. (1982). <u>Mina ord i bild-fallstudie av Blis</u> [<u>My words in pictures: Case study in Bliss</u>]. Broma, Sweden: Handikappinstitutet.

Maharaj, S. (1980). <u>Pictogram ideogram communication</u>. Regina, Canada: The George Reed Foundation for the Handicapped.

Malone, J. (1962). The larger aspects of spelling reform. <u>Elementary English, 39</u>, 435-445.

Marko, K. (1967). Symbol accentuation: Application to classroom instruction of retardates. <u>Proceedings of the First Congress of the International Association for the Scientific Study of Mental Deficiency</u> (pp. 773-775).

Matthews, M. (1966). <u>Teaching to read, historically considered</u>. Chicago: University of Chicago Press.

McDonald, E. (1980). Teaching and using Blissymbolics. Toronto: Blissymbolics Communication Institute.

McNaughton, S. (1975). Symbol secrets. Toronto: University of Toronto Press.

McNaughton, S. (1976). Bliss symbols: An alternate symbol system for the non-vocal pre-reading child. In G. Vanderheiden & K. Grilley (Eds.), Nonvocal communication techniques and aids for the severely physically handicapped (pp. 85-104). Baltimore: University Park Press.

McNaughton, S. (1981). Personal computers and Blissymbolics. Toronto: Blissymbolics Communication Institute.

McNaughton, S. (1982). Augmentative communication system: Blissymbolics. In Bleck & Nagel (Eds.), Physically handicapped children - A medical atlas for teachers. New York, NY: Grune & Stratton.

McNaughton, S. (Ed.) (1985). Communicating with Blissymbolics. Toronto: Blissymbolics Communication Institute.

McNaughton, S., & Kates, B. (1980). The application of Blissymbolics. In R. Schiefelbusch (Ed.), Nonspeech language and communication: Analysis and intervention (pp. 303-321). Baltimore: University Park Press.

McNaughton, S., Kates, B., & Silverman, H. (1975). Teaching guidelines. Toronto, Canada: Blissymbolics Communication Foundation.

McNaughton, S., Kates, B., & Silverman, H. (1976). Provisional dictionary: Revised edition. Toronto, Canada: Blissymbolics Communication Foundation.

McNaughton, S., & Warrick, A. (1984). Picture your Blissymbols. Canadian Journal of Mental Retardation, 34(4), 1-7.

Meador, D., Rumbaugh, D., Tribble, M., & Thompson, S. (1984). Facilitating visual discrimination learning of moderately and severely mentally retarded children through illumination of stimuli. American Journal of Deficiency, 89, 313-316.

Miller, A. (1967). Symbol accentuation: Outgrowht of theory and experiment. In E. Meshorer (Chair), A new approach to language development with retardates. Symposium presented at the First International Congress on the Scientific Study of Mental Deficiency, Montpellier, France.

Miller, A.  (1968).  Symbol accentuation:  A new approach to reading.  New York: Doubleday Multimedia.

Miller, A., & Miller, E. (1968).  Symbol accentuation:  The perceptual transfer of meaning from spoken to printed words.  American Journal of Mental Deficiency, 73, 202-208.

Miller, A., & Miller, E.  (1971).  Symbol accentuation, single-track functioning and early reading.  American Journal of Mental Deficiency, 76, 110-117.

Morris, D., Collett, P., Marsh, P., & O'Shaughnessy, M. (1979).  Gestures:  Their origins and distribution.  London:  Jonathan Cape Ltd.

Musselwhite, C., & St. Louis, K.  (1982).  Communication programming for the severely handicapped:  Vocal and nonvocal strategies.  San Diego, CA:  College-Hill Press.

Naisbitt, J. (1982).  Megatrends.  New York:  Warner Books.

Nelson, J., Park, G., Farley, R., & Cote-Baldwin, C. (1981).  Providing access to computers to physically handicapped persons:  Two approaches.  Proceedings of the Fourth Annual Conference on Rehabilitation Engineering (pp. 140-142). Washington, DC:  RESNA.

Norton, S., Schultz, M., Reed, C., Braida, L., Durlach, N., Rabinowitz, W., & Chomsky, C. (1977).  Analytic study of the Tadoma method:  Background and preliminary results.  Journal of Speech and Hearing Research, 20, 574-595.

Orcutt, D. (1984).  World Sign:  A kinetic language.  Communicating Together, 2(3), 17-19.

Paget, R. (1951).  The new sign language.  London:  The Wellcome Foundation.

Paget, G., & Gorman, P. (1968).  A systematic sign language.  London:  Royal National Institute for the Deaf.

Paget, R., Gorman, P., & Paget, G. (1971).  An introduction to the Paget-Gorman Sign System with examples.  Reading, Berkshire, England:  A.E.D.E.  Publications Committee.

Paget, R. Gorman, P., & Paget, G.  (1972).  A systematic sign language.  London: Mimeographed.

Paget, R., Gorman, P., & Paget, G. (1976). The Paget-Gorman sign system (6th ed.). London: Association for Experiment in Deaf Education, Ltd.

Parnwell, E. (1977). Oxford English picture dictionary. Oxford, England: Oxford University Press.

Premack, D. (1970). A functional analysis of language. Journal of Experimental Analysis of Behavior, 14, 107-125.

Premack, D. (1971a). Language in chimpanzee? Science, 172, 808-822.

Premack, D. (1971b). On the assessment of language competence in the chimpanzee. Behavior of Non-human Primates, 4, 1985-228.

Premack, D., & Premack, A. (1974). Teaching visual language to apes and language-deficient persons. In R. Schiefelbusch & L. Lloyd (Eds.), Language perspectives: Acquisition, retardation, and intervention (pp. 347-376). Baltimore: University Park Press.

Ricks, D., & Wing, L. (1975). Language, communication, and the use of symbols in normal and autistic children. Journal of Autism and Childhood Schizophrenia, 5, 191-221.

Riekehof, L. (1963). Talk to the deaf. Springfield, MO: Gospel Publishing House.

Rinard, G., & Rugg, D. (1978). Application of the ocular transducer to the Etran (1) communicator. Proceedings of the Fifth Annual Conference on Systems and Devices for the Disabled (pp. 164-166). Houston: Baylor College of Medicine, Texas Institute for Rehabilitation and Research.

Rohner, T. (1966). Fonetic English spelling. Evanston, IL: Fonetic English Spelling Associates.

Romski, M. (1986, April). Acquisition of symbolic communication in persons with severe mental retardation: Presentation at Purdue University. (55 minute color videotape).

Romski, M., Sevcik, R. & Joyner, S. (1984). Nonspeech communication systems: Implications for language intervention with mentally retarded children. In J. Kemp (Ed.), Retardation and language intervention. Topics in Language Disorders, 5, 66-81.

Romski, M., Sevcik, R., Pate, J., & Rumbaugh, D. (1985). Discrimination of lexigrams and traditional orthography by nonspeaking severely retarded persons. American Journal of Mental Deficiency, 90, 185-189.

Romski, M., Sevcik, R., & Pate, J. (1986). The establishment of symbolic communication in persons with severe mental retardation. Manuscript in preparation.

Romski, M., Sevcik, R., & Rumbaugh, D. (1985). Retention of symbolic communication skills by severely mentally retarded persons. American Journal of Mental Deficiency, 89, 441-444.

Romski, M., White, R., Millen, C., & Rumbaugh, D. (1984). Effects of computer-keyboard teaching on the symbolic communication of severely retarded persons: Five case studies. Psychological Record, 34, 39-54.

Rubino, F., Hayhurst, A., Guejlman, J., Madson, W., & Plum, O. (1975). Gestuno: International sign language of the deaf. Carlisle, England: The British Deaf Association.

Rumbaugh, D. (Ed.). (1977). Language learning by a Chimpanzee: The Lana project. New York: Academic Press.

Rumbaugh, D., Gill, T., & von Glaserfeld, E. (1973). Reading and sentence completion by a chimpanzee (Pan). Science, 82, 731-733.

Rutter, M. (1965). Speech disorders in a series of autistic children. In A. Franklin (Ed.), Children with communication problems. London: Pitman.

Sanders, D. (1976). A model for communication. In L. Lloyd (Ed.), Communication assessment and intervention strategies. Baltimore: University Park Press.

Savage, R., Evans, L., & Savage J. (1981). Psychology and communication in deaf children. Sidney: Grune & Stratton.

Schiefelbusch, R. (1980). Nonspeech language and communication: Analysis and intervention. Baltimore: University Park Press.

Silverman, F. (1980). Communication for the speechless. Englewood Cliffs, NJ: Prentice-Hall.

Silverman, H., McNaughton, S., & Kates, B. (1978). Handbook of Blissymbolics. Toronto: Blissymbolics Communication Institute.

Skelly, M. (1979). Amer-Ind gestural code based on universal American Indian hand talk. New York: Elsevier.

Skelly, M., Schinsky, L., Smith, R., Donaldson, R., & Griffin, J. (1975). American Indian Sign: A gestural communication system for the speechless. Archives of Physical Medicine and Rehabilitation, 56, 156-160.

Skelly, M., Schinsky, L., Smith, R., & Fust, R. (1974). American Indian Sign (AMERIND) as a facilitator of verbalization for the oral verbal apraxic. Journal of Speech and Hearing Disorders, 39, 445-466.

Sutcliff, T. (1981). Sign and say. London: The Royal National Institute for the Deaf.

Sutcliff, B. (1983). "Total Communication" or total confusion. Journal of the British Teachers of the Deaf, 5(7), 134-136.

Sutter, E. (1983). An oculo-encephalographic communication system. Proceedings of the Sixth Annual Conference on Rehabilitation Engineering (pp. 242-244). RESNA.

Sutton, V. (1981). Sign writing for everyday use. Newport Beach, CA: The Center for Movement Writing. (P.O. Box 7344, Newport Beach, CA 92658-0344)

Tebbs, T. (Co-ordinator). (1978). Ways and means. Houndmills, Basingstoke, Hampshire: Globe Education.

Topper, S. (1974). Gesture language for the severely and profoundly mentally retarded. Denton, TX: Denton State School.

Topper, S. (1975). Gesture language for a non-verbal severely retarded male. Mental Retardation, 13, 30-31.

Van Adestine, F. (1932). An evaluation of the Tadoma method. Volta Review, 34, 199.

van Oosterom, J., & Devereux, K. (1982). REBUS at Rees Thomas School. Special Education: Forward Trends, 9(1), 31-33.

van Oosterom, J. & Devereux, K. (1984). Rebus glossary. Blackhill, England: EARD.

Vanderheiden, G. (in press, a).   Overview of basic selection techniques for augmentative communication:  Present and future.  L. E. Bernstein (Ed.), The vocally impaired:  Clinical practice and research.  New York:  Academic Press.

Vanderheiden, G. (in press, b).   A quantitative modeling approach for analysis of augmentative techniques and aids.   In L. E. Bernstein (Ed.), The vocally impaired:  Clinical practice and research.  New York:  Academic Press.

Vanderheiden, G., & Grilley, K.  (1976).  Non-Vocal communication techniques and aids for the severely physically handicapped.  Baltimore: University Park Press.

Vanderheiden, G. & Kelso, D. (1982).  The talking Blissapple.  Madison, WI:  Trace Research and Development Center.

Vanderheiden, G. (1982).  Hybrid optical headpointing technique.  Proceedings of the Fifth Annual Conference on Rehabilitation Engineering (p. 24).   Houston: RESNA.

Vanderheiden, G. (1983).  Curbcuts and computers:  Providing access to comuters and information services for disabled individuals.   Excerpted from the keynote speech at the Indiana Governor's Conference on the Handicapped, October 13, 1983.  (Available from Trace Research and Development Center, Room S-151, Waisman Center, 1500 Highland Avenue, Madison, WI  53705)

Vanderheiden, G. (1984).   A high-efficiency flexible keyboard input acceleration technique:  SPEEDKEY.  Proceedings of the Second International Conference on Rehabilitation Engineering (pp. 353-354).  RESNA.

Vanderheiden, G. (1985).   A unified quantitative modeling approach for selection-based augmentative communication systems.  University Microfilms.

Vivian, R. (1966).   The Tadoma method:  A tactual approach to speech and speech reading.  Volta Review, 68, 733-737.

Wampler, D. (1971).  Linguistics of visual English.  Unpublished manuscript.

Warrick, A.   (1982).   Blissymbolics for preschool children  (2nd ed.).   Toronto: Blissymbolics Communication Institute.

Washington State School for the Deaf.  (1972).  An introduction to manual English. Vancouver: Washington State School for the Deaf.

Watson. D. (1973). Talk with your hands. Menasha, WI: George Banta.

Watts, M., & Llewellyn-Jones, M. (1984a). Teachers handbook: Hands on. Nottingham, England: Signit Project, Arnold Derrymount School.

Watts, M., & Llewellyn-Jones, M. (1984b). User manual: Hands on. Nottingham, England: Signit Project, Arnold Derrymount School.

Webster, C., McPherson, H., Sloman, L., Evans, M., & Kaucher (1973). Communicating with an autistic boy with gestures. Journal of Autism and Childhood Schizophrenia, 3, 337–346.

Wendon, L. (1979). Exploring the scope of a picture code system for teaching reading and spelling. Remedial Education, 7(3), 33–42.

Wilbur, R. (1976). The linguistics of manual languages and manual systems. In L. Lloyd (Ed.), Communication assessment and intervention strategies (pp. 423–500). Baltimore: University Park Press.

Wilbur, R. (1979). American sign languages and sign systems. Baltimore: University Park Press.

Woodcock, R. (Ed.) (1965). The rebus reading series. Nashville: George Peabody College, Institute on Mental Retardation & Intellectual Development.

Woodcock, R., Clark, C., & Davies, C. (1968). Peabody rebus reading program. Circle Pines, MN: American Guidance Service.

Wundt, W. (1973). The language of gestures. The Hague: Mouton.

# CHAPTER 4

## ASSESSMENT PROCEDURES

KATHRYN M. YORKSTON

*Department of Rehabilitation Medicine*
*University of Washington, Seattle*


GEORGE KARLAN

*Department of Special Education*
*Purdue University*
*West Lafayette, Indiana*

## OBJECTIVES

- Define assessment as a process during which communication problems are identified and described and a systematic plan for communication intervention is designed or reevaluated.

- Discuss the multidisciplinary, transdisciplinary, and interdisciplinary team approaches to assessment of individuals who use or may potentially use augmentative communication components.

- Provide guidelines for assessment that will lead to the selection of the most appropriate aids, techniques, symbols, and strategies to meet

This preparation of this chapter was supported in part by Grant #G008200020 from the National Institute of Handicapped Research, Department of Education, Washington, DC. The authors wish to thank David Beukelman and Patricia Dowden for their assistance.

163

current and future communication needs, including:  approaches to assessment; assessment of communication needs; capability assessment; and performance trials.

- Provide guidelines for assessment that will lead to the development of appropriate short- and long-term intervention objectives and procedures.

- Discuss the relationship between assessment, intervention, and measurement of outcomes.

## INTRODUCTION

### *Purpose of Assessment*

Assessment is a process during which information is gathered in order to make clinical, educational, or vocational management decisions.  Assessment of severely speech- and writing-impaired individuals may involve gathering enough information (a) to make decisions about the need for augmentative communication aids and techniques, (b) to select appropriate communication interventions for meeting the communication needs of the individual, and/or (c) to plan and implement appropriate intervention programs.  This chapter focuses on assessment as a decision-making process that occurs at critical points throughout the clinical management of persons with severe expressive communication disorders.  During this process, a team of specialists will be involved in the initial evaluation of the individual, the development of a management plan or intervention program, and the on-going or follow-up evaluations needed to successfully implement the management plan or intervention program.

### *Assessment "Triggers":  Critical Decision-Making Points*

Critical decision-making points occur when communication needs are unmet, have changed, or will change substantially in the near future.  For example, a critical decision-making point may occur when individuals enter or change educational programs.  At these points, the capabilities, skills, and needs of severely speech/language- and writing-impaired individuals must be assessed, along with the resources and constraints of the environment.  For a young child, a critical point may be reached when speech has not developed and the child appears frustrated when attempting to express specific messages (e.g., requesting a favorite toy from another room). A second critical point may occur when a child prepares to enter a preschool program or, later, when a change in educational programs has occurred or is contemplated. For a mentally retarded adolescent, the need to reevaluate the individual's educational or communication needs may be related to a change from a secondary educational program to a vocational or sheltered workshop placement. For the young adult who is making the transition to community college, assessment may revolve around evaluation of environmental needs and the selection of an augmentative aid that would allow access to portable note-taking and text-editing capabilities. Upon graduation, the same individual may need to be reevaluated so that an optimal work station, for use in a specific employment site or setting, can be developed. For the individual with recent onset of quadraplegia who wishes to return to a previous vocational setting, assessment may have as its goal the selection of an appropriate writing system or development of a work station in the former job site. For the adult with a progressive neurological disorder, assessment may take place when speech is no longer intelligible or efficient enough to serve as a functional means of communication. An augmentative approach may be considered that permits conversational exchanges related to self- or health-care and telephone communication. In summary, impetus for assessment is provided by factors related to change. This may involve either changes in the capabilities of the nonspeaking and/or nonwriting individual or changes in the individual's communication needs.

## *The Ongoing Nature of Assessment*

At a very basic level, assessment is a process by which an individual's communication needs are determined, the components of the individual's existing communication system are evaluated, and potential augmentative components are selected to meet these needs. The components that are selected are then evaluated using performance trials. These components include the devices, techniques, symbols, and strategies that are required to enhance or augment the individual's system in order to provide, to the greatest extent possible, an "optimal communication system." An optimal communication system would ideally permit normal conversational exchanges (i.e., those that are as efficient and effective as speech). The optimal communication system would also include additional tools and strategies specific to the individual's communication needs. Thus, the optimal system for one individual will be different from the optimal system for others and will change over time. For example, a college freshmen's optimal communication system will include speech as the primary component of the system, but will require the use of additional tools that permit the student to take notes, to access information systems, to use word processing for term papers, to calculate math problems, and so on.

As discussed in the previous chapter, individuals with severe expressive communication disorders need special aids, symbols, and techniques in order to communicate. The optimal system for these individuals is constrained not only by their cognitive, socio-communicative, sensory, or motor skills, but also by features of available augmentative aids and techniques and their use under various conditions. The "constrained-but-optimal" system of today should not be considered the only one the individual will need. Instead, team members involved in assessing and designing an individual's communication system should plan ahead and, in addition to planning a system for the present, should design at least two or three successively more advanced constrained-but-optimized systems that the individual might utilize in the future. In this way, today's communication system can facilitate skill acquisition in the areas in which the individuals are limited at different developmental points (Reichle & Karlan, 1985). For example, intervention with a cognitively limited older child who currently uses only a small number of gestures may focus upon expanding the child's communicative behavior through expressive manual sign training. It may also include teaching recognition and production of graphic symbols. As the child becomes involved in community settings (where the use of manual or gestural systems is not understood), a communication board or speech output aid will be necessary to permit successful interactions. Thus, early introduction of graphic symbols may facilitate the child's later use of a communication board or speech output aid. Another example might involve a severely physically handicapped young child for whom a scanning strategy appears to be cognitively too difficult. For the present, this child may be limited to a very small number of symbols/messages that can be accessed through direct selection. However, a structured training program to teach step-scanning might be included in the initial intervention program, along with direct selection training, because a combination of these strategies appears to be the most optimal long-term approach. Over the short term, direct selection should be stressed while the scanning skills are being learned; when they are learned, the additional technique can be incorporated into the child's communication system.

Having a functional communication system is likely to permit continued development of the individual's cognitive, socio-communicative, educational, vocational, and even motor skills. Therefore, after an initial network of components is established (i.e., the constrained-but-optimized system), periodic reevaluations must be undertaken to determine whether subsequent changes have occurred that would necessitate redefining the system and recommending additional or alternative components. Thus, the outcome of the assessment process is the design of an intervention program that seeks to reduce current disability (by compensating for those impairments that are present today) and to reduce future disability (by improving skills that are essential for later development of more effective communication). In this way, goals for the present and the future are set.

## Communication Needs

Critical to the selection of augmentative aids and techniques is the identification of communication needs. Needs assessment involves the identification of specific communication tasks that the individual must perform in order to function optimally in particular communication environments. Such needs statements are often quite specific. Examples of specific areas of needs statements appear in Table 4-1 and are adapted from those in Beukelman, Yorkston, and Dowden (1985). A review of this table suggests that the needs can be categorized under a number of headings, including positioning, communication partners, locations, message needs, and modality of communication. The needs list in Table 4-1 is not an exhaustive one. Rather, it is intended to serve as a model for identifying the needs of a particular individual or population. For example, when addressing the needs of young children, a series of unique developmental requirements may be added.

The information required to complete statements about communication needs can be obtained easily by interviewing the client, family members, and primary communication partners (e.g., teachers, therapists, etc.) Each of the needs on the individually prepared list can be categorized as:

1. Currently met - A need is currently met if the individual already has a satisfactory means of accomplishing a task (e.g., headshake/headnod as a yes/no response).

2. Mandatory - A mandatory need is necessary for communication today, and priority is given to selection of communication components that have the potential of meeting this need. The success of an augmentative communication aid or technique can be assessed by documenting the number of mandatory needs that are met (e.g., ability to print messages).

3. Desirable - A desirable need is important but not essential; therefore, a lower priority is given to meeting that need (e.g., use of the telephone).

4. Unimportant - An unimportant need is not considered in the selection of augmentative aids and techniques to meet present needs. Of course, an unimportant need may become desirable or mandatory in the future when either the communication environment or the capabilities of the individual change.

## TABLE 4-1.  EXAMPLES OF COMMUNICATION NEEDS STATEMENTS

POSITIONING

In bed:
- while supine
- while sitting
- in a variety of positions

In adaptive therapeutic positioning:
- side-lying
- in a prone stander
- prone over a bolster

Related to mobility:
- carrying the system while walking
- in a manually controlled wheelchair
- with a lapboard

Other equipment:
- eating devices (cups, spoons, feeding devices)
- orally intubated
- with electric wheelchair controls
- with environmental control units
- with adaptive toys or microcomputer work/learning stations

COMMUNICATION PARTNERS

- someone who cannot read or who has cognitive delays or deficits
- someone who is unfamiliar with the system
- someone who is across the room or in another room
- someone who is an augmentative system user

LOCATIONS

- single room with multiple activity locations
- noisy rooms
- multiple rooms/settings
- car or van
- work station

MESSAGE NEEDS

- call attention to/initiate an interaction
- carry on a conversation or take turns in play or social interaction
- take class notes
- respond to teacher's questions
- participate in academic or vocational activities
- construct messages and prepare written text

MODALITY OF COMMUNICATION

- communicate across a distance
- prepare printed message
- talk on the telephone
- access other equipment (e.g., environmental control units)

5. <u>Future</u> - A future need is one that is predicted to be important or mandatory in the foreseeable future. This category of needs is particularly important when selecting communication aids and techniques for children. Decisions regarding present needs should allow for easy transitions to future needs (e.g., text editing).

The needs assessment interview process serves four different functions. First, a list of communication needs is compiled and a priority rating for each of these needs is determined. Then, guided by the client's needs, a second list is created that contains those augmentative aids, techniques, symbols, and strategies that may potentially meet the client's needs. Compiling the second list, of course, requires a thorough knowledge of currently available aids, devices, symbol sets and systems, techniques, and intervention strategies. The reader is referred to the previous chapter for characteristics of a large number of system components and to Kraat and Sitver-Kogut (1984) for a summary of features of commercially available communication aids.

The second function of the needs assessment interview is to provide information that can be used to establish a series of specific, objectively defined intervention goals (see chapter 5). These goals also provide an important avenue by which intervention outcomes can be measured (see chapter 7).

The needs assessment interview also enables team members, and those they serve to reach a consensus with regard to goals and expectations. Often, potential problems are avoided by detailing where, when, with whom, and for what purpose(s) each augmentative component may be used; thus, unrealistic expectations may be avoided. Finally, the interview is educational. It is often easy for the team to highlight the multimodalities approach to communication by emphasizing that certain communicative functions are most easily and effectively performed with one communication mode and others with another. The needs assessment interview serves to acquaint expressively impaired individuals and their families with communication possibilities that they had not previously considered. For example, the wife of an individual with a progressive neurological impairment came to an evaluation session asking to see "some portable typing systems." During the course of the needs assessment interview, she realized that a communication aid that had speech output as well as printed output would allow her husband to communicate with her when she was across the room. She and her husband decided that this feature would be increasingly important to them and added it to their list of mandatory needs.

## THE ASSESSMENT TEAM

The team approach to management has a long-standing history in medical and educational settings, and has been a hallmark in the area of augmentative communication. The team, composed of individuals with widely differing skills, is brought together to make decisions. The goal of the team is to enhance and/or facilitate communication in the broadest sense. Since the ability to communicate is a fundamental aspect of one's daily life, the assessment team must understand the capabilities of the individual as well as the social and physical factors and constraints that exist in the environment. These factors include aspects of the social environment, such as the number of communication partners, communication modes utilized by actual and potential communication partners, communication roles available, and frequency of communication interaction. Physical factors include arrangement of the environment, light and noise levels, distance at which communication interaction occurs, availability of adaptive equipment for sensory impairments or physical disabilities, and degree of mobility (frequency, distance, level of independence). Having access to this information is essential to the assessment team, especially when cognitive deficits are present that limit the speech/language-impaired individual's ability to participate in or direct the development of the communication system.

### *Multidisciplinary, Transdisciplinary, and Interdisciplinary Teams*

The augmentative communication team functions in either a multidisciplinary, interdisciplinary, or transdisciplinary capacity. For purposes of this discussion, a *multidisciplinary team* is one in which the members of the professional team make independent decisions related to their areas of expertise. By sharing their plans, an intervention program is formulated. For example, as part of a stroke rehabilitation team, a speech-language pathologist would evaluate and plan treatment in the area of communication, a psychologist would evaluate and plan in the area of cognitive function, and physical and occupational therapists, under the direction of a physician, would develop programs for intervention in the areas of mobility and activities of daily living. Although a multidisciplinary team cannot function adequately without sharing information, the basic approach to intervention is one of independent decisions made by professionals in mutually exclusive areas of interest.

At times, the augmentative communication team may function as a multidisciplinary team. For example, when undertaking long-term planning in the area of academic, social, communication, and motor development of a severely handicapped youngster, each team member may develop an intervention program for their particular area. When taken as a whole, these separate intervention sequences are presumed to form a program that will foster maximum development. This approach may be problematic for individuals with multiple or severe deficits, such as the person with a degenerative condition, the severely multiply handicapped person, or the severely mentally retarded person. The chief disadvantage of independently conceived and executed programs is that they may not result in an adequate level of integration. Any specific task that an individual must perform every day requires motoric, visual, cognitive, communicative, and social abilities. The particular skills needed for a specific task to be performed successfully will form a cluster for that task (Sailor & Guess, 1983). Assessment teams must take into consideration the cluster of skills, the interaction between skills, and the skill integration required to be successful in a specific task. Such integration is more difficult to achieve when each discipline is, in essence, individually responsible for program planning and implementation.

In the *transdisciplinary team* approach professionals acquire knowledge of related disciplines and incorporate that knowledge into their own practice. Thus while still consulting with professionals from other disciplines, one professional on the assessment team assumes primary responsibility for direct client contact. The disadvantage of this model, as it applies to augmentative communication assessment teams, is that the specific expertise needed to treat multiple disorders adequately may not be available on a regular basis or may be at an unsophisticated level and, therefore, ineffective (Blackstone & Painter, 1985).

An *interdisciplinary team* makes decisions in a somewhat different style (Valletutti & Christoplos, 1977). Like the multidisciplinary team, it is made up of individuals who possess expertise in widely divergent areas. In addition, a formal mechanism exists so that information is shared by the team members. Unlike the multidisciplinary team, decisions are not made independently. Rather, the team makes decisions as a whole based upon shared information. Augmentative communication teams often function as an interdisciplinary team when making decisions about the selection of communication system components. Ideally, in an interdisciplinary team, the decision-making process facilitates the development of integrated assessment and intervention plans.

## Expertise of Team Members

While the list of potential experts that may serve as team members is a long one, not all decisions must be made by the entire team. The team manager may call upon experts as needed; thus, the core of the team may be quite small. For example, the core members of a team serving severely speech-impaired children often include a speech-language pathologist, a special educator, an occupational therapist, and the family. Consultative support must also be available from audiologists, rehabilitation engineers, psychologists, physical therapists, computer programmers, and engineers, among others. In addition to expertise in their respective disciplines, these individuals must have knowledge and skills in the augmentative communication area. The family is also an important resource when making appropriate and time-effective decisions. Often, family members not only have a clear understanding of the capabilities of nonspeaking individuals in a variety of natural communication settings, but are also invaluable in establishing intervention goals and in carrying out whatever training may be necessary in order to achieve these goals. Educational, vocational, and medical histories, and the results of formal testing performed over the years, also provide useful data to the team.

Table 4-2 contains a listing of the areas of knowledge and skills needed on an augmentative communication team. Please note that team members include not only augmentative communication specialists, who always function as members of a specialized assessment team, but their counterparts in the community as well. Those who implement recommendations and who live and work directly with severely speech- and/or writing- impaired individuals each day provide valuable information that increases the efficiency of the specialized team.

## *Levels of Professional Involvement*

In general, professionals from various disciplines who take part in the assessment process function at three levels. Each level entails varying degrees of direct client contact and responsibilities. At the primary level, the professional serving a general caseload in a school or hospital setting carries out assessments that require observations over time. In addition to being responsible for assisting in the development and implementation of intervention plans, the primary professional is responsible for appropriate referral; thus, this individual must have a general knowledge of the area of augmentative communication and the ability to apply principles of assessment and intervention to those with severe expressive disorders. The various tasks that are carried out by professionals at this level include in-depth testing modified to meet the cognitive and motoric needs of the client and ongoing observations of behaviors related to the use of augmentative aids and techniques.

Rather than handling the general caseload of the primary clinician, the secondary level professional plays the role of a local specialist. A local specialist may serve as manager for a number of nonspeaking clients and as the local resource in consulting with other professionals. This consultation may involve helping professionals to (a) modify standard assessment approaches in accordance with the cognitive and motor control limitations of the client, or (b) develop appropriate nonstandard assessment approaches. The local specialist may also take part in the development of intervention programs or curricula for severely speech/language- and/or writing-impaired individuals.

## TABLE 4-2. AREAS OF EXPERTISE ON AN AUGMENTATIVE COMMUNICATION TEAM

A. SPEECH-LANGUAGE PATHOLOGY

- communication sciences
- normal & disordered communication
- receptive and expressive language development & disorders
- speech development & disorders
- alternative & augmentative aids, symbols, techniques, & strategies
- management of communication interventions

B. MEDICINE

- management of therapeutic programs
- natural course of the disorder
- medical intervention
- management of medication regimes

C. PHYSICAL THERAPY

- mobility aids
- motor control & motor learning
- positioning to maximize functional communication in all environments
- maintenance of strength & range of motion
- physical conditioning to increase flexibility, balance, & coordination

D. OCCUPATIONAL THERAPY

- activities of daily living
- positioning to maximize functional communication in all contexts
- adaptive equipment
- mobility aids
- access to aids, computers
- splints, etc.

E. ENGINEERING

- application & modification of existing electronic or mechanical aids & devices

F. COMPUTER TECHNOLOGY

- evaluation of software programs for potential use by clients
- modification of existing software programs
- developing programs to meet existing communication needs

G. EDUCATION

- planning for appropriate social & academic experiences
- development of cognitive/conceptual objectives
- assessment of socio-communicative functioning
- integration of augmentative components in the classroom
- development of an appropriate vocational curriculum

H. PSYCHOLOGY

- documentation of level of cognitive functions
- selection of appropriate learning styles
- estimation of learning potential

I. SOCIAL SERVICES

- evaluation of total living situation
- identification of family & community resources
- provision of information about funding options

J. VOCATIONAL COUNSELING

- assessment of vocational potential
- identification of vocational goals
- education of coworkers
- identification of augmentative components in vocational settings

K. OTHER AREAS OF CONSULTATION

- audiology
- ophthamology
- orthopedics
- neurology
- rehabilitation nursing
- prosthetics

At a tertiary level, professionals work as members of a specialized augmentative communication team, which can often be found at regional centers. These individuals should be at the leading edge of service delivery to nonspeaking/nonwriting individuals. They should possess a comprehensive, up-to-date knowledge of augmentative communication aids, techniques, symbols, and strategies. At this level, their role often includes: (a) comprehensive assessment of complex cases, (b) personnel training, including both the clinical training oportunities for students and continuing education opportunities for practicing clinicians at the primary and secondary levels, (c) research that involves, for example, the development of outcome measures, (d) advocacy, and (e) consultative service related to funding and intervention programs. Case management may be included among the duties of individuals at this level. However, in most instances, geographic distance from their clients precludes tertiary specialists from being heavily involved in the implementation of the programs that they recommend.

*Role of the Speech-Language Pathologist*

The speech-language pathologist, in collaboration with other professionals, is able to observe subtle changes in communication behaviors over time in a variety of communication situations and to share this information with the assessment team. A comprehensive discussion of the speech-language pathologist's role and necessary competency areas is available (ASHA, 1981, p. 270). The various tasks that are carried out by the speech-language pathologist will include:  in-depth language testing modified to meet the cognitive and motoric needs of the client; evaluation of interaction skills with primary communication partners in various communication settings; evaluation of speech motor control and articulation; evaluation and selection of the aids and techniques in order to develop an effective repertoire of communication modes; identification and selection of lexical items for augmentative communication vocabulary displays; understanding the communication needs of the individual; and assessment of the client's potential for learning language, speech, and communication skills. A description of the speech-language pathologist's responsibilities with regard to the dispensing of products, including prosthetic devices, can be extrapolated from the ASHA Code of Ethics (ASHA, 1979). As the communication specialist on an augmentative communication assessment team, the speech-language pathologist must be prepared to provide leadership and to function as a case manager.

## ASSESSMENT OF CAPABILITIES

To assess the capabilities of individuals with severe expressive communication disorders, it is necessary to:  (a) identify the cognitive, linguistic, motoric, sensory, and perceptual skills the individual brings to communication; (b) select augmentative communication components and recommend intervention strategies that optimize performance within the constraints of the individual's capabilities; and (c) determine whether the components selected are likely to address the communication needs effectively and efficiently.  This chapter offers guidelines for assessing individual capabilities and identifying and selecting appropriate augmentative communication components (through performance measures), taking into consideration both present and future communication, educational, and vocational needs (Coleman, Cook, & Meyers, 1980; Owens & House, 1984).  For purposes of this discussion, assessment approaches have been divided into three different categories:  comprehensive capability profiling, criteria-based profiling, and predictive profiling.

*Comprehensive capability profiling*. Capability profiling involves identification of an individual's maximum level of performance in critical areas of interest (e.g., cognition, language, spelling, fine motor skills, etc.). This approach results in a unique profile of each individual's capabilities and skills. The capability profiling approach to assessment is a comprehensive one, involving not only an understanding of the severely speech- and/or writing-impaired individual's performance on any number of standard and nonstandard measures of capability, but also involves an attempt to understand functional communication performance in natural settings.

The strength of the capability profiling approach to assessment is, of course, its thoroughness and its appreciation of the individual's unique skills. The detailed information arising from a comprehensive capability profile has broad application for adults with acquired or degenerative conditions and in the education of children (particularly the multihandicapped). Each professional discipline may contribute unique information about skills and abilities that relate to communication, thus providing an excellent means of developing short- and long-term clinical, educational, and vocational goals and objectives. The advantages of the capability profiling approach to assessment must be weighed against the extensive time commitment and expense required for the completion of such a comprehensive assessment.

*Criteria-based profiling*. The criteria-based approach, as described by Beukelman, Yorkston, and Dowden (1985), is typically used when selecting augmentative aids and techniques to meet current needs. When using this approach, the assessment team is interested in identifying whether the client meets minimal levels of performance or exceeds the threshold of performance necessary for successful use of a specific aid or technique. The team frequently has at its disposal some basic information regarding the client. This information is usually obtained through a screening procedure that may involve a survey of the broad areas of cognitive and language function, hearing, and speech as well as environmental factors. Based on this screening, a decision is generally made not to conduct a comprehensive assessment. For example, when the goal of assessment is to select a portable writing/text editing system for an individual who has successfully attended a community college, in-depth assessment to identify the specific grade level in spelling or grammatical composition may not be necessary.

The criteria-based assessment approach is used to expedite assessment because it is based on a series of branching decisions that allow the team to exclude a large number of possible questions and proceed to critical decisions. For example, when selecting the most appropriate interface by which an individual can access an augmentative communication device, one of the first questions asked is, "Can this individual access the aid in a direct selection mode?" If the answer is no, then a number of scanning options are explored in more detail. However, if the answer is yes, then a large number of scanning options are eliminated from consideration, and attention is focused on selecting the most appropriate direct selection option. Dowden, Honsinger, and Beukelman (1986) used this approach when attempting to select augmentative communication aids for individuals in an intensive care unit. In that situation, the patient's fragile medical condition may prevent the assessment team from obtaining a complete profile of skills. Therefore, the question that must be posed is criteria-based (i.e., "Does this individual have spelling skills to communicate day-to-day messages using a typing-based aid?"). If a capability profiling approach were being used, the question posed might be, "What is the maximum level of performance on graded spelling tasks?" One of the obvious advantages of the criteria-based assessment is that it allows the assessment team to survey areas of interest very quickly when detailed capability skill profiles are not required. The criteria-based approach is frequently used when selecting specific augmentative communication aids, symbols, and techniques.

*Predictive profiling*. The predictive approach to assessment is in some ways an extension of the criteria-based approach in that it has been applied when decisions regarding device selection must be made. The capabilities of the communicatively handicapped individual are assessed on a number of carefully constructed tasks. Performance on these tasks is then used to predict the efficiency with which the individual would be able to use a given aid or technique. This approach to assessment is a sophisticated one and requires, in addition to carefully constructed assessment tasks, a detailed understanding of the requirements of a particular augmentative aid or technique. Goodenough-Trepagnier and Prather (1981) suggested that it would be possible to develop an approach to motor assessment involving the measurement of the speed and accuracy of performance on tasks that vary target location, direction of movement, key force, and key travel. In later work, Goodenough-Trepagnier and Rosen (in press) have developed an "off-device" measurement technique in which a clients' performance is assessed on structured tasks not involving the augmentative aid. They suggest that performance on these tasks can be used to predict eventual output rates. Although much longitudinal research will be needed to develop the tasks necessary to incorporate information about environmental factors and to establish both concurrent and predictive validity of the predictions, this approach has the potential of streamlining and standardizing some aspects of the assessment process.

## Assessment Tools

Measurement of an individual's capabilities and skills is required in a number of areas related to communication. Such measurement is fundamental to selection of optimal communication system components and to planning appropriate intervention programs. Since the number of available augmentative components is steadily growing, it is not practical to take a trial-and-error approach in their selection. Instead, assessment teams must rely on a variety of assessment tools that allow them to determine a person's ability to use certain approaches to communication. Typically, the assessment team will obtain information about a number of functional areas in order to determine whether an individual can use a particular symbol system, aid, or technique.

Before proceeding to a discussion of specific assessment tools, a general word of caution related to testing is warranted. As is the case in educational and clinical assessments, there is a fundamental but easily overlooked distinction between testing and assessment that must be recognized when undertaking an evaluation. Tests are standardized tools that are used to obtain certain information; testing, then, is the process of using these tools to obtain this information. "Standardized" should not be confused with norm-referencing; rather, it means that certain defined procedures must be administered in prescribed ways using particular materials. Standardized tests may then be referenced to normative data (norm-referenced) or to criterion levels (criterion-referenced).

In addition to tests, there are many other ways of collecting specific information required by the assessment team. One example of an assessment protocol developed to assist the augmentative communication team in their evaluations is the Augmentative Communication Assessment Resource (Goossens' & Crain, 1986). Assessment data may be gathered using checklists, rating scales, interview protocols, direct observations, and videotaped samples. Thus, assessment involves the collection and interpretation of data using standardized and nonstandardized, formal and informal, or direct and indirect procedures, techniques, and instruments.

*Applications of standardized tests*. At present, there are no generally accepted test batteries available that provide a comprehensive description of the cognitive, language, motor control, visual, hearing, motor, speech, and academic capabilities of nonspeaking individuals. If the assessment team needs either normative or criterion-referenced information, it will need to rely on tests specifically designed to measure selected capabilities of nonspeaking individuals (Bolton & Dashiell, 1984; Huer, 1983; Single-Input Control Assessment, 1983) or on standard tests that can be easily modified to meet the needs of individuals with severe expressive communication disorders. For example, there are a number of tests of receptive language, cognition, reading, and spelling in which responses can be made in a multiple-choice format. Thus, the severely physically handicapped individual can participate by pointing, eye-gaze, or yes/no indications. Tests that require minimal motor performance include the Peabody Picture Vocabulary Test (Dunn, 1965), Test of Auditory Comprehension of Language (Carrow, 1973), Raven's Progressive Matrices (Raven, 1960), Gates-MacGinitie Reading Test (Gates & MacGinitie, 1969), the spelling and reading subtests from the Peabody Individual Achievement Test (Dunn & Markwardt, 1970), and the Parsons Visual Acuity Test (Parsons Acuity Research Project, 1980). It is the task of the assessment team to interpret the results of these tests in order to determine whether an individual is capable of using a particular technique; however, these interpretations may be problematic.  For example, in the area of spelling, research data are not yet available that describe the spelling skills of "successful" users of augmentative communication techniques who rely on letter-by-letter spelling.  Further research documentation will be necessary before predictive validity between performance on standardized tests and successful use of augmentative approaches for a particular population can be established.  Until such research is available, professionals must depend on their clinical judgments when making decisions.

Often, standardized tests are interpreted within the framework of the criteria-based assessment model described earlier.  In this case, it might be appropriate to ask, "Does this individual have the spelling skills to use a typing system for ordinary written or spoken communication?"  Research data suggest that most of the vocabulary used by individuals with spelling-based augmentative communication aids were at a spelling level ranging from second to fifth grade (Beukelman, Yorkston, Poblete, & Naranjo, 1984).  If standardized tests, adapted to compensate for any perceptual, sensory, motor, or physical deficits, show that the individual is functioning at the eighth-grade level, it is clear that the minimal criterion has been achieved.  Conversely, if an individual is functioning at the first grade level on adapted spelling tests, it is obvious that sufficient spelling skills are not available to support the use of typing systems to meet ordinary communication needs.

*Alternatives to standardized tests*.  Even modified standard tests do not always provide an adequate description of capabilities.  One reason for this may relate to the inadequacy of test norms.  With the severely developmentally delayed or mentally handicapped individual, this inadequacy may be due, in large part, to the fact that this group was not represented in the original validation of the test, thereby resulting in a "floor effect" (i.e., the test does not extend to a low enough level to permit a base or floor to be established for the individual).  Second, inadequacies may relate to test content.  For example, for severely speech- and/or writing-impaired individuals who have normal intellectual ability and who communicate but have severely limited spoken language, the available tests may yield an inadequate description of their ability to communicate due to language-biased item content; that is, the items have been selected for the purpose of establishing the individual's semantic or grammatical level of expressive language rather than for the purpose of establishing the variety, quality, or frequency of acts of communication.  As a result of these inadequacies, other measures must always be used.

For example, ordinal scales derived from formal theories of child development assume that early behaviors form the basis for later behavioral developments. Examples of such ordinal scales used with young children and adapted for use with severely physically multiply handicapped children and adolescents include, in the area of cognitive development, the Ordinal Scales of Psychological Development (Uzgiris &

Hunt, 1975) and, in the area of socio-communicative development, the Early Social Communication Scales (Seibert & Hogan, 1982a,b). Ordinal scales are not norm-referenced; they do not predict an age at which behaviors should develop. They are concerned with establishing a sequence of theoretically related behaviors that must occur in a particular progression regardless of age. In addition, in the assessment of cognitive or socio-communicative ability, the behaviors of interest are typically ways of responding to particular situations and are not specific behaviors. For example, in assessing cognitive development according to Piagetian theories, it is important to know how an individual attempts to get an interesting event to reoccur or continue. It is not important that all children demonstrate a specific behavior (e.g., vocalization), but rather that the particular individuals always perform what is for them a characteristic response (e.g., shaking their fist and smiling when a person who has been making a spectacle of himself pauses during such activity). The fact that a "restart" signal is used in the context of a person to person game is significant. Thus, ordinal scales do not typically use standardized test situations with standardized materials and instructions; rather, they describe a situation or a context in which various types of problem-solving behaviors could occur. The particular type of solution used by the individual in that situation becomes the scaled response. Some behaviors indicate an early stage of cognitive development, while other behaviors indicate a more advanced stage. The particular eliciting situation, materials, and instructions are selected for each individual by the evaluator.

## *Other Areas of Assessment*

In order to obtain additional information required for the augmentative communication assessment, it is necessary to measure the communicative interaction between severely speech-impaired individuals and their primary communication partners in various communication settings and to assess motor control in an effort to determine the optimal means of accessing a communication aid and/or to determine the constraints of using gestural communication.

*Measurement of interaction*. Measurement of interaction often involves the sampling of behaviors in two general contexts: observation of spontaneous conversational exchanges in natural settings, or observation of performance during structured tasks designed to elicit certain types of behavior. The team member responsible for the assessment of communicative interaction will have expertise in language, speech, and nonverbal communication behaviors. For children, free play and story retelling are frequently employed in spontaneous and structured tasks, respectively. For adults, direction-giving and decision-making tasks may be used to elicit information about interaction skills (Farrier, Yorkston, Marriner, & Beukelman, 1985). Spontaneous or structured observations can be made for any number of behaviors not typically sampled in standardized testing. For example, videotaped segments of structured interaction tasks can be used to sample the various modes of communication used, the number of communication breakdowns, the resolution strategies employed, or the patterns of initiation and response. Measures of performance can be obtained from these samples in a number of ways. For example, checklists of behaviors can be obtained, selected behaviors can be tallied during *in situ* observation (Calculator & Luchko, 1983), or videotaped samples of spontaneous interactions can be analyzed using frequency counts of specified behaviors (Beukelman & Yorkston, 1980; Calculator & Dollaghan, 1982; Harris, 1982). More complex analysis of interactions can also be obtained from transcription of structured or unstructured interaction (Buzolich, 1984; Fishman, Timber, & Yoder, 1985; Light, Collier, & Parnes, 1985; Wexler, Blau, Leslie, & Dore, 1983; see chapters 5 & 7 in this book for further discussion).

*Motor control assessment*. Assessment of motor control is undertaken to identify the optimum means of accessing an augmentative communication aid or to determine possible constraints of using a gestural communication approach. For the severely physically handicapped individual, the team member involved in motor assessment may include the case manager and those with expertise in motor control, positioning, and access to augmentative communication aids. Assessment of motor control is often delayed until an optimal seating system has been acquired because positioning will affect a physically impaired individual's access to an aid.

Comprehensive testing of all motor control options for a nonspeaking individual may be both time-consuming for the assessment team and exhausting for the individual; therefore, a streamlining of the process is necessary. The following principles may be brought into play when attempting to streamline the assessment of motor control.

1. *Screening to exclude the inappropriate*. The first assessment principle involves rapid exclusion of a number of options that are clearly unacceptable. For example, direct selection techniques are faster and less cognitively demanding for some individuals than scanning techniques. Therefore, when an individual demonstrates the motor capability for direct selection, further testing in single switch control can be eliminated. Conversely, if the motor control assessment suggests that direct selection is not an acceptable option at this time, then attention must be focused on a variety of single- and multi-switch options.

2. *In-depth testing of selected options*. During motor assessment, it is important to evaluate, in-depth, a small number of options that potentially offer access to the augmentative communication aid or technique, rather than to evaluate, perhaps in less detail, all possible

options. In-depth testing may be followed by an extended period of practice (or field testing) with one or two of the most promising options. The need for this phase of the assessment can be illustrated by considering the differences between cognitive learning and motor learning. For example, the conceptual learning needed for switch use may take place in a single trial when the user understands that activating the left switch moves the scanning light to the left and the right switch to the right. The motor learning required for switch activation cannot be accomplished in one or two trials. Instead, switch activation that is accurate, consistently reproducible, and automatic may take literally thousands of trials. The term *motor thinking* describes the ability to predict the consequences of motor activity. It is clear that motor thinking needs to be developed for adequate augmentative system use. At times, when motor options are being selected, a training period is necessary in order to make the final selection decisions. Such a training period would be of particular importance with the young, severely developmentally delayed or mentally handicapped individual. It is very likely that, with these individuals, introducing switch-activated toys for motor skill development will also provide opportunities for the development of cognitive skills. The child is not merely learning motorically how to operate the switch, but may also be learning the basic relationship between touching a switch and having the toy reproduce an interesting event that the child has just witnessed.

The in-depth assessment involves a number of informal tasks. For example, if initial testing suggests that a single-switch option is most appropriate, then a small number of switches might be assessed at various anatomical sites. Activation, release, and reactivation of the switch might be tested by counting at metered pace and asking the individual to activate at a given count, to release several counts later, and to reactivate still later. Thus, it is possible to assess rate and accuracy of switch activation and release as well as the effects of anticipation on motor performance. Indepth motor testing may also be accomplished via computer software. For example, a computer-based assessment package has been developed that includes the assessment of reaction time, scanning rate, and hold-release time (Single-Input Control Assessment, 1983). This approach uses a model (referred to as the MSIP model) that specifies single-input switch control as a function of movement (M), anatomical site (S) for making the movement, interface (I) or switch used, and positioning (P) of the individual and switch. Computer programs have also been developed in order to assess direct selection access with keyboard devices

(Goodenough-Trepagnier & Rosen, in press; Rosen & Goodenough-Trepagnier, 1983).  For young children and adolescents, a number of motor control games (Schwejda, 1984) are available that can be used to examine a child's capability to control selected switches.  With individuals who have limited comprehension of the required instructions, switch control can be assessed using adapted toys (Karlan, 1985).

Also included among the tasks used for in-depth assessment of selected motor control options are those that are referred to as fatigue drills.  These drills are designed to sample extended periods of performance.  Fatigue is particularly critical for certain individuals with weakness associated with degenerative neuromotor diseases, such as amyotrophic lateral sclerosis.  These individuals may reliably control a movement for a brief period of time but, once fatigued, are no longer able to do so.  Fatigue may also be of concern for those individuals who will need to use the aid for extended periods of time (i.e., for communication or writing systems in the workplace).

The identification of size and location of direct selection displays is another form of in-depth motor control testing.  A threshold testing approach can be utilized to accomplish this.  Using the models for physical response parameters outlined by Coleman, Cook, and Meyers (1980) and for single-input control assessment discussed above, Karlan (1985) has presented a threshold testing approach to determining size and location parameters for direct selection displays.  Range of motion has been used to describe the distance, in given directions, that an individual can move a particular body part; for direct selection displays, this would refer to the surface area that can be covered by individuals when moving their hand and arm or when moving head pointers or mouth sticks.  One method commonly employed for determining the range of motion is to mark on a grid those areas that an individual can reach when instructed to do so for the various grid "cells."  This does not take into consideration, however, the degree of accuracy in reaching those locations, nor does it work well with the severely mentally handicapped individual who has limited comprehension of the instructions involved.  An alternative would be to use a switch-activated toy or device that the individual has already demonstrated the ability to use.  The switch used to activate the toy/device is systematically moved to varying locations corresponding to the locations of interest in the direct-selection grid.  By counting the frequency of both successful and unsuccessful attempts at switch activation, the accuracy of responding at a particular location can be determined. To insure continued performance by the severely handicapped young child or the mentally retarded individual, a threshold approach to selecting the response location is used. Using this approach, the first location selected is one where the individual can be expected to have a high degree of accuracy. With successive locations, if the individual maintains the high degree of accuracy, a new location is selected without necessarily returning to an old location. If, however, the individual is successful three or fewer times in five attempts, then an old location, where a high degree of accuracy was achieved, is reassessed in order to provide a return to assured success. In this way, the process of evaluating accuracy at various locations moves back across the threshold for success whenever this threshold has been exceeded and the individual has failed. This technique yields a measure of accuracy at each potential location on the selection grid. Optimal size of target locations or cells of the direct selection matrix can be assessed in a similiar fashion. If a programmable expanded keyboard is available, the threshold procedure could be conducted using software programs that provide contingent feedback for each different location.

3. *Planning for the future*. Motoric complexity refers to the type of movements required to use augmentative communication aids or techniques, including gestures and manual signs. It is nearly impossible to establish a general hierarchy of motoric complexity because the impairments vary so extensively from person to person depending on underlying neuropathology. For example, a motoric hierarchy for an individual recovering from a brain stem cerebral vascular accident may be sequenced as follows: a single, head-activated switch, a single hand-activated switch, direct selection from a small keyboard, and direct selection from a standard keyboard. This hierarchy is constructed to reflect the expected course of recovery that involves gradual return of function (i.e., head control, followed by function in the upper extremity; gross movements, followed by fine movements). The hierarchy is also based on the nature of the motor control impairment. In the case of the individual with a brain stem cerebral vascular accident, the impairment is characterized by weakness, slowness, and limited range of movement rather than problems with movement patterning seen, for example, in some individuals who have cerebral palsy. Thus, a hierarchy of motoric complexity for switch control or access to an augmentative communication aid must be individualized. However, all hierarchies are based on the general rule that progression through the sequence

results in increased communication efficiency. A hierarchy of motoric complexity may also be applied to gestural systems (Kohl, 1981; Shane & Wilbur, 1980). Some signs require complex motor planning in the execution of fine sequential movements. Others involve fewer sequences and grosser movements. The motoric complexity of manual sign and gestural systems has been approached through the grouping of signs according to the motor components required to produce them (Shane & Wilbur, 1980) and, more recently, through consideration of developmental models for the order of acquisition of the various motor movements of handshape configurations needed to produce manual signs and gestures (for a review, see Doherty, Daniloff, & Lloyd, 1985).

4. *The final decisions*. In some cases, decisions about the most appropriate control options are clear cut. In other situations, however, the final decisions represent a compromise. Among the factors that must at some times be considered when making final selections is the effect of an interface control on other reflex patterning. For example, some cerebral palsied individuals experience undesirable reflex patterning when attempting to control a switch with their hand but not when they are using a head switch. In addition, the cosmetic aspects of the interface are an important consideration for some individuals (e.g., some might consider a tongue-controlled switch unacceptable regardless of its superiority over other options in terms of rate and accuracy of activation). At other times, the team will make selection decisions based on the possibility of future development. For example, a young child with cerebral palsy may be more accurate in activating four switches with four different anatomical sites (hand, foot, knee, head) than when attempting to activate multiple switches using a single site (e.g., the hand). The team might choose the option of a single anatomical site despite inferior rate and accuracy because they believe that it will afford greater potential for future progression in multi-switch or direct-selection access.

## INITIAL VOCABULARY SELECTION

Selection of vocabulary for gestural training, for inclusion on communication boards, or for programming into the memory of electronic communication augmentation devices is frequently the last phase of an augmentative communication assessment. Kraat (1982) lists restricted vocabularies as one of the features of aided communication systems that limits interaction. Among the consequences of restricted vocabularies are limitations on how and what can be said. Further, messages generated from small vocabularies may be ambiguous or not readily understood. The burden of communication is placed on the partner, who must expand and interpret the limited message. Kraat suggests that "observations of infrequent initiation of conversation and topics by some of our aid users may have a basis in the limited lexical repertoire and the demands for listener expansion" (p. 84).

## *Prereading or Prespelling Vocabulary*

Normally developing children have access to an unrestricted vocabulary acquired in response to new or expanding experiences and concepts. Consider, on the other hand, the restrictions placed on a 3-year-old, physically handicapped, nonspeaking child who uses a communication board with a vocabulary set of 25 symbols. First, the number of items is, because of motor and cognitive limitations, small. Further, new items, whether they are pictures, printed words, or other symbols, must be added by others. Usually, this addition does not take place immediately in response to the demands of the situation.

Augmentative communication aids used by nonspellers require the selection of customized vocabularies. Carlson (1981) suggests that inadequate vocabulary selection may account for many of the failures of augmentative communication aids. Describing her experiences in attempting to select vocabularies for nonspeaking children, she states:

> . . . the lexicon suggested by parents, teachers, and others usually consisted of words that the adult wanted or needed to have the child communicate, rather than those that would have emerged out of the activities and interests of the children. (p. 241)

In response to the difficult problems of vocabulary selection, Carlson suggests a format that utilizes caregivers in vocabulary selection. This format involves two steps: (a) identification of environments in which communication occurs and (b) development of corresponding vocabulary lists within the child's developmental experience and interest level. As the vocabulary for one environment is established, other environments are added. Caregivers are encouraged to continually update vocabulary selection in an effort to mimic, as closely as possible, the self-selected lexicon of the normal child.

Holland (1975) listed the following criteria for evaluating the adequacy of vocabulary selection when teaching children spoken language: (a) using child language as a model, (b) emphasizing what is important to the child, (c) stressing communication rather than simply language skills, and (d) focusing on objects that are present and events that are happening. Lahey and Bloom (1977) added the following considerations: (a) the relative ease with which a concept can be demonstrated in context, (b) the eventual usefulness to the child of particular words--their potential for combination to convey meaning, and (c) the organization of lexical items according to the ideas they encode (concept categories).

Fristoe and Lloyd (1980), using the criteria suggested by Holland (1975) and Lahey and Bloom (1977), evaluated approximately 50 signs that are most frequently taught to retarded and autistic individuals. From this work, they suggest a basic list and recommended additions for an initial expressive sign lexicon. Karlan and Lloyd (1983) extended this work by reporting social validation data related to this lexicon. Each item was rated according to how essential it was determined to be by two groups (one group having contact with elementary-aged, severely handicapped persons and the other having contact with adolescents and adults with severe handicaps). Table 4-3 contains a list of the items considered essential in the elementary and adult surveys.

## *Selection of Spelling- or Reading-Based Systems*

Customized vocabularies for spelling- or reading-based systems are needed for a variety of reasons. (a) Rate of communication is increased when a word, phrase, or sentence can be retrieved in its entirety rather than spelled in a letter-by-letter fashion. (b) Users of augmentative communication who have reading recognition skills more advanced than their spelling skills communicate more effectively and rapidly when aids have a message retrieval capability. (c) Message retrieval capability is often available in aids with synthesized speech output.

Despite the importance of vocabulary selection, little research has been done in this area. Kelly and Chapanis (1977) studied the impact of restricted vocabulary size on the performance of nonimpaired subjects participating in problem-solving tasks. They found that small vocabularies (300-500 words), with words appropriate to the task, did not limit performance of a number of variables, including time to solve the problem and errors made. Their study would suggest that large vocabularies are not essential if items are appropriately selected for specific tasks.

Research reported by Beukelman, Yorkston, Poblete, and Naranjo (1984) suggests that reliance on the traditional data obtained by word frequency counts of

## TABLE 4-3. ESSENTIAL LEXICAL ITEMS

Items are rank ordered according to the proportion of judges who rated them as essential (from Karlan & Lloyd, 1983)

| ELEMENTARY SURVEY | ADOLESCENT/ADULT SURVEY |
|---|---|
| bathroom/toilet/potty | bathroom/toilet/potty |
| eat/food | eat/food |
| name sign (I, me, my) | no |
| drink | drink |
| no | stop |
| help | name sign (I, me, my) |
| Mother/Mommy | help |
| more | water |
| Father/Daddy | go |
| water | bed/sleep |
| stop | cold |
| bed/sleep | hot |
| look/watch | you |
| milk | coat |
| go | good |
| happy | more |
| hot | work |
| good | come |
| coat | wash |
| | clean |
| | in |
| | sad |
| | shoes |
| | walk |
| | angry/mad |
| | open |
| | shirt |
| | milk |

written prose may not accurately reflect the vocabulary used by nonspeaking individuals in natural communication settings. These authors studied the actual vocabulary of five nonspeaking adults with intact language who were using the Canon Communicator in natural settings. Data regarding frequency of word occurrence suggest that a relative small core vocabulary list (500 words) accounted for 80 percent of the total words used by these language-intact individuals. However, the ability to generate unique words was essential because only 33 percent of the messages produced by the subjects were communicated in their entirety when subjects were restricted to words in the core vocabulary lists.

Goodenough-Trepagnier and Prather (1981) circumvent the problem of vocabulary selection by using syllables rather than words as the unit of retrieval. SPEEC (Sequences of Phonemes for Efficient English Communication) contains frequently occurring sequences of sound that can be combined by the user to form messages with unrestricted vocabularies. WRITE, a similar system by the same authors, contains frequently occurring sequences of letters and can be used for writing.

*Planning for the future.* When selecting vocabulary, the team must consider the future communicative needs of the client. A hierarchy in the area of symbolic load (complexity) may help professionals to make appropriate decisions. Symbolic load refers to the extent to which written symbols, signs, or gestures are arbitrary symbols for the concept they convey. Table 4-4 contains an example of such a hierarchy. A review of this table suggests that the hierarchy of printed material begins with concrete material, such as photographs of objects, and progresses through a number of slightly more abstract symbols, such as line drawings, Picsyms (Carlson, 1985), and Blissymbols (Kates & McNaughton, 1975). The most highly symbolic printed material is standard orthography (or printed words), which are arbitrary symbols for the concepts they convey. Gestural approaches may also be ordered in a hierarchy according to symbolic load (Griffith, Robinson, & Panagos, 1981; Daniloff, Noll, Fristoe, & Lloyd, 1982; Katz, LaPointe, & Markel, 1978; Skelly, 1979; see chapter 3).

Message flexibility (potential of the communication system to generate unique messages) must be considered when selecting lexicons and designing vocabulary displays. The least flexible systems are those in which each symbol has a restricted range of representation. For a particular concept, that symbol represents only one of a number of possible meanings. An example of such a system component might be a photograph of a child drinking a glass of water to indicate, "I'm thirsty." Slightly more flexible are those approaches that allow combinations of elements in order to generate a finite number of different messages. For example, a word/picture board may contain items representing "I want" and "drink." These items can be combined to indicate, "I'm thirsty," or can be combined with other items to generate different

### TABLE 4-4. HIERARCHY OF SYMBOLIC LOAD

PRINTED MATERIAL

    Standard orthography (written words)

    Abstract symbols (some Blissymbols)

    Iconic symbols (Pisyms, linedrawings, and Blissymbols)

    Referential symbols (photographs)

GESTURAL SYSTEMS

    Arbitrary or codified (American Sign Language)

    Iconic (American Indian Sign Language)

    Referential gestures (pointing to objects)

    Nonsymbolic gestures (coverbal behaviors)

---

messages. The most flexible approaches are these with unlimited potential to generate unique messages. Examples of such approaches are orthographic English, American Sign Language, Blissymbolics, and syllable-based systems, including SPEEC and WRITE (Goodenough-Trepagnier & Prather, 1981).

## PERFORMANCE TRIALS

At the completion of the assessment process, two lines of information come together. The first involves identification of potential approaches that will meet the individual's communication needs within specific environments. The second line involves identification of the system components that the individual is capable of using. Performance trials involving actual use of the augmentative communication system components are needed before final judgments about the adequacy of selection can be made.  Although many of the activities carried out during performance trials may be considered a part of intervention, they may also be appropriately viewed as the last phase of the assessment process.  These are described in more detail elsewhere (Beukelman, Yorkston, & Dowden, 1985.)  Briefly, they involve actual use of the communication aid, symbols, and techniques in a variety of functional settings.  Performance trials serve a number of functions.  First, they provide extended periods for motor learning to occur.  A nonspeaking individual cannot be expected to communicate with maximum effectiveness until motor access to the aid or movement involved in gestures are so well learned that they are nearly automatic.  Performance trials may also serve as a time to select additional vocabulary.  In addition, they may be used to document improvement in communication skills.  This information can then be used when submitting requests for funding.  After these trials, the team often becomes active in identifying sources of funding and providing funding sources with documentation of (a) the need for augmentative components; (b) the results of performance trials or evidence of user capability and potential for successful use of the technique; and (c) a description of the potential impact of the augmentative aid or technique on communicative, educational, or vocational functioning.  See chapter 8 for a further discussion of funding.

## ASSESSMENT-INTERVENTION-OUTCOME MEASURES

Assessment is closely related to two other phases of management:  intervention and measurement of outcomes, which are discussed in chapters 5, 6, and 7.  While assessment is defined as a process during which decisions are made at critical points when either capabilities or communication needs have changed, intervention is a process during which these plans are carried out, and measurement of outcome is a process during which the impact of intervention is documented.  The common thread that runs through each of these phases of management relates to measurement.  Each phase is dependent on similiar information.  Areas of interest include communication needs and capabilities of the individual as well as communication performance itself.  During assessment this information is used to select optimal system components to meet current needs and to develop educational and vocational programs that will advance the severely speech/language- and/or writing-impaired individual through a hierarchy toward more effective communication.  During intervention, information is used to monitor training activities and to modify plans when goals are not being achieved.  In outcome measurement, information is used to document changes in communication and to compare the efficacy of various intervention approaches.  Measurement is a critical element of all phases of management.  Research, development, and verification of measurement tools are critical to continued advancement of the augmentative communication area.

# SUMMARY

Assessment is a process during which a team is brought together to make clinical and education/vocational decisions when an individual's communication capabilities or needs have changed. Selection of the components of a communication system to meet current needs is one important outcome of assessment. Selection is accomplished by matching nonspeaking individuals' needs and capabilities with augmentative system components that meet these needs and are compatible with current capabilities. The second important outcome of assessment is a plan for the future. Setting goals for future intervention involves (a) identification of current levels related to a series of general hierarchies; (b) establishment of goals that advance the individual through these hierarchies, and (c) development of intervention plans by which the goals can be achieved. Three general approaches to assessment were described--comprehensive capability profiling, criterion-based profiling, and predictive profiling. Specific assessment techniques were discussed, including the needs assessment interview, use of standard and alternatives to standard testing when assessing cognitive, linguistic, communicative, and motoric capabilities of nonspeaking individuals, and use of performance trials as the final phase of assessment.

# STUDY QUESTIONS

1. Describe factors that may necessitate or trigger assessment.

2. Compare and contrast the activities of a multidisciplinary, transdisciplinary, and an interdisciplinary assessment team.

3. What are the functions of the needs assessment interview?

4. Why are alternatives to standard tests so important in capability assessment for nonspeaking individuals? Describe some alternative areas requiring assessment, and measurement testing techniques.

5. What assessment approaches would be used to assess:

   a. a six-year-old nonspeaking child with cerebral palsy and normal intelligence;

    b.   a 30-year-old with a recent onset, high-level spinal cord injury (client is able to speak but not write);

    c.   a 12-year-old severely retarded, ambulatory individual.

## REFERENCES

American Speech-Language-Hearing Association. (1979, January). Code of Ethics of the American Speech-Language-Hearing Association. Asha, 22(4), 267-272.

American Speech-Language-Hearing Association. (1981, August). Position statement on nonspeech communication. Asha, 23(8), 577-581.

Beukelman, D., & Yorkston, K. (1980). Nonvocal communication: Performance evaluation. Archives of Physical Medicine and Rehabilitation, 61, 272-275.

Beukelman, D., Yorkston, K., & Dowden, P. (1985). Augmentative communication: A casebook of clinical management. San Diego: College-Hill Press.

Beukelman, D., Yorkston, K., Poblete, M., & Naranjo, C. (1984). Frequency of word occurrence in communication samples produced by adult communication aid users. Journal of Speech and Hearing Disorders, 49(4), 360-367.

Blackstone, S., & Painter, M. (1985). Speech problems in multihandicapped children. In J. Darby (Ed.), Speech and language evaluation in neurology: Childhood disorders (pp. 219-242). Orlando: Grune & Stratton.

Bolton, S., & Dashiell, S. (1984). INteraction CHecklist for Augmentative Communication (INCH). Huntington Beach, CA: INCH Associates.

Buzolich, M. (1984). Interaction analyses of augmented and normal adult communicators. An unpublished doctoral dissertation, University of California, San Francisco.

Calculator, S., & Dollaghan, C. (1982). The use of communication boards in a residential settings: An evaluation. Journal of Speech and Hearing Disorders, 47, 281-287.

Calculator, S., & Luchko, C. (1983). Evaluating the effectiveness of a communication board training program. Journal of Speech and Hearing Disorders, 48, 185-191.

Carlson, F. (1981). A format for selecting vocabulary for the nonspeaking child. Language, Speech, and Hearing Services in Schools, 12(4), 240-245.

Carlson, F. (1985). Picsyms: Categorical dictionary. Lawrence, KS: Baggeboda Press.

Carrow, E. (1973). Test of auditory comprehension of language. Austin, TX: Learning Concepts.

Coleman, C., Cook, A., & Meyers, L. (1980). Assessing non-oral clients for assistive communication devices. Journal of Speech and Hearing Disorders, 45, 515-526.

Daniloff, K., Noll, J., Fristoe, M., & Lloyd, L. (1982). Gesture recognition in patients with aphasia. Journal of Speech and Hearing Disorders, 47, 43-47.

Doherty, J., Daniloff, J., & Lloyd, L. (1985). The effect of categorical presentation on Amer-Ind transparency. Augmentative and Alternative Communication, 1(1), 10-16.

Dowden, P., Honsinger, M., & Beukelman, D. (1986). Serving non-speaking patients in acute care settings: An intervention approach. Augmentative and Alternative Communication, 2(1), 25-32.

Dunn, L. (1965). Expanded manual for the Peabody Picture Vocabulary Test. Circle Pines, MN: American Guidance Service.

Dunn, L., & Markwardt, F.C. (1970). Peabody individual achievement test. Circle Pines, MN: American Guidance Service.

Farrier, L., Yorkston, K., Marriner, N., & Beukelman, D. (1985). Conversational control in non-impaired speakers using an augmentative communication system. Alternative and Augmentative Communication, 1, 65-73.

Fishman, S., Timler, G., & Yoder, D. (1985). Strategies for the prevention and repair of communication interactions with communication board users. Augmentative and Alternative Communication, 1, 38-51.

Fristoe, M., & Lloyd, L. (1980). Planning an initial expressive sign lexicon for persons with severe communication impairment. Journal of Speech and Hearing Disorders, 45, 170-180.

Gates, A., & MacGinitie, W. (1969). Gates-MacGinitie reading test (2nd ed.). New York: Teacher's College Press, Columbia University.

Goodenough-Trepagnier, C., & Prather, P. (1981). Communication systems for the non-vocal based on frequent phoneme sequences. Journal of Speech and Hearing Research, 24, 322-329.

Goodenough-Trepagnier, C., & Rosen, M.J. (in press). Predictive assessment for communication aid prescription: Motor-determined maximum communication rate. In L.E. Bernstein (Ed.), The vocally impaired: Volume II basic research and technology. New York: Academic Press.

Goossens', C., & Crain, S. (1986). Augmentative communication assessment resource. Lake Zurich, IL: Don Johnston Developmental Equipment.

Griffith, P., Robinson, J., & Panagos, J. (1981). Perception of iconicity in American Sign Language by hearing and deaf subject. Journal of Speech and Hearing Disorders, 46, 388-397.

Harris, D. (1982). Communicative interaction processes involving nonvocal physically handicapped children. Topics in Language Disorders, 2, 21-37.

Holland, A. (1975). Language therapy for children: Some thoughts on context and content. Journal of Speech and Hearing Disorders, 40, 514-523.

Huer, M. (1983). The nonspeech test. Lake Zurich, IL: Don Johnston Developmental Equipment.

Karlan, G. (June, 1985). Transitions in technology: Introduction of medium and high technology into educational programs for young, multiply handicapped children. Instructional course presented at the 8th Annual Conference on Rehabilitation Technology, Memphis, TN.

Karlan, G., & Lloyd, L. (1983). Considerations in the planning of communication interaction: Selecting a lexicon. Journal of the the Association for the Severely Handicapped, 8, 13-25.

Kates, B., & McNaughton, S. (1975). The first application of Blissymbolics as a communication medium for non-speaking children: History and development, 1971-1974. Toronto: Blissymbolics Communication Institute.

Katz, R., LaPointe, L., & Markel, N. (1978). Coverbal behavior and aphasic speakers. Clinical Aphasiology Conference Proceedings (pp. 164-173). Minneapolis: BRK Publishers.

Kelly, M., & Chapanis, A. (1977). Limited vocabulary natural language dialogue. International Journal of Man-Machine Studies, 9, 479-501.

Kohl, F. (1981). Effects of motoric requirements on the acquisition of manual sign responses by severely handicapped students. American Journal of Mental Deficiency, 85(4), 396-403.

Kraat, A. (1982). Training augmentative communication use: Clinical and research issues. In K. Galyas, M. Lundman, & U. Lagerman (Eds.), Communication for the severely handicapped (pp. 76-93). Bromma, Sweden: Swedish Institute for the Handicapped.

Kraat, A., & Sitver-Kogut, M. (1984, August). Features of commerically available communication aids. (Available from Prentke Romich Co., 1022 Heyl Road, Wooster, OH 44691)

Lahey, M., & Bloom, L. (1977). Planning a first lexicon: Which words to teach first. Jounal of Speech and Hearing Disorders, 42, 340-349.

Light, J., Collier, B., & Parnes, P. (1985). Communicative interaction between young nonspeaking physically disabled children and their primary caregivers: Part I - Discourse patterns. Augmentative and Alternative Communication, 1, 74-83.

Owens, R., & House, L. (1984). Decision-making processes in augmentative communication. Journal of Speech and Hearing Disorders, 49, 18-15.

Parsons Acuity Research Project. (1980). Parsons visual acuity test. South Bend, IN: Bernell Corp.

Raven, J. (1960). Guide to the standard progressive matrices. London: H.K. Lewis.

Reichle, J., & Karlan, G. (1985). The selection of an augmentative system in communication intervention: A critique of decision rules. Journal of the Association for Persons with Severe Handicaps, 10, 146-156.

Rosen, M., & Goodenough-Trepagnier, C. (1983). Development of a computer-aided system for prescription of non-vocal communication devices. A progress report.

Proceedings of the RESNA 6th Annual Conference on Rehabilitation Engineering (pp. 191-193). San Diego, CA.

Sailor, W., & Guess, D. (1983). Severely handicapped students: An instructional design. Boston: Houghton-Mifflin.

Schwejda, P. (1984). Motor training games. Seattle: Washington Research Foundation.

Seibert, J., & Hogan, A. (1982a). A model for assessing social and object skills and planning intervention. In D.P. McClowry, A.M. Guilford, & S.O. Richardson (Eds.), Infant communication, development, assessment and intervention. New York: Grune & Stratton.

Seibert, J., & Hogan, A. (1982b). Procedures manual for the early social-communication scales (ESCS). Miami: University of Miami, Mailman Center for Child Development.

Shane, H., & Wilbur, R. (1980). Potential for expressive signing based on motor control. Sign Language Studies, 29, 331-347.

Single-Input Control Assessment. (1983). Microcomputer applications programme, The Hugh MacMillan Medical Centre. Lake Zurich, IL: Don Johnston Developmental Equipment.

Skelly, M. (1979). Amer-Ind gestural code based on universal American Indian hand talk. New York: Elsevier North Holland.

Uzgiris, I., & Hunt, J. (1975). Assessment in infancy: Ordinal scales of psychological development. Urbana: University of Illinois Press.

Valletutti, P., & Christoplos, F. (1977). Interdisciplinary approaches to human services. Baltimore: University Park Press.

Wexler, K., Blau, A., Leslie, S., & Dore, J. (1983). Conversational interaction of nonspeaking cerebral palsied individuals and their speaking partners, with and without augmentative communication aids (Final Rep. R-313-80). New York: UCP Research & Education Foundation.

# CHAPTER 5

## DEVELOPING INTERVENTION GOALS

ARLENE W. KRAAT

*Speech and Hearing Center*
*Queens College of the City University of New York*

## OBJECTIVES

- Discuss the different applications of augmentative communication interventions.

- Outline some of the differences between using augmentative techniques or natural speech to communicate.

- Delineate some of the adaptive strategies and patterns observed during interactions involving individuals who use augmentative aids and techniques.

- Discuss the evaluation of interaction in augmentative communication.

- Identify areas of intervention planning.

- Discuss the process of defining user-specific goals.

## INTRODUCTION

A 4-year-old child with severe spasticity and neuromuscular impairments is added to your caseload. The augmentative assessment team has recommended using eye-pointing, an Etran, and picture symbols as a means of expressive communication. An adult with a neuromuscular disease acquires a sophisticated piece of communication technology, and you are asked to provide him with appropriate training. A severely retarded child requires the use of formal signs paired with spoken language to facilitate language comprehension and expression. These intervention needs can appear quite foreign to the clinician accustomed to treating children and adults through more traditional spoken language techniques.

The questions are many. How does one go about constructing an eye-pointing chart and creating symbol displays? What language items should be selected for the communication system? How does one introduce and teach a 5-year-old to use eye-pointing and the number/color coding involved in an Etran? What skills should be taught to the adult using a computerized communication aid, and how might the large memory storage in the device be programmed to assist him in achieving effective and efficient communication exchanges? How might signs be taught? Should all the words spoken be signed, or just the primary ones? These important questions reflect areas of intervention that speech-language pathologists and other professionals on an augmentative communication team must become familiar with and competent in if they are to adequately meet the needs of these individuals.

After a client is provided with special augmentative components, can the clinician then proceed to facilitate the client's language and communication skills in the same way that those skills are developed in speaking children and adults? Can the same decision-making process and goals be applied to the child using a scanning chart of 200 words as would be applied to a speaking child of a comparable developmental level? Do the language and communication goals for a 6-year-old child with autism change whether signs or spoken language are used? Does the adult with acquired neuromuscular disease need specialized training beyond acquisition of the augmentative techniques? We have slowly come to realize that intervention with augmentative clients is in many ways different from conventional treatment, and some adaptations to the usual decision-making process are necessary.

Intervention with clients who have severe communication disorders requires much more than specialized competencies in symbol and sign selection, device construction, language selection and programming, and transmission techniques. It also requires a knowledge of how communication that is achieved through the use of augmentative symbols, aids, techniques, and strategies may be similar to, as well as different from, conventional spoken language exchanges. In this chapter, we will explore the inherent differences between standard and special augmentative components, how these differences affect communication potentials and possibilities, and how people typically react and interact when augmentative communication aids and techniques are involved. This will provide a framework for understanding special needs in augmentative interventions and how the conventional intervention planning process often needs to be altered. The evaluation of communicative interaction will be discussed, along with considerations for establishing appropriate intervention goals. Chapter 6 will focus on specific procedures for implementing these goals. In both chapters, the emphasis will be on those aspects of the intervention process that appear unique to individuals who use augmentative components. Although differences will be highlighted here, readers need to recognize that augmentative intervention also shares many aspects of the communication and language training processes used with speaking persons with various communication disorders.

## THE GOALS OF AUGMENTATIVE INTERVENTIONS

Intervention planning must begin with a clear understanding of why augmentative communication is being considered for a client. Possible reasons may include: (a) to enhance daily communication when spoken language abilities are inadequate; (b) to serve as a *bridge* leading to the development of natural speech or spoken language comprehension; or (c) to ascertain whether language skills can be acquired using augmentative components when they have not been acquired in spoken language use. The primary purpose in the first instance is to improve daily functional communication and interaction; in the second, to facilitate the acquisition of speech production and comprehension; and in the third, to answer a diagnostic question. These purposes are quite different, and each significantly affects the planning and implementation of intervention goals and procedures. It is important to note that these applications are not mutually exclusive, and may occur in a singular, serial, or parallel fashion. While this chapter focuses on the most frequently used application (i.e., enhancing daily communication), the three applications and their major differences are briefly described to provide a framework for the discussion of intervention that follows.

### *Application #1: Improve Daily Functional Communication and Interaction*

In this application, augmentative aids and techniques are typically used to assist severely impaired individuals in daily communication when the comprehension or production of natural speech is inadequate. For example, a dysarthic adult might reminisce with a friend by using an alphabet board or by printing words across a visual display.   A child might ask a parent for another cheese doodle by using gestures, signs, or a Blissymbol board. A parent, through a combination of signs and speech, may tell a language-impaired child that she cannot go swimming.   Whether addressing the comprehension or production of language, intervention goals and procedures focus on the *interactive* use of augmentative components for daily communication and on the development of language and other skills necessary for that interaction.  Illustrative examples of the use of augmentative applications to facilitate daily communication can be found in the case studies of Beukelman and Yorkston (1980), Beukelman, Yorkston, and Dowden (1985), Carlson (1981), Calculator and Luchko (1983), Davis and Wilcox (1985), and Vicker (1974).

### *Application #2:  Serve as a Bridge to the Development of Natural Speech and Spoken Language Comprehension*

In this application, the primary goal and emphasis of augmentative intervention is to acquire or reacquire natural speech and/or to understand spoken language.  To that end, augmentative language forms and techniques are used as *stepping stones*. Consider these examples.  An adult with aphasia might be able to verbally name an object when a natural gesture related to that object is produced (e.g., a gesture for unlocking a door facilitates the production of the spoken word *key*).  Over time, the use of gestures to facilitate spoken speech might be phased out or maintained as a strategy for eliciting spoken language.  A 3-year-old child at an early preoperational cognitive level is not speaking.  Signs may be introduced into this child's treatment program, along with speech, to facilitate the development of spoken language.  A child with severe cognitive limitations or a language disorder may not have acquired the notion that spoken words represent objects and actions in the environment.  Nonspeech signs and symbols (e.g., natural iconic gestures, objects) might be used alone or in conjunction with speech to develop the idea of symbolic representation.  These may be deemphasized once language comprehension or spoken language appears, or may be used to develop new spoken language forms and concepts.

This application is based on the assumption that nonspeech symbols and signs are less complex and abstract than speech and, therefore, may be acquired more easily. Augmentative symbols, aids, techniques, and strategies can be used to *facilitate* the understanding and/or production of spoken language.  Illustrative examples of this application can be found in the case studies of Bricker (1972), Fulwiler and Fouts (1976), Miller and Miller (1973), and Schaeffer (1980).

*Application #3:  Determine Whether Language Skills Can Be Acquired Using Augmentative*
*Components*

Augmentative communication can also be used to determine if an individual
with a language disorder can acquire or reacquire language skills in a visual or
gestural modality when they have been unable to acquire conventional spoken
language production and comprehension.  This diagnostic exploration assumes that the
underlying language disorder does not affect all learning modalities equally, and/or
that visual or gestural representation might be more easily acquired because it is less
abstract and complex than spoken speech.

In this application, data regarding the client's ability to acquire specific
nonspeech forms and to use those language forms in a meaningful way are compiled.
Results of this diagnostic training process determine whether augmentation will be
pursued further.  In some cases, results indicate little differential learning between
nonspeech forms and natural spoken language.  For example, a child with autistic
behaviors may exhibit the same pragmatic problems in both modes.  In this case,
augmentative interventions would not be pursued.  In another case, an augmentative
aid may appear to facilitate communication or language reacquisition in a specific
area.  For example, an adult with severe, nonfluent aphasia may demonstrate equal
impairment in the use of speech and graphic modes in spontaneous interactions.
However, that individual's ability to respond to learned question-answer routines (e.g.,
biographical information) may improve significantly when written words are available
for communication.  Intervention in this case might include the use of symbols for
limited purposes and continuation of spoken language training procedures.  In another
example, a school-age child with severe verbal dyspraxia may demonstrate the ability
to communicate effectively during diagnostic training sessions using sight words.  In
this case, postdiagnostic goals might include the development of a language board for
use in daily communication in conjunction with continued articulation therapy.
Illustrative examples of diagnostic applications can be found in the work of
Bonvillian and Nelson (1976), Carrier (1976), DeVilliers and Naughton (1974), Glass,
Gazzaniga, and Premack (1973), and Skelly (1979).

Subsequent sections of this chapter focus on the major application of
augmentative communication interventions (i.e., for daily communication).  Although
the other two applications are of equal interest and importance, improving functional
communication skills and interaction is selected for further discussion because of its
frequent use and the need to limit the chapter's scope and length.

# A FRAMEWORK FOR APPROACHING INTERVENTION PLANNING
## (FOR DAILY COMMUNICATION)

It is generally recognized that while augmentative communication has many similarities to spoken communication, many unique differences exist.  Clinicians facilitating communication, language development, and interaction with persons using augmentative components need to be keenly aware of these differences when developing intervention plans and in evaluating performance.  As an introduction to communication through these techniques, note some atypical language and interaction behaviors in the following examples:

Example A.  An 8-year-old using a 100-symbol board and a headpointer is communicating with her father.  She keeps looking toward the television and indicating the symbol *me* and the letter *C*.  A lengthy negotiation follows in which the father attempts to guess what his daughter is trying to say.  After many yes/no questions and unproductive guesses (e.g., "Did you see something that begins with a *C*?"), the intended utterance becomes clear.  His daughter was trying to ask if she might get a computer.

Example B.  A 4-year-old child with severe cerebral palsy is being cared for by a baby sitter while the parents are out for the evening.  Before putting him to bed, the baby sitter begins to read a Dr. Seuss book to the child.  When the child begins to fuss and flex his knees, the baby sitter tries to find out what is wrong by asking a series of yes/no questions (e.g., "Does your knee hurt?," "Do you want another book?").  The child gives no observable response to these questions and continues to flex his knees.  Much frustration follows for both of them.  The baby sitter is not aware that flexing the knees is a gesture for asking to go on a person's lap, nor is she aware of the child's idiosyncratic gestures for yes and no (i.e., a broad smile for *yes*; lack of a response for *no*).

Example C.  An adult with an acquired neuromuscular disease joins a family gathering in the living room.  He recently acquired a portable communication device and can type out what he wishes to say and have it either spoken by a speech synthesizer or printed on a small calculator tape.  The conversation turns to a discussion of a house that his son and daughter-in-law would like to buy.  As they discuss a possible legal problem with the title, the father begins to type on his device.  The lively discussion continues and moves on to stories of how the parents bought their original house.  Because of the noise in the room, the father's attempts at entering into the conversation via his synthesizer are not understood.  He then prints his message.  When he finishes, his wife walks over to his chair and reads his message aloud, which says, "You should really check with Bill Truscott about that."  Each member of the family looks puzzled.  They then realize that his message has nothing to do with the current topic (i.e., the parents' house buying), but is a suggestion relative to the earlier topic, a title search.

Example D.   A child with an extensive symbol vocabulary board, but no wheelchair mobility, is mainstreamed into a regular kindergarten class.  One day the class makes chocolate cupcakes, and the teacher attempts to involve the child in the activity by asking what they should do next.  As the words *mix*, *stir*, *pour*, *oven*, *pan*, and *bake* are not on the child's current language board, the teacher asks a series of yes/no questions (e.g., "Should we pour the milk in?," "Should we put it in the pan like this?").  When asked about whether cupcakes go in the oven, or whether the powder and milk need stirring, the child does not give appropriate answers. The well-meaning teacher suspects that the child is retarded.   However, this child has never before observed or participated in cooking or baking.  He has rarely been in his family's kitchen or watched the family meals being prepared.

Example E.   A teenager using an Etran chart with alphabet spelling is approached by a student in her new ninth grade class.  The classmate begins talking to her in short, simple sentences using an intonation pattern that would be appropriate for a second grader.   The teenager, using her communication aid, attempts to participate in and upgrade the level of the conversation.  She does this by staring at a section of her Etran to indicate the first letter of a message.  Her classmate continues to talk *at* her, not expecting her to be able to participate in the conversation and assuming that she needs to be spoken to like a young child.

These examples illustrate just a few of the common problems and differences that are inherent in communicating through augmentative modes.  If these children and adults were able to speak naturally and clearly, the interactions would have been quite different.   For example, the adult would have made a comment during the family conversation that was clear and appropriately timed and that did not require another individual in close proximity to him.  The child wanting the computer would have had the vocabulary words and form that she needed to make the request.  The teenager could have provided her classmate with an immediate indication of her peer status and participated in the conversation when she wished.  The communications of the 4-year-old child would have been clear to the baby sitter. The kindergartener in the wheelchair would probably have been watching his mother or father cook for years, asking questions and demanding some participation in the process. All of these individuals would have been less dependent on their partners for elaboration, guessing, and an opportunity to communicate.

In developing augmentative communication intervention plans, clinicians often tend to (a) transfer verbatim the decision-making process and language/communication goals used in spoken language interventions to persons using augmentative systems, or (b) train the child or adult in the technical aspects of augmentative components only (e.g., sign or symbol acquisition, indication techniques, device operations), with the expectation that, given a means of expression, linguistic and communication competencies will naturally follow. Both approaches mirror spoken language interventions. Neither approach is adequate.

Interventions that do not take into account the differences between individuals who use augmentative components and those who speak, or that assume that aids and techniques can accomplish what normal speech and language interactions do, are based on erroneous assumptions, including: (a) the person will receive sufficient communication experiences, reaction, interaction, and modeling from the environment to acquire communicative and conversational competence; (b) the language forms, content, and uses that surround the child or adult and that they are familiar with can easily be produced using augmentative components; (c) the productive use of these aids and techniques is the same as the productive use of speech; and (d) the person using augmentative communication techniques does not have a language disorder or delay requiring special intervention.

These assumptions need to be very carefully examined. First, children using augmentative components are not necessarily exposed to a sufficient number of communication experiences or to appropriate modeling in the environment. The work of Calculator (1985), Harris (1978), Light, Collier, and Parnes (1985a,b), and Shere and Kastenbaum (1966), among others, has indicated that the amount, frequency, and variety of communication experiences and overall interactions are often severely reduced in this population. Second, it is often difficult for individuals using gestures, signs, or an aided device to duplicate the use of language learned from the speakers around them. For example, a child may want to ask the question, "Can we go to McDonalds on the way home?" That child may understand information-seeking as a function and the semantic notions coded, and may have knowledge of the form and content used by others to express it. However, that child needs to ask this question with the language repertoire and techniques available. The child may need to gain the adult's attention through an attention-getting buzzer and point to *?* and *McDonalds* on a language board, or vocalize to gain attention and then sign *eat* and *car*. This requires the use of unique linguistic forms and content that are not consistent with language used by others in the child's environment. Such discrepancies would appear to have a significant impact on incidental learning in natural environments. Third, by applying a spoken language intervention model, little or no consideration is given to the differences involved in communicating through modes other than speech. Communication aids, in particular, cannot begin to match the speed and flexibility of spoken language. Although they may provide a means of linguistic interaction, they are by no means a substitute for natural spoken language. Obvious differences include the rate of communication (e.g., 6 words per minute) and the restricted language available to a prespelling child (e.g., 300 language items), even though the child's linguistic knowledge and communication needs are much greater. It is not realistic to expect a 7-year-old child with a 300-word vocabulary display and a slow rate of communication to communicate like an able-bodied child at the same developmental level. It is also not realistic to expect an adult using an alphabet board at a rate of 15 words per minute to accomplish the same communication and discourse behaviors that were accomplished previously with natural, spoken speech. Finally, persons using augmentation may have severe mental retardation, aphasia, autism, or other language disorders and delays. These problems will not be addressed if the acquisition of symbols/signs and techniques is the sole emphasis of the intervention effort.

## Characteristics of Standard and Special Augmentative Components

In this section, differences between special and standard augmentative components and spoken communications will be further explored. It is important that clinicians recognize these differences as they dramatically shape the language and communication behaviors that are possible and effective, and those that are difficult, ineffective, and even impossible. Knowledge of these similarities and differences assists the clinician in selecting intervention goals that are realistic and appropriate for an individual using augmentation. For an expanded discussion of this area, readers are referred to Musselwhite and St. Louis (1982) and Yoder and Kraat (1983).

### *Characteristics of Nonverbal Behaviors*

Face-to-face communication is a complex interweaving of spoken language, silences, and the use of multiple nonverbal behaviors, such as eye gaze, facial expressions, body postures, pointing, hand gestures, traditional head nods, and symbolic gestures, all of which can convey meaning (see chapter 1). For example, eye contact (or the lack of it) accompanies the turn-taking structure in conversation and serves to regulate turn-taking options (Craig & Gallagher, 1982; Duncan & Fiske, 1977; Sachs, Schegloff, & Jefferson, 1974). Pleasure, anger, and boredom are sensed through body postures, facial expressions, or a person's fidgeting or doodling. Expected and important feedback is often provided to a speaker through a smile or head nod from the listener. A gesture in the direction of an object or place makes a referent clear, even though it may not be explicitly labeled in speech (e.g., *it*, *there*). The list goes on. Most of us are not consciously aware of these communicative signals unless they are brought to our attention or violated in some manner. A summary of several of these normal nonverbal communication behaviors can be found in the writings of Duncan and Fiske (1977), Higgenbotham and Yoder (1982), Preisler (1983), and Wood (1981).

Physical disability can affect a person's eye gaze, facial expression, body movements and postures, as well as traditional head nods and pointing/reaching behaviors.  Consequently, the nonverbal communication behaviors of these individuals may be atypical, reduced ork, in some cases, absent.  These differences may limit that person's ability to produce the conventional range of nonverbal behaviors used to convey meaning and regulate discourse, and can lead to multiple communication misunderstandings.  Partners frequently interpret the nonverbal behaviors observed (or their absence) as if these were produced by an able-bodied person.  For example, an excited child may go into a hyperextension or an asymmetric tonic reflex pattern as a tub of water is brought to him for a water play activity.  His turning away or pushing away of the tub may easily be interpreted as a rejection of the activity by a caregiver unfamiliar with that child's reflex patterns.  An adult with facial paralysis may be unable to maintain continued eye contact, smile, or show facial expression when approached by another individual.  This atypical social response may be interpreted as disinterest and the interaction quickly terminated.  Communication partners may also fail to recognize idiosyncratic nonverbal behaviors, such as eye-pointing or an atypical gesture for *yes*.  Limitations and differences within a person's repertoire of nonverbal behaviors need to be recognized and taken into account when evaluating communication interaction and planning intervention goals.

The augmentative team may intervene and attempt to reduce some the most interfering nonverbal behaviors and/or work toward the development of more normalized movements and expressions.  These changes are often not possible and adaptive or compensatory strategies are needed to convey meaning and intentions in another manner.  These strategies might include:  (a) providing the user of the communication aid with linguistic content to counteract or clarify the nonverbal messages being sent (e.g., "I really like this," "I didn't mean to push it away," or "I can look at you better if you sit facing me"); (b) training the various people who frequently communicate with the child or adult to interpret nonverbal behaviors appropriately; or (c) providing some direct means of conveying this information to partners who do not receive training (e.g., through written instructions on a communication aid).

## *Characteristics of Communication Aids and Selection Techniques*

*Rate*.  One of the most striking differences between spoken and aided communication is the rate of that communication.  Natural spoken communication occurs at a very rapid rate of between 126-172 words per minute (Foulds, 1980).  In contrast, the productive rates of communication aids are extremely slow, ranging from 2 to 26 words per minute, with most rates falling below 12 words per minute (Kraat, 1985a).  These figures were obtained primarily from individuals using alphabet arrays with direct-selection and row-column scanning techniques.  Although the use of whole words and other rate enhancement techniques can increase the speed of message transmission, the overall rates of communication remain considerably below that of spoken language. This reduced rate of communication affects many aspects of communication and conversation. The natural speaker is dominant during interactions, being able to speak at about 150 words per minute and capable of taking a speaking turn in less than a second. This discrepancy can change the normal balance within a conversation and reduce the communication participation of the person using augmentative techniques. The slow rate of communication also has an impact on what can efficiently be said by the person using an augmentative device and how it might best be expressed. A simple question such as, "Do you suppose he knows what he is doing" may take as long as four or five minutes to convey through a scanning technique. A different mode (e.g., nonverbal gesture) or language form may need to be used to reduce the communication time to a minute or less. Other time-dependent remarks (e.g, humor, a comment about on-going action) may even be impossible.

The intervention process must take into consideration the impact of a reduced rate of communication and optimize the speed of communication when possible. Increased rates of communication may be achieved by selection of augmentative aids and techniques that allow the fastest rates of communication, thoughtful placement of language items, the development of optimal physical indication skills, and the use of communication strategies. In making decisions about the rates of communication possible across devices and selection techniques, one must consider many factors, including: (a) the rate of communication output possible from the aid; (b) the user's probable rate of communication with training; (c) the rate at which primary listeners will probably receive that communication and interpret it; and (d) any time needed for a partner to come to the user to note mesages. The speed of communication may also be enhanced by the strategies of the person using an aid and their partners. Partners may facilitate by predicting and expanding utterances or attempting to guess the meaning of the message using a quick series of yes/no questions. Persons using augmentative aids may increase communication rates by changing and shortening the wording of an utterance, using available stock phrases and sentences, or incorporating multiple communication modes (e.g., vocalization, facial expression, gestures) when appropriate and effective.

*Language form and content*. Communication aids can also vary from spoken language in vocabulary size and the nature of the language forms and content available to an individual. For those who cannot spell, communication is limited by the symbols available on a language board, chart, or communication aid. This content generally has been provided by someone else (e.g., speech-language pathologist). The language array may contain as few as 25 items, or as many as 600 language forms. As previously noted in this text, although 300 to 600 language items may seem like a large lexicon, in reality, this is fewer items than an average 3-year-old uses. Limited vocabularies restrict what a person can say and how it can be said. This can make even basic communication difficult.  For example, a child may want to tell others that his pet fish died.  He may not have any language items available to convey that message, or he may have a limited number of symbols that can relay only part of the message (e.g., animal, sad, swim).  The meaning must be developed through the guesses, associations, and questions of others.  Language restrictions may also reduce the flexibility and style with which an idea can be expressed.  For example, a school-age child may want to politely ask the class aide to stop calling him "Heckman" and to address him by his first name.  The form/content is not available that would allow the child to manipulate the situation politely (e.g., "I'd rather you call me by my first name. . .I hate "Heckman!"  Do you mind?").  Instead, available vocabulary gives the child only two options (i.e., "Stop it," and "Don't say that!").  Although this may convey the message, the child may have to take the consequences of using an impolite style or of having the aide misunderstand his statement.  Finite language sets not only affect the communication potentials of the person using augmentative aids, but often alter the role and requirements of the communication partner as well.  Partners are no longer just reacting and interacting with another person.  They are often placed in the role of elaborating, guessing, and clarifying an intended message with minimal cues from the communication aid user.  People vary in their ability to fulfill this role.  Limited skills on the part of the partner will further reduce the communication that is possible.

As a limited number of language items is generally available for communication, the language content and symbol forms selected are critical.  The largest and most powerful set of language elements possible needs to be provided.  This requires some adaptive decisions about how to maximize daily communication and interaction with a limited number of language units.  Problems associated with finite vocabulary sets also suggest the need for development of literacy skills as early as possible so that communication can be supplemented with partial or full spelling.

Both the users of augmentative communication aids and techniques and their partners need to acquire adaptive strategies for communicating within restricted lexicons.  For partners, this may require learning how to effectively expand on communication efforts or to ask productive, information-seeking questions.  For the user, this may involve (a) learning how to use available symbols effectively in given communication situations; or (b) acquiring vocabulary expansion techniques (e.g., using multiple modes of communication or providing topic or vocabulary hints such as "similar to," "about news," or "sports - tall- win").

*Mode of expression*.  Communication exchanges between persons using communication aids and their partners are accomplished through symbols, written orthography, and/or synthetic speech.  These messages are transmitted through a variety of high-tech output modes, such as visual displays (liquid crystal and light emitting diode displays), print, Braille, and synthetic speech, and low-tech symbol displays in which the user selects language elements and the partner visually notes each element. None of these options offers the independence, intelligibility, and environmental flexibility of natural speech, the medium that is generally used in face-to-face interactions. In developing intervention plans, the clinician needs to understand how a particular mode of expression can influence and shape the communicative interactions that do and do not occur, and the adaptive strategies that might be needed in conversing through nontraditional modes.

Some forms of output (language boards, eye-pointing charts, and scanning arrays) require the active participation of another person for communication to take place at all. That is, the partner must be physically next to the individual to note the items or codes selected one by one or, in the case of a scan chart, actually present the item or row options to the user. This dependency upon another person for expression is atypical of spoken language exchanges, where individuals can express themselves independently whenever they wish to. In dependent communication modes, the partner's behaviors greatly influence the interactions and levels of communication that take place. The ability to communicate from a distance or independently participate in a group conversation may also be limited by the characteristics of the communication output mode being used. Although communication across distances can be independently accomplished by a person using synthetic speech, a display facing outward, or an Etran (if the partner is highly familiar with the codes), other communication modes (e.g., print, pointing, or a language board) require a person near the aid or device to receive the communication. These modes limit a person's ability to independently participate in a group conversation without an "interpreter" or to communicate with persons at a distance, unless the device user has independent mobility. The need to come to the person communicating through augmentative aids can limit opportunities for linguistic communication in a classroom, worksite, or living room.

The level of communication and interaction is further shaped by the fact that messages conveyed using augmentative components are not as universally intelligible as natural spoken language. For example, a person using an orthographically based printout or visual display will not be able to communicate directly with nonreading or nonspelling children and adults. Persons using abstract symbols or symbol strategies may also be limited to communicating with particular partners who have reading ability or knowledge of those symbol representations and strategies. Intelligibility may also be reduced by characteristics of the communication modes themselves. Synthetic speech, for example, is frequently not as intelligible as natural speech. This difference may cause communication difficulties with partners who are unfamiliar with this mode, with some of the utterances, or in situations that are noisy.

Intervention often needs to address the use of adaptive strategies to accommodate the differences in modes of expression. Persons using augmentative aids may need to acquire strategies for getting partners to come to them or to assume collaborative roles in augmentative techniques when indicated.   The person using augmentative components may also need to learn how to accommodate different partners and physical situations by selecting the optimal mode for a particular situation (e.g., using nonverbal or vocal behaviors from a distance or with a nonreader; not using Blissymbolic combination strategies with persons unfamiliar with Bliss). Characteristics of output modes may also require alterations in the conventional form and content used to express some meanings and communicative functions.   For example, spoken language uses paralinguistic features (e.g., rate, stress, pausing, and intonation) to convey meaning.  The absence of these features in symbol boards, print, and synthetic speech may create misunderstandings (e.g., humor or sarcasm may not be understood), or make the intentions of early symbol users (e.g., single-word level) ambiguous.   Consequently, communication aid users often must convey nuances of meaning in an explicit manner through direct wording (e.g., joke) or obvious nonverbal behaviors.  In devices not having speech output, the language form and content used to express some communicative functions may need to be altered because of the differences between spoken and visual/graphic modes.  For example, a speaking child might say "Mommy" to get her mother's attention; "look" to get someone to notice something in the environment; or "car" to begin a communication about a toy car when the partner is not paying attention or looking.  Although a child may have these forms on a language board, pointing to them will not be particulary effective at achieving these same functions, particularly if the partner is not looking.  That child may need to use vocalization, nonverbal behaviors, or a buzzer to gain attention, get someone to notice something, or to establish "car" as a topic focus.

## *Characteristics of Gestures/Signs*

Inherent constraints in gestures and signs also may lead to differences in daily communication and need to be recognized and considered in generating intervention programs.  Although one frequently assumes that sign and gesture systems provide a larger language repertoire than aided systems, the language symbols available are very much tied to what has been taught to the individual and what is understood by their communication partners. In contrast to children of signing, deaf parents, most individuals who learn gesture and sign systems for augmentative communication purposes are not surrounded by peers, family, or teachers who are fluent in sign. Consequently, nonspelling individuals using signs and gestures are often limited in the messages they can produce.  It is commonly reported in the literature that language-impaired clients use less than 200 signs or gestures for communication purposes.  That limited language pool may reflect the person's reduced ability to learn signs rapidly and/or their lack of appropriate models for incidental learning.

The rate of communication when gestures and signs are used by individuals who are language disordered or delayed has not been reported in the literature. Clinical experience would suggest, however, that the overall rates of communication are rather slow and may only approximate whole word use by persons using direct-selection techniques. These slow rates are influenced by the rate of sign production, the time between signs, and the time it takes receivers to comprehend the message. Frequently, both individuals who use gestures/signs and their partners lack high-speed fluency.

Although communicating across distances and within a group may not be a problem for a person using typical gestures, intelligibility appears to be a critical problem for persons using idiosyncratic or translucent/opague signs. Signs, signals, and gestures are not as universally intelligible and independent as spoken speech and frequently are not understood by persons untrained in these language forms. This severely reduces the number of individuals that the unaided speaker can communicate with and the extent to which they can communicate. Many of the communication and intervention implications discussed for persons using aided language components and techniques also apply to individuals using gesture and signs. The reduced rate of communication, the available lexicon, and characteristics of the output mode affect the nature of communication and interaction, and must be addressed in intervention planning.

## Interaction Characteristics

Given the inherent differences in augmentative components, what might the communicative interactions between users of augmentative techniques and others look like? How do speech-impaired individuals and their partners adapt to unconventional communication components? Which compensatory strategies of both partners appear to be most successful?

Most of what is currently known about interactions involving persons using augmentative aids and techniques comes from the reports and observations of clinicians and a small but growing number of formal studies. This research has predominantly focused on communication interactions observed between physically disabled children or young adults and adults who are familiar with these individuals. Most of these young people have used a variety of symbol and alphabet boards with a direct-selection technique. Minimal information is available about interaction between persons using other techniques or computerized devices or about the interaction patterns of their communication partners. A detailed summary and integration of published and unpublished research in aided interactions to date can be found in Kraat (1985a).  Studies of interaction between persons who primarily use signing or gesture modes are sparse, however.  Although the literature contains several case studies on sign training or sign acquisition, these studies generally have not extended to observations of interaction patterns between these dyads in natural environments.

## Observed Patterns in Discourse

Studies and observations in natural or quasi-natural environments have begun to provide some understanding of a few of the frequent discourse patterns that occur in interactions that involve the use of augmentative aids and techniques.  A frequent pattern reported in the literature is one in which the unimpaired speaker extensively dominates the interaction and controls much of the conversation (Calculator & Dollaghan, 1982; Calculator & Luchko, 1983; Collquhoun, 1982; Culp, 1982; Farrier Yorkston, Marriner, & Beukelman, 1985; Harris, 1978, 1982; Kraat, 1985a; Light et al., 1985a,b; Wexler, Blau, Leslie, & Dore, 1983).  It has been observed that unimpaired speakers frequently initiate the conversational sequence, dominate topic initiation and extension, produce many more utterances per turn, and often terminate the exchange.  This domination and control is quite understandable given the slow rate of communication, possible lexical constraints, and some characteristics of the expressive modes.  Of interest is how unimpaired speakers use their dominant position, how communication opportunities and participation on the part of the speech-impaired person may be adversely affected, and how the adaptive behaviors of both partners can optimize those interactions.

In some of the communication samples studied, partners dominate the exchanges in ways that appear detrimental to the overall interaction and impede the participation of the individual using communication augmentation.  In some cases, partners limit participation by controlling the interaction and asking multiple questions.  Partners may not pause long enough for the person using augmentative components to take a turn, or may interrupt after one or two words, thus taking away the individual's speaking opportunities (Harris, 1978, 1982).  Partners, given the dominant position, may also limit the augmentative user's participation to that of a primary responder (versus initiator and responder) through use of continuous questions.  These questions are rarely open-ended.  They include yes/no questions, simple choices, or *wh* questions that require single-word answers.  Research findings also suggest that persons using augmentative techniques may not, at times, be given an opportunity to participate at all.  In the studies of Blackstone and Cassatt-James (1984) and Light (1984), both studying the interactions between mothers and children, it was observed that some mothers never provided communication opportunities for their children who used communication aids, even on a nonverbal level.

Such patterns severely limit the contributions to a conversation that can effectively be made by the augmentative communication user, and may also have an impact on the language/learning process for developmentally disabled, speech-impaired children. They are observed not only in the interactive behaviors of individuals who use rudimentary augmentative aids and techniques, but also in the interactions of persons with more advanced systems and capabilities (Beukelman & Yorkston, 1980; Calculator & Luchko, 1983; Farrier et al., 1985; Kraat, 1979; Light et al., 1985a,b; Wexler et al., 1983). Some of these behaviors (i.e., continuous yes/no question asking and interrupting) are illustrated in the following conversation. (Note: In the following examples, *P* is used to refer to the communication partner, and *C* is used to refer to the individual who uses a communication aid):

P:  What did you do last night?

C:  (Begins to formulate a response using communication device.)

P:  Did you go home?  Did you watch TV?  Did you see Walt Disney?
    Did your brother come home? (Harris, 1978, p. 135).

An imbalance in an interaction may also be created by the communication behaviors of the person using augmentative components. In some observations, communication aid users fail to respond to a partner's communication advances or do not take advantage of available communication opportunities (Light et al., 1985a). The user may place the communicative burden on the unimpaired speaker, even though linguistic forms are available to assist that communication (Harris, 1978; Kraat, 1979). For example, in the next conversation, the client knows that his Medicaid card is in a notebook in the back pocket of his wheelchair bag. Even though the client has spelling capability and a device with a paper printout, he places the communication burden on his partner.

P:  Do you have a Medicaid card?

C:  Yes (gesture).

P:  Is it in here? (Pointing to the wheelchair bag.)

C:  Mm.

P:  I'll start looking. . . I don't think you have one in here. . . . You
    certainly have a lot of things in here! . . . Wait, you might have one.
    Maybe it is back here. (Starts removing the contents of the bag.)

C: (Picks up the notebook and hands it to her.)

P: Check this?

C: Yes (gesture).

P: (Leafs through notebook and envelopes). . . . There we go!

C: Mm. (Kraat, 1979)

Exchanges have also been observed in which the communication needs of the individual using a communication aid dominate the conversation (particulary for individuals who have limited language forms available and are nonspellers). In these interactions, the able-bodied partner serves more like a message elaborator than a participant in the conversation.

C: Home (word on language board).

P: Home? What about home? Something about your sister?

C: No (gesture).

   Day of the week (board).

P: Something about home and Saturday? Are you going home on Saturday?

C: Man (board).

P: A man? Someone special is coming?

C: No (gesture).

P: I should find out who the man is?

C: Yes (emphatic gesture).

P: A relative? A friend? Someone in the hospital?

C: Yes (gesture).

P: Someone in the hospital. Let me see. A doctor? Therapist? Friend? Can you give me another hint?

C: (Eye points to top of partner's head.)

P: Head. Part of the head? Brains? He works with the head?

C: Color (board).

(Negotiation continues for approximately 100 turns and 20 minutes until . . . )

P: Oh, can Carl (a security guard) possible take you home on Saturday in the hospital van?

C: Yes (gesture).

P: He's not allowed to do that. (Conversation ends.)     (Kraat, 1985a, p. 81).

In this example, repeated questions had to be asked because the user had a very restricted lexicon (50-word board) available for communication. The lengthy negotiation ended with a quick answer to C's question, and the interaction was terminated. The partners did not elaborate on the topic or continue the conversation beyond two completed utterances (i.e., Can Carl take me home on Saturday in the hospital van?; He's not allowed to do that.).

The excessive use of any of these patterns is detrimental to communication development and to the quality of an interaction. In one, the individual using an augmentative aid is not given a sufficient opportunity to respond, get into the conversation, or make an extended contribution. In another, the individual does not participate in the interaction at a level commensurate with his capabilities. In the last example, conversation in the traditional sense does not occur.

Interactions involving severely speech/language-impaired individuals who use augmentative aids and techniques may never duplicate the patterns and more equalized participation seen in spoken conversations. However, conversations can achieve some balance when particular strategies are employed by both partners. Note the following conversation involving a young student and two familiar staff members (P1 and P2). The student uses a direct-selection alphabet and word communication board, communicating primarily through sight words and some beginning spelling skills. All of C's utterances were made through the board.

(Woman in adjoining office comes out, asks if the group took her chair, and returns to her room.)

C:  Off with the head.

P1:  We should have given her your wheelchair.

C:  Ha-ha!

P1:  I think it would be a great idea.

C:  Dream on, sister.

P1:  Are you calling me "sister?"  That's fresh.

C:  I know . . . sister.

P1:  I've got to think of a name for you.

P2:  I know one (whispers it to P1).

C:  What did she say?

P1:  She called you a very polite word.

C:  Like what?

P1:  (Mouths word.)

C:  No, talk it.

P1:  (No response.)

C:  Look, Big Ear, say it or else. . . .

P1:  She said "blabbermouth."

C:  (looks at P2)  You should talk. (Potter & Kraat, 1986).

Although the contributions of the person using the communication aid took longer, both the adults and the child made accommodations to each other.  Partners expected participation, waited for responses, and reacted to the contributions made by the child using his communication aid. Rather than asking a series of questions and controlling the topic, the adults made comments, expanded on the utterances of the board user, and made contributions. The student used the aid to introduce ideas of his own, demanded responses from the adults, and expanded on topics through comments, humor, and questions.

## *Communication Opportunities*

Persons using augmentative aids and techniques appear to have reduced levels of interaction when compared to their able-bodied counterparts. Regardless of the types of augmentation used, these individuals often have fewer communication partners, less frequent opportunities for interaction, and reduced participation in many exchanges. People may avoid interaction with a person using an augmentative technique because they feel uncomfortable with this communication difference or they may interact on a superficial social level, not expecting a conversational exchange or response (e.g., lousy weather today). Opportunities to communicate are often restricted to one or more partners (e.g., a parent, family member, or professionals working with the speech/language-impaired individual). Consequently, the person communicating through augmentative components may have infrequent experiences interacting with peers, a variety of partners, or persons not very familiar with them.

It has also been observed that individuals using augmentative techniques often have fewer communication opportunities within the interactions that do take place. Several researchers have noted that attempts to initiate an interaction or utterance on the part of the speech-impaired individual may go unrecognized or may not be acknowledged by others (Beukelman et al., 1985; Calculator & Dollaghan, 1982; Light, 1984). These efforts included nonverbal behaviors, vocalizations, or getting a partner to read printed output. Possible reasons for this lack of response to initiation attempts include differences in the output medium and the time and effort sometimes required to actualize or respond to those utterances. As discussed earlier, individuals using augmentative techniques may also have fewer communication opportunities within the interactions that do take place because of the communication behaviors and strategies of a partner. Research studies also suggest that the overall length of many of these interactions may be reduced. In the interactions observed by Calculator and Dollaghan (1982), Calculator and Luchko (1983), and Harris (1978), the average length of an exchange was frequently no more than three turns or utterances.

Individual users of communication aids and augmentative techniques also vary in their ability to make and take communication opportunities. Although this area has been given little attention, some initial observations are of interest. Reports suggest that some individuals appear to take little initiative in communicating and may react sporadically or not at all to communication opportunities that are afforded (Light et al., 1985a).   That is, they (a) minimally use their opportunities following a silence, comment, or other nonobligatory utterances, (b) rarely interrupt, or (c) infrequently expand on a topic beyond what is minimally required.   Other individuals, regardless of the techniques utilized, will use or create communication opportunities.


## Communicative Breakdowns

Communication breakdowns are frequently observed in augmentative interactions.   They occur among speakers of various cognitive abilities and developmental levels who use a variety of augmentative components.   It has been reported that during mother-child interactions, as much as 25 percent of the child's utterances were unrecognized, unclear, or unintelligible (Culp, 1982; Light, 1984).   In a classroom setting, the user's initiation efforts may go unrecognized as often as 39 percent of the time (Calculator & Dollaghan, 1982).   Even adults with normal cognitive abilities and acquired disabilities (e.g., ALS) find communication difficult. In one dyad studied by Beukelman and Yorkston (1980), 20 percent of the interactions between an adult nonspeaker with a scanning, spelling technique and her nurse-attendant were unsuccessful.   Communicative breakdowns can be caused by limitations in the aids and techniques themselves (e.g., insufficient vocabulary, rate, intelligibility of the symbols, etc.), the adaptive strategies of the user, or the behaviors of the partners.


## Atypical Partner Roles

Partners do not necessarily have the competencies needed to effectively communicate with a person who uses augmentative components.   In conversing with these individuals, the temporal aspects of turn-taking may be different, the conventional signals for turn bids and acceptances may be atypical, and the accompanying nonverbal behaviors may be altered.   Communication partners cannot use the usual overt verbal behaviors to estimate the cognitive level of the person with whom they are speaking.   Partners may have little idea of how to communicate with individuals who are unable to speak, who speak quite unintelligibly, or who use unfamiliar symbols, strategies, or techniques, or who have a concomitant language disorder.

The nature of augmentative communication exchanges often require partners to assume atypical listener roles.   In spoken conversation, one person generally completes an utterance while the other listens; then, the speaker role may change, with the person who was the listener taking a turn at speaking while the other person becomes the listener. These traditional speaker-listener roles may be kept when using high-tech aids with independent communication output (e.g., print or synthetic speech). In communicating with a person using a low-tech aid or a limited sign/gesture repertoire, however, the traditional role of the partner changes. Partners often cannot passively wait for a turn or utterance to be completed, but must actively participate in many of the user's turns. This participation may take the form of repeating or noticing each item selected, presenting a scanning array and decoding items selected, guessing or elaborating on associated or limited cues, and confirming each element identified. This participation may also extend into the resolution of communicative breakdowns. Again, this is an atypical role for partners communicating with older children and adults. Generally, once a listener signals difficulty, it is the responsibility of the speaker to clarify and resolve the misunderstanding. With restricted language sets, the listener's role is not only to signal breakdowns, but often to actively assist the augmentative speaker in resolving the situation.

## *The Multi-Component Nature of Augmentative Communication*

Individuals communicating through augmentative techniques use multiple modes of communication to a greater extent than able-bodied speakers. Topic introductions, message-bearing elements, and whole propositions may be conveyed through nonverbal behaviors, residual speech or vocalization, gestures and formal signs, and/or graphic symbol forms. This use of multi-components (or modes) has been observed in the interactions of adults who spell and/or use advanced communication aids, as well as in the interactions of nonspellers with limited vocabularies. Individuals shift among these multiple communication techniques as different communication situations arise. The modes of expression selected often reflect the need for communication efficiency, the partner's distance from the user and ability to comprehend a specific form or mode, and the limited language forms that may be available in a sign/symbol repertoire. Clinicians working with this population need to view communication behaviors holistically, rather than solely focusing on the communicative use of a communication aid or formal signs.

Interaction research has described individuals who use nonverbal behaviors, vocalization/speech, and gestures more frequently than their augmentative devices (Blackstone & Cassatt-James, 1984; Calculator & Dollaghan, 1982; Calculator & Luchko, 1983; Colquhoun, 1982; Culp, 1982; Kraat, 1979; Light, Collier, & Parnes, 1985c; Wexler et al., 1983), as well as individuals who communicate primarily through an augmentative aid (Beukelman & Yorkston, 1980; Wilson, 1982). Differences in the percentage of aid use may be attributed to: (a) the communicative functions frequently expressed by an individual (e.g., answering yes/no questions); (b) the nonverbal and speech abilities available to a specific person: (c) limitations within the language content available to a particular individual; or (d) longstanding communication styles.  In the last instance, an individual may not be using an optimal mode for a given situation or partner.  For example, a person may point in a general direction to introduce a topic of conversation, even when this gesture is ambiguous to the partner and a clear form of communication is available.  Or, an individual may fail to switch modes appropriately across listeners and contexts (Huschle & Staudenbaur, 1983; Reichle & Ward, 1985).  For example, an individual may attempt to use dysarthric speech with a partner who is unable to understand that speech pattern, even when other options are open to them.

## *Altered Use of Language Form*

We all use many incomplete and fragmented language forms in daily communication.  However, individuals who use augmentative techniques frequently use telegraphic forms to a greater extent (e.g., signing *bathroom* rather than use an elaborated form such as *May I go to the bathroom?*).  It has been suggested that these truncated and telegraphic forms are used for efficiency due to the effort and time it takes to complete an expanded utterance.  The conventional use of language content and form may also be altered in augmentative communication for reasons other than efficiency.  As mentioned earlier, the necessary lexical items or lexical diversity may not be available to the speaker.  Or, the characteristics of the communication aid or technique may shape the forms that are successful in varying social contexts (e.g., nonverbal behaviors may be needed in communicating from distances, paralinguistic features are absent, partners may not comprehend formal signs, and so on).

## *Rhetorical and Remedial Patterns*

Conversations between nonspelling individuals and others may involve many question-and-answer sequences in which the information is already known to both parties (Colquhoun, 1982).  For example, a person who is asked "What is your favorite TV show?" or, "Who lives with us in the house?" is expected to sign, gesture, or point to a specific written word or symbol in response, even when the answer is already known to both individuals.  It has been suggested that rhetorical sequences are used by partners to simulate a normalized conversation and/or to demonstrate the facility of an individual who uses a language board or a sign repertoire.

Remedial patterns (e.g., teaching sign/board use) are also observed in interactions with parents, teachers, aides, and therapists.  A child may point to a desired object or to a single word on a language board.  Instead of responding to the child's request, the adult may say "Tell me on your board," or  "Say it in a sentence," even though the message has been understood.  Clearly, this is not a typical interaction pattern beyond the early stages of language development. Obviously, while there is a need for teaching and modeling, this pattern is inhibitory to comunication and interaction when it extends into all conversational interactions or occupies a large portion of exchanges.

## *Adaptive Strategies*

The communication patterns that are observed are a composite of the characteristics of augmentative components and the communication choices made by each of the partners involved. Given specific symbols, aids, or techniques and a communication context, people may act and react very differently as conversation unfolds. Some adaptive communication behaviors are facilitory, while others may have a negative influence on the message exchange or may create communication breakdowns. Note the strategies used by clients and partners in the following examples:

*Adaptive strategies - Augmented speakers*. Two children with severely dysarthric speech, gestures, and a small sign vocabulary attempt to tell a neighbor about buying a new puppy. Given the same communication repertoire, one may be successful and the other not. One child may attempt this communication by signing *dog* and *home* to the neighbor who has no sign experience. The other child, aware of his neighbor's limitations, may point to his neighbor's dog, himself, and his house. This is accompanied by nonverbal expressions and vocalizations showing his excitement. The second child is more successful at conveying his meaning to the neighbor.

*Adaptive strategies - Partner*. An adult using an alphabet board may begin to make a request of his attendant by spelling *my head*. . . . One attendant may immediately respond by moving the man's head to various positions on the pillow or in an annoyed manner say, "I just fixed your head." The communication is misunderstood. A second attendant may respond quite differently. That person may not interrupt, or may guess and then ask the man to agree or disagree with that elaboration. In this exchange, the man's request, "My head needs two pillows," will probably be successful.

Although we have begun to outline some adaptive strategies employed by persons using augmentation and their partners, many more behavioral observations are needed in this area. The adaptive strategies that facilitate communication and interaction in a variety of communication situations, or that optimize the communication possible using specific aids and techniques, are of particular importance.

## Language/Learning Environments

Most theories of language development take into account the input and reactions of persons who interact with the language learner as an important aspect of the acquisition process. One needs to ask what the learning environments for the severely speech/language-disabled individual might be like, how they might differ from the environments surrounding able-bodied, speaking children, and how those environmental factors might affect the language and communication behaviors that are observed in these individuals. Beginning research and observations suggest that the input and feedback given to many developmentally disabled children may, in fact, be quite different from that of other children (Harris & Vanderheiden, 1980; Light, 1984; Morris, 1981; Shere & Kastenbaum, 1966; Wilcox & Campbell, 1985; Yoder & Calculator, 1981; Yoder & Kraat, 1983). These differences extend across many areas of learning and development, including cognitive, social, and linguistic (semantic, syntactic, and pragmatic) areas.

Parents and caregivers confronted with an atypical child do not necessarily know how to compensate for this abnormality in their daily interactions. Shere and Kastenbaum (1966), in their study of mothers and their severely speech and physically impaired preschoolers, noted that some mothers spoke infrequently to their children. Many of these children also lacked stimulation and exposure to a range of cognitive experiences. Observations of object play in these mother-child dyads, for example, suggest an emphasis on developing physical capabilities (e.g., controlled movement of the upper extremity), rather than on exploring objects and the associated semantic notions involved.

It has also been observed that "everyday" experiences may be reduced, particulary for physically disabled children. Harris and Vanderheiden (1980) report that many of these children may experience life from a single room or static physical position. Experiences that would naturally evolve for a child through crawling to objects, manipulating them, and engaging adults and siblings in demonstrating, interacting with, and talking about them are not possible without assistance. As children develop, experiences outside the home may also be limited. It is quite possible that these children may not have visited a supermarket, seen a cash register, felt grass, turned on a light switch, tasted sugar, or joined the family at the dinner table. Severely speech-impaired children who have no adequate means of linguistic communication at an early age are also unable to seek further information about the world through the use of language.

Communication experiences may also be reduced by the interaction patterns of partners and other environmental factors. Language learners may have a history of unsuccessful communication and interaction, and may not receive consistent and clear feedback during the acquisition process. Wilcox and Campbell (1985) observed that families and professionals who were very familiar with persons primarily using nonverbal and vocal behaviors for communication respond to these behaviors in an inconsistent manner. Their research found that caregivers did not necessarily identify and respond to the same signals as being "communicative," nor did they assign the same meaning to them.

As discussed previously, some of the interaction patterns observed in nonspeaking dyads provide little opportunity for communication participation. Others promote the use of some language forms and functions over others (e.g., answering questions). The language environments that surround severely speech-impaired individuals may also be atypical in other ways. These environments may (a) be very routine with few new topics to talk about (Harris & Vanderheiden, 1980; Shane, Lipschultz, & Shane, 1982); (b) place minimal demands or expectations on the speech-impaired person (Calculator, 1985); and/or (c) have a large number of other individuals with severe communication disorders who are unable to provide appropriate language and communication models.

Parents of young, able-bodied speaking children frequently expand on their children's utterances to provide them with a learning model or point out the inappropriateness of particular language usage. Parents also frequently simplify their language input to a level close to the emerging language skills of the child when speaking. To date, there is a paucity of information on the input, modeling, and expansion that caregivers provide to individuals who use augmentative components. It appears that many augmentative language/communication learners may be given spoken language models and expansion, but may have minimal experiences in how symbols or nonverbal behaviors might be used to communicate and interact in everyday environments. Culp (1982) tabulated the number of times a parent modeled use of the child's symbols and nonverbal behavior. Of the five mother-child (communication aid users) dyads observed, only nine of the 839 utterances by the mothers contained any use of the child's communication repertoire (most of these were nonverbal gestures). In a more recent study of 11 similar dyads, Culp and Stahlecker (1986) found no occurrences of modeling in the parental utterances. Bruno and Bryen (1985) examined the communication modeling that occurred in the interactions between speech-language pathologists and children using augmentative aids and techniques. Prior to intervention with these therapists, observations of modeling were also infrequently observed. One might anticipate that persons who use signs are exposed to more modeling of signs than persons who use aids are exposed to the use of graphic symbols. However, modeling for these individuals is frequently limited because of the reduced sign fluency of many partners.

## Implications for Intervention Planning

Characteristics of augmentative communication necessitate some alterations or adaptations to conventional intervention processes. Decision-making must take into account the inherent differences in augmentative components, the patterns of conversation exchange frequently observed, and the possible deficits created by the inability or reduced ability to communicate and interact. Previous sections of this chapter have suggested ways in which augmentative components differ from conventional spoken communication and how those differences might affect communication, interaction, and intervention planning. Several intervention needs and directions were outlined for nonverbal communication behaviors, communication efficiency, adaptive strategies (augmentative communicators and their partners), the use of restricted language content and form, and the effective integration of multiple modes of communication. Additional considerations and guidelines for intervention planning based on frequently observed interaction and language learning patterns include:

1. Early referral and intervention (with all types of disorders) is important to insure that optimal communication patterns and social interaction are achieved.

2. The language and learning environments of persons with developmental disabilities need to be evaluated and often modified or expanded.

3. Language and interaction samples cannot necessarily be judged in a traditional manner to determine a client's language levels and the immediate intervention goals for that client.

4. Intervention areas that are identified as being problematic in augmentative interactions should be carefully evaluated and addressed. These include, among others: (a) discourse styles, (b) availability and use of communication opportunities, (c) communication breakdowns, and (d) effective expression of communicative meanings and functions.

5. The communication behaviors of partners are important to assess and shape (e.g., partners may require assistance in recognizing and interpreting atypical communication signals and forms, providing appropriate communication opportunities, adapting interaction styles to accommodate differences described earlier, or acquiring the ability

to elaborate and expand on the communication efforts of the severely speech/language-impaired individual).

6. Communication goals should be realistic, given the augmentative aids and techniques involved. (<u>Note</u>: Persons who use augmentative components are unlikely to achieve the conversational competencies and/or flexibility of unimpaired speakers.)

7. Intervention goals may include the acquisition of conventional form, content, and use of language as well as unique alterations and strategies to maximize augmentative communication components.

8. Effective conversational and interaction skills for daily communication often need to be taught so that clients learn how to accomplish communication tasks in a unique manner (e.g., use a prestored utterance or create a novel utterance, gain someone's attention) and how to do so across diverse social contexts (e.g., group activities or discussion, peer interactions, and so on).

## EVALUATION OF COMMUNICATION INTERACTION

Central to any intervention decision is an assessment of a person's communication abilities and performance. This is not unique to this area, but is a process that is used across the field of speech and language pathology. Chapter 4 suggests several ways in which these abilities might be assessed in a person with a severe communication disorder. This section further explores the evaluation of communication interaction, focusing on how language and communication behaviors are actually being used in the communication exchanges that occur every day between persons using augmentative components and their partners.

Speech-language pathologists are accustomed to taking a language sample and analyzing the language form and content, as well as the speech acts, used by a client. That same clinician may also be familiar with evaluation procedures for assessing discourse skills or examining a dyad's interactive style for purposes of identifying positive and negative discourse patterns that inhibit or facilitate language learning and participation. This clinician, however, faced with an evaluation of the communication behaviors of a person using augmentative components, often feels awkward. The behaviors exhibited by a 6-year-old child communicating through a small repertoire of natural gestures, or those of an adult using a computerized communication aid and his partner, seem unfamiliar and atypical. Evaluation of interaction with individuals who use augmentative communication components raises many questions. Among them are: (a) Does an evaluation of communication and interaction differ from the procedures used with speaking clients and, if so, how? (b) How does one transcribe and code nonverbal behaviors and augmentative signs and symbols? (c) Can the taxonomies and coding systems used with conventional speakers be applied? (d) How can these conversational samples be evaluated to determine whether or not intervention is needed and to outline intervention goals? In this section, we will explore the process of sampling interaction as it applies to individuals who use augmentative communication and their partners.

### Assessment Differences

Until recently, augmentative communication interactions were sampled and evaluated in the same manner as spoken communication samples. That is, known conversational parameters were observed, available taxonomies and coding schemas were used, and judgments were made using a normal, spoken conversational model. Minor alterations in the procedures were generally made to accommodate the augmentative components that were used. Differences were identified based on a comparison with normal conversational performance; inadequacies that were identified became the focus of intervention programs.

As the inherent constraints in augmentative aids, symbols, and techniques are better understood, the use of standard sampling procedures for this population has been questioned (Harris, 1982; Kraat, 1984, 1985a; Yoder & Kraat, 1983; see also chapters 7 & 9). Of particular concern is the appropriateness of judging augmentative interactions in a conventional manner. Protocols based on normal spoken language models and discourse rules judge these individuals against a standard that may not be effective, functional, or possible. Such judgments can lead to intervention programs that focus on unrealistic goals or on the development of behaviors that do not necessarily improve the functional communication skills of clients using augmentative components.

Although it appears that sampling procedures need to be adapted for this population, the nature of those modifications has not yet been outlined (see chapters 4, 6, 7, & 9 for related discussions). However, some of the differences that must be recognized during the evaluation process are beginning to be understood. Specifically, speech-language pathologists need to: (a) observe communication behaviors that are unique to or take on greater importance in augmentative interactions; (b) modify and adapt the transcription coding schemas used with other populations to fit these interactions; (c) recognize the atypical variables present in these samples when making judgments about language and communication behavior; and (d) ask questions about the data that are functionally appropriate to augmentative interactions. These differences will be explored in subsequent sections of this chapter, along with a discussion of procedures for obtaining samples of interaction behavior.

## *Collecting a Sample*

Presently, communication samples are planned in a similar manner whether those observations involve natural speakers or an individual using augmentative components. Speech-language pathologists and other professionals need to recognize, however, that the field of communication disorders is currently struggling with the broad question of how best to collect a language sample that is representative, valid, and clinically useful. Until recently, it was thought that any conversation that was spontaneous could provide a representative sample of a client's language and communication capabilities. This assumption has been questioned over the past few years, as research has shown that contextual variables influence the behaviors that are observed (Gallagher, 1983). Different language and communication profiles of the same person can be obtained, depending on the partner(s), topics, and/or physical environments involved. This awareness of contextual influences has made representative sampling a much more difficult process. The current challenge is to obtain samples of communicative interaction that are, in fact, typical or representative of a person or dyad's daily interaction.

There currently is no standard or standardized way of obtaining a representative sample of interaction performance for a person or dyad. A variety of sampling techniques are proposed in the literature (Bolton & Dashiell, 1984; Calculator & Luchko, 1983; Dollaghan & Miller, 1986; Farrier et al., 1985; Gallagher, 1983; Holland, 1982; Kraat, 1985a; Light, Collier, & Parnes, 1985b; Light et al., 1986; Miller, 1981). Several of these are discussed further in chapters 4 and 7. The speech-language pathologist must decide which sampling approach to use and what interactions and contexts to examine. Dollaghan and Miller (1986) suggest that the contexts and sampling procedures used should be selected on the basis of the questions being asked and the purposes for which the information is being collected. Toward that end, it is helpful for clinicians to consider the following questions:

*1. What is the main purpose of the observation?* The augmentative communication team must decide whether they are interested in obtaining an overall impression of the person's communicative interaction or more in-depth information about specific interaction behaviors (e.g., with a familiar or unfamiliar partner, particular language or discourse behavior, or behaviors that occur in a specific environment). Each purpose suggests different contexts and procedures for an observation. Global assessments, which are generally required as part of an initial assessment and, subsequently, during periodic reevaluations, necessitate observation of a variety of interactions (across partners, environments, situations), either in the natural environment or in multiple contrived or naturalistic contexts in the clinic (Bloom & Lahey, 1978; Gallagher, 1983; Miller, 1981).

At times, the speech-language pathologist may wish to investigate a narrower, or more specific aspect of interaction behavior. This assessment might examine an area of communication or interaction that is important or problematic to establish specific intervention needs or goals. Or, a narrower assessment might be conducted to provide baseline information prior to the implementation of a treatment program or to evaluate the success of that intervention. In-depth observations might be made to explore the interaction that takes place between the speech/language-impaired individual and a partner (e.g., wife, teacher, aide, unfamiliar person) or in a specific environment (e.g., work site, at the bus stop, during morning care). Or, the focus might be on investigating one or more language or communicative behaviors (e.g., initiating conversation, communication breakdowns and their repair, requesting information). The situations selected for these observations should be directly related to the communication behaviors, dyad(s), or environments under investigation or those that will be addressed in training. Behaviors of interest may be assessed in natural environments, or during structured or unstructured tasks in the clinic, depending on the communication behaviors of interest.

2. *What communication and language behaviors should be observed?* In setting up observations, speech-language pathologists should first define the communication behaviors that they are most interested in observing or knowing about. The context(s) selected for observation are dictated by the linguistic and pragmatic behaviors that are of interest. For example, if a speech-language pathologist is interested in how an individual's initiations are being responded to, the context selected for sampling would need to evoke a high frequency of initiations under a variety of environmental conditions. Initiation behaviors could occur during open-ended conversations; however, these behaviors are more likely to occur during mealtimes, free play and other recreational activities, or when others are busy and little attention is being paid to the individual. The communication situations that are most likely to elicit the behaviors of interest are selected for observation, or the clinician may choose to set up contrived situations in an effort to increase the occurrence of those behaviors (e.g., the clinician might place interesting toys out of reach, have necessary items for an activity unavailable, or violate a familiar routine [Constable, 1983]). Some of the communication behaviors of special interest in interactions involving a person using augmentative techniques are discussed later.

3. *What level of performance is of interest--The client's typical performance, the client's best performance, or both?* In observing interaction behavior, the team is generally most interested in "typical" behaviors (i.e., what usually occurs in the individual's daily life), even though these behaviors do not necessarily reflect what

that person or dyad is capable of doing with maximum effort under optimal conditions or their knowledge of linguistic and pragmatic rules. Observations of "typical" behaviors reflect an individual's average performance. This performance level may be examined by observing situations that are reported by others to be typical (Gallagher, 1983; Light et al., 1986), or by examining a broad range of communicative situations in natural environments.

In setting intervention goals, both typical and optimal performance levels are of interest. Optimal levels of performance (i.e., what the client or dyad is capable of under ideal conditions) are important to the speech-language pathologist, as they may reveal emerging language skills or behaviors that a person is capable of but not typically using. Intervention then may be directed toward increasing the frequency of behaviors observed at the optimal level. Sampling techniques to observe optimal performance include: (a) using elicitation scripts designed to examine performance under ideal conditions (Cassatt-James, chapter 6; Light et al., 1986), (b) observing interactions reported to be optimal (Gallagher, 1983), or (c) probing particular communication skills during interactions with the client.

4. *What contexts (partners, environments, activities), sampling techniques, and sample lengths best provide the desired information?* Clinicians need to plan observations carefully. The contexts typically used (e.g., an "open conversation" in the clinic, or a parent and child interacting during free play with a group of toys) may or may not be appropriate observational contexts within which to collect a communication sample. By more clearly defining the communication behaviors of interest, the overall purpose of the observation, and the levels of performance desired, the particular contexts and sampling procedures to be used are more clearly defined. The observational plan should specify: (a) how many and which partners will be observed, (b) where those observations should be made, (c) the activities that are most likely to elicit the desired behaviors, (d) how long the observation should be in order to obtain a representative sample, and (e) what data collection methods (i.e., transcription and analysis, a checklist) are required.

Speech-language pathologists may find one of the published research or clinical protocols appropriate to the questions they are asking, or may wish to develop their own sampling protocol for a specific client. Currently, there are several published clinical protocols that might be used in making global assessments of interaction. Some of these have been developed for sampling interaction in natural speakers, while others are specific to augmentative communication. Gallagher (1983) outlines a sampling protocol for clinical use with children who have speech and language disorders. A preassessment interview is used to select two sampling contexts (i.e., an optimal and a typical performance) based on a child's pattern of language use and variability. The protocol specifies the communication partners, time of day, physical location, and objects and activities involved. A third sampling context (one of the two selected) uses the clinician as a conversational partner to probe particular behaviors of interest in more depth.

Published clinical protocols developed specifically for interactions involving a person using augmentative components include those of Bolton and Dashiell (1984), Calculator and Luchko (1983), and Holland (1982).   These protocols are all directed toward making global communication assessments in the natural environment.  Bolton and Dashiell recommend that at least three partners and situations be observed, and that the partners include persons who are familiar-trained, familiar-untrained, unfamiliar-trained, and unfamiliar-untrained.   Calculator and Luchko, in their interaction study of an adult within a nursing home, selected an environment and time of day, rather than specific partners, to obtain a representative sample of interaction. A segment of each morning, during which most interactions reportedly occurred, was repeatedly observed across days.  Holland, in examining the communication behavior of aphasic adults in their home environments, used a time segment of two hours for observations.

To examine discrete aspects of communication interaction involving augmentative components, the reader is referred to protocols outlined in  Farrier et al. (1985), the unpublished research reported in Kraat (1985a), and Light et al. (1986). The protocol of Light et al. may be helpful to those interested in examining one dyad in more depth.  This sampling procedure focuses on eliciting typical and optimal performance in a specific dyad (i.e., a caregiver and person using augmentative communication techniques) during interactions involving both basic needs and social interactions.

Language sampling protocols often suggest that 100 utterances, or a 30-minute time frame, constitute a sample length (Bloom & Lahey, 1978; Miller, 1981).  Further research is needed, however, to determine the sample length that is required to obtain an adequate and representative sample of discourse or interaction behaviors for both speaking clients and augmentative dyads.  As interactions within these dyads are often slower and/or require multiple turns to achieve a communication message, it is probable that the sample length for those dyads may need to be longer.  It is important that the sample length be long enough to provide sufficient and representative data to answer the clinical questions being asked.

Issues of reliability and validity need to be considered, as well.  When possible, observations should be made across days or sessions to insure that behaviors observed are, in fact, typical of a dyad, the person using augmentative components, and the context.   Clinicians also must be concerned about validity issues; that is, how representative is the sample of the interaction behaviors in comparison to what actually occurs daily.  Some of these concerns can be reduced by sampling a sufficient number of behaviors, including multiple contexts or partners, and by carefully selecting the activities or contexts observed. Hopefully, additional research efforts will assist us in identifying the contexts that provide a representative range of behaviors and in delineating those in-clinic tasks that reflect this range in a reliable and valid manner (see chapters 7 & 9 for further discussion).

## *Communication Behaviors of Particular Interest*

Augmentative and spoken interactions share many general discourse characteristics and mutual rules involving the social use of language. For example, whether a person is using spoken language, signs, a language board, a coded alphabet chart, or a combination of these, participants will take turns at "speaking"; topics will be introduced and elaborated; various types of speech acts or communicative functions will occur as initiations and responses; and so on. Obviously, these general aspects of interaction are important to observe in augmentative users, as well. The reader is referred to Bedrosian (1985); Blank and Franklin (1980); Blank, Gessner, and Esposito (1979); Coggins and Carpenter (1981); Davis and Wilcox (1985); Miller, (1981); Prutting and Kirchner (1983); Van Kleek and Carpenter (1980); Wiig (1982); and Wollner and Geller (1982) for a review of some of the communicative behaviors currently evaluated in clinical protocols with speaking clients.

Although normative communication behaviors are an important starting point, some conversational characteristics are more critical, problematic, or unique to the investigation of augmentative interaction, and it is these behaviors that warrant special investigation by speech-language pathologists. Table 5-1 lists the communication behaviors that are of special interest, including some communication behaviors examined in standard protocols, conventional behaviors not routinely examined but of importance, and behaviors that are unique to augmentative interactions. This composite list is based on research findings, observations of clinicians, and behaviors felt to be important by persons developing clinical evaluation protocols (Bolton & Dashiell, 1984; Eddins & McDowell-Fleming, 1984; Light, McNaughton, & Parnes, 1986).

The communication behaviors listed were selected because they are either particularly problematic in augmentative interactions or appear to take on greater significance in this type of communication exchange. For example, the ability to gain attention to communicate is frequently included in general observations of language use, but appears to take on greater importance in augmentative interactions. Unimpaired speakers gain attention as an utterance is spoken ("Hey, got a minute?"; "I don't want to"). When a problem exists, the speaker does something to get a partner's attention (e.g., goes over to the partner, taps the partner on the shoulder). Physically disabled persons who use visually based symbols (e.g., signs, language board displays) have a more difficult time obtaining a partner's attention in order to deliver a message (Calculator & Dollaghan, 1982; Light, 1984).  For these individuals, attention-getting and message transmission is not an integrated process.  Consequently, this communication function (attention-getting) is of concern to the augmentative communication team.

Table 5-1 also outlines communicative behaviors that, while not routinely examined in the clinical practices of most speech-language pathologists, are of particular importance in augmentative communication.  For example, several of these behaviors are related to the communication opportunities that are provided to, used, or created by persons using augmentative communication components and the overall communicative balance that is achieved during interactions.  Finally, Table 5-1 lists behaviors that are unique to augmentative exchanges.  These "unique" behaviors may include, among others, the nontraditional roles assumed by communication partners, accommodation to proxemic differences, a partner's ability to "read" idiosyncratic communication behaviors, or the unique adaptive strategies used by both partners during these exchanges.

Obviously, the behaviors that are of interest will depend on the developmental/cognitive levels of both partners, the purpose of the observation, and the augmentative components being used.  The behaviors observed will also be affected by the nature of any language or cognitive disorders that are present (e.g., memory abilities are of particular interest in postcoma clients).  Regardless of the differences among clients, speech-language pathologists need to observe the behaviors of both partners in the interaction and must consider all components of an individual's communication system, including speech.

## *Transcribing and Coding Behaviors*

Observations can be made quite informally, or may involve a summary checklist of behaviors observed and not observed (Bolton & Dashiell, 1982; Light et al., 1986).  In some instances, a more in-depth analysis is appropriate.  This generally involves transcribing the behaviors that occur and/or synthesizing that information into some meaningful taxonomy or coding schema for analysis.  Some practical suggestions for that process are outlined below, as well as some of the problems that might be encountered (see also chapter 9).

*Transcriptions*.  Speech-language pathologists who are used to transcribing samples of natural speakers are often confronted with new behaviors when transcribing augmentative interactions.  For example, in spoken language, utterance boundaries are typically defined by intonation contours, pauses, grammatical

## TABLE 5-1. COMMUNICATION BEHAVIORS OF PARTICULAR INTEREST

**BEHAVIORS EXAMINED IN STANDARD PROTOCOLS**

- Ability to gain attention to communicate
- Ability to open a conversation/begin an interaction
- Initiation & response roles of all partners
- Communication breakdowns (nature, signaling, repair)
- Topic: Frequency of topic initiations; variety; maintenance of topic (both partners)
- Communicative acts or functions: Variety of functions & forms to express a function; complexity

**BEHAVIORS NOT ROUTINELY EXAMINED IN STANDARD PROTOCOLS, OF IMPORTANCE**

- General communication opportunities (number, characteristics and variety of partners; frequency of new partners)
- Frequency of interactions, partner initiating
- Opportunities within conversations

    - turn opportunities available to client (obligatory; optional)
    - adequate time available for client to take turn/respond
    - % of turn opportunities taken by client
    - # of utterances exchanged
    - % of client initiation efforts responded to
    - % of times client is interrupted and consequences of these interruptions
    - % of times client obligates a response from partner

- Level of interaction

    - partner speaks at appropriate cognitive level
    - % of rhetorical questions asked by partner
    - % of client turns filling minimal requirements only
    - % of topics self-oriented/other-related

- Feedback from the client during partner's speaking turn
- Ability to adapt to fluctuations in partners and contexts
- Overall interaction pattern

**BEHAVIORS UNIQUE TO AUGMENTATIVE INTERACTIONS**

- Partner's participation in augmentative techniques (e.g., ability to participate in scanning or decoding; note selections, etc.)
- Partner's participation in actualizing intended utterance of nonspellers
- Partner's use of efficiency strategies (e.g., guessing, completing)
- Partner's participation in the resolution of nonspeller's communication breakdowns
- Participation rules clear to partners
- Intelligibility of client's available modes of expression (e.g., nonverbal; signs and symbols; pointing responses; synthetic speech)
- Adaptation to mobility restrictions (e.g., getting partner to come; communicating at a distance)
- Accessibility of aided techniques - across environments and situations
- Adaptive strategies used by the client (e.g., to convey meaning, achieve various discourse functions; repair breakdowns; adapt to partner and context; maintain participation)
- Adaptive strategies used by partners (e.g., to actualize or clarify meaning; provide opportunities for interaction; increase the rate or efficiency of communication; handle breakdowns)

completeness, or segments that function as a communicative unit. In using augmentative components, intonation contours are not present, pauses may be related to the rates of communication possible rather than utterance segmentation, and communication behaviors and turns may not reflect grammatical completeness. In transcribing samples from persons using augmentative techniques, it has been suggested that utterance boundaries be segmented by definitions of a communicative unit (Marriner, Yorkston, & Farrier, 1984), a conversational act (Wexler, Blau, Leslie, & Dore, 1983), or a completed message (Fishman, Timler, & Yoder, 1985). For some individuals (e.g., persons using alphabet boards or those with a limited number of language forms available), an utterance boundary may extend over several speaking turns. These turns may contribute individual elements to the overall message and may involve partner confirmations, guesses and elaborations, and the resolution of message breakdowns. Examples of these multiple turn and multipartner utterances can be found in Fishman et al. (1985), Harris (1978, 1982), Kraat (1985a), Marriner et al. (1984), and Wexler et al. (1983). The research of Light et al. (1985a) has also brought to our attention the need to document the temporal aspects within the interactions that occur. In augmentative communication, short pause times are often viewed by partners as a "no response" or as a cue to take another turn. Of particular interest is whether or not sufficient time was provided for the augmentative partner to respond, and whether "within turn" pauses are misinterpreted as completed turns by others.

While most speech-language pathologists are unaccustomed to transcribing multiple nonverbal and vocal parameters beyond the prelinguistic or preoperational stages of language development, transcriptions need to include these behaviors, as they are important components in augmentative communication repertoires. In noting these behaviors, it is helpful if the person transcribing is familiar with the client. Without some shared knowledge of which movements, idiosyncratic behaviors, or vocalizations are intentional communication efforts, behaviors that are unrelated to a communication exchange can be mistakenly transcribed and analyzed. Table 5-2 lists some of the nonverbal/vocal behaviors that might be communicative and of interest.

*Coding*. Given a reliable transcription, analysis can proceed. Currently, several taxonomies are available in the research and clinical literature for analyzing communicative functions or intentions, discourse structure, and communicative breakdowns and repairs of natural speakers. Far fewer taxonomies exist that code other aspects of communicative interaction or those behaviors specific to augmentative communication. Coding schemas have generally been developed for a specific developmental level (e.g., a child's early use of language) and type of investigation (e.g., mother-child dyads). Dollaghan and Miller (1986) and Chapman (1981) caution clinicians and researchers against using an available coding schema without first investigating its appropriateness with regard to the persons and situation being

### TABLE 5-2. NONVERBAL AND VOCAL COMMUNICATION BEHAVIORS OF INTEREST

**NONVERBAL BEHAVIORS**

- Mutual eye gaze toward or away from speaker or object/action; ability to maintain eye gaze

- Facial expression - affective states (e.g. smile, displeasure, excitment, disinterest)

- Turning of head or body toward interest focus; away from what is not of interest

- Movement and tone of body and extremities; affective state signaled

- Pointing or designating focus of interest through eye-pointing, reaching toward, touching, giving object to partner, or actions (e.g., taking partner's hand to request something); rejecting by pushing, shoving, and throwing

- Gaining attention through tugging, touching

- Moves toward and away from partners

- General body posture and alignment

**VOCAL/AUDITORY SIGNALS**

- Auditory/vocal means of gaining attention (e.g., click, vocal noise, attention buzzer or bell)

- Differentiated vocalization (e.g., meaning conveyed by pitch, duration, prosodic patterns, loudness)

- Giggle or laughter

- Vocal means of providing feedback to listener (e.g., "uh," "m-m")

**NONVERBAL OR VOCAL SIGNALS POTENTIALLY INTERFERING WITH COMMUNICATION**

- Involuntary or reflexive movements

- Bizarre or atypical nonverbal behaviors

- Lack of or reduced facial expression

- Unintentional vocalizations or vocal characteristics

studied.  Clinicians need to thoughtfully evaluate the validity and adequacy of available taxonomies, use those that appear productive and appropriate for answering their assessment and intervention questions, and/or construct their own taxonomies.

Standard taxonomies and definitions often do not easily accommodate the unique behaviors observed in augmentative interactions.  Questions often arise with regard to coding "technical" turns, partner elaborations, and communicative intentions.  Transcriptions may contain multiple turns in which a partner repeats or confirms a language element (e.g,, a-a, n-n), assists with the technique itself (e.g., "Is it this row?"), or attempts to complete the message given some of the elements (e.g., plant - "You want me to water it?").  Marriner et al. (1985) suggests that persons coding and analyzing augmentative interactions separate the turns directed at actualizing the utterances (i.e., technical utterances) from those that are completed communicative units or messages (i.e., communicative utterances).  In doing so, the behaviors involved in actualizing a message (e.g., multiple confirmations and questions) are analyzed separately and do not weight the communication analysis in those directions.  Coding schemas are also needed to accommodate the fact that partners frequently interrupt the person using augmentative techniques and guess or expand on message elements.  Coding communication behaviors involves some subjective decision-making, particularly with regard to communicative intentions and functions.  These are not observable phenomena.  This coding becomes even more difficult during augmentative interactions, because nonverbal behaviors, single-word utterances, and partner-collaborated behaviors lend themselves to much ambiguity (Harris, 1978).  For example, arm pointing toward a record in a group of objects or indicating the single symbol "record" may be a request for music, a comment on a song, or even a request for some information about a new singing group.  The syntactic form and paralinguistic features often used to make inferences about communicative intentions may be absent.  Therefore, judgments are even more subjective.

### *Recognizing Atypical Behaviors in the Data*

Prior to making judgments about the communicative behaviors observed and coded, clinicians must be aware of atypical variables in those samples.  Some of these variables are reviewed briefly below.

1.  *Influence of available augmentative components on language performance.*  In samples of spoken language performance, the communication behaviors that are spoken by a child or adult are generally viewed as representative of that person's developmental level and knowledge about language and language use.  This is not necessarily the case in samples involving persons using augmentative techniques.  What occurs may not be representative of what that person knows and understands about language and communication; rather, it may reflect how that person is attempting to

communicate through language components that are limited and quite atypical. In making judgments about a child or adult using augmentation, this potential knowledge-use gap needs to be kept in mind.

    2. *Effect of augmentative components on pragmatic possibilites.* Each client has a specific repertoire of language units and augmentative aids and techniques through which to communicate. To evaluate the communication behaviors of a client or dyad, the speech-language pathologist must first be aware of: (a) the repertoire that is available to the client; and (b) the pragmatic possibilities that repertoire allows. This provides the clinician or researcher with an understanding of the communication options open to severely speech/language-impaired individuals and enables their performance to be observed more appropriately.

- Expressive Repertoire. To develop a composite picture of a person's communication repertoire, the clinician needs to list: (a) the vocabulary set available in any communication board or device (e.g., stored words, sentences); (b) the language units available in the signs and symbolic gestures acquired; (c) spoken language that can be understood; (d) alphabet and spelling capability; and (e) the vocal and nonverbal behaviors used by that individual to convey meaning. Table 5-2 outlined some of the nonverbal/vocal behaviors that may be communicative or that may interfere with communication. In outlining these nonverbal or vocal behaviors, the specific behaviors of the client that convey meaning to others should be specified, along with the meaning and the functions they appear to represent. This is not always an easy task, particularly with persons with severe physical disability. This is further complicated by possible fluctuations in vocal and physical abilities that result from changes in muscle tone or physical positioning. In outlining these behaviors, it is helpful to get input from all members of the team, make informal observations, and/or to use protocols developed for young children for this purpose (Carlson, 1981; Morris, 1981, 1982; Wilcox & Campbell, 1985).

    It is also important to note specific transmission characteristics associated with techniques and aids that could affect interactions. Of interest is the rate of communication, how communications can or cannot be made across distances, whether or not active participation is required from the partner (e.g., scan or encoded language chart), and the intelligibility of the augmentative components to the partners involved.

● <u>Pragmatic Possibilities</u>.  What individuals can do in a given communication situation is shaped by the expressive repertoire available to them.  Consider the following example.  Two children, Child A and Child B, want to participate in a group discussion about a fight that took place on the playground.  Both want to say that "John started it."  Child A, with his synthetic speech device and orthographic vocabulary display, says *John start fight*.  Child B, with his eye-coded chart, tries to get the teacher over to read his eye-pointing signals.  Unfortunately, the teacher does not hear his vocalizations because of the chatter in the classroom, and does not come over to him.  Even if he had, Child B does not have the necessary vocabulary to express his thoughts independently as the words *fight, John, first* are not on his vocabulary display.  To communicate his message, he needs to select an associated word (e.g., *boy, outside*) or depend on the teacher to ask the right "twenty questions."  The communication options and potentials available to these two boys are quite different.  When evaluating an interaction, it is important to take into account the capabilities inherent in the augmentative symbols, aids, or techniques that are specifically available to that client.  Of interest is what the interactants are accomplishing, given the potentials in a specific repertoire, and how effectively they are doing it.

The field has only begun to examine the pragmatic differences between various language arrays/lexicons and certain augmentative aids and techniques (Buzolich, 1984; Goossens' & Kraat, 1985; Kraat, 1985b).  Clinicians may find it useful to attempt to interact in a variety of situations using a client's repertoire, or to conceptualize how a person of comparable age and cognitive ability might be able to accomplish specific communicative acts, given a particular expressive repertoire.  These exercises should provide some insights into how repertoires differ, how specific characteristics affect the everyday communication interactions of a given individual, and what communicative options and strategies are open to a particular client.

3.  *Adaptive strategies used by clients and partners*.  A nonverbal gesture may be used to make a comment about some on-going action, rather than a specific linguistic form.  Or, an individual may take very short turns and use only single-word utterances as a result of elaborations and guessing on the part of an adept partner.  These behaviors are not necessarily regressive or deficient, but are different and adaptive.  Behaviors observed frequently reflect how individuals in the dyad adapt to unconventional modes of communication.  Although these adaptive strategies are

atypical, behaviors need to be judged with regard to their communicative efficiency and effectiveness, rather than against the conventionalities of spoken language use.

4. *Interrelationship of partner behaviors*. Research in pragmatics has given us an understanding of how partners influence each other, both within and across speaking turns (e.g., a predominance of responding behavior may be the by-product of frequent obligatory questions by a partner). In augmentative communication, the behaviors of partners have an even more pervasive and stronger influence on the communicative behaviors that are observed because of the imbalance between communicating through augmentative components and natural speech. This necessitates that the communication profiles of clients are examined with respect to their communicative styles and to the demands and behaviors of persons with whom they are interacting.

## *Interpreting the Sampling Data*

The speech-language pathologist must make some judgments about the strengths and weaknesses within the interactions observed and begin to form hypotheses about intervention directions and procedures. The following questions should assist the clinician in making clinically relevant decisions about the interactions observed.

1. *How well is each member of the dyad interacting, given the augmentative repertoire available?* In evaluating observational data, three questions need to be asked: (a) How effectively is the user of augmentative communication components interacting given the constraints and capabilities of the available repertoire, within or across dyads? (b) How effectively are partners communicating with the user of augmentative communication components, given the available augmentative repertoire? and (c) Would the interactions improve if changes were made in the available augmentative aids, techniques, or language content? The first two questions assess the quality of the interactions given a person's *present* system. The last question relates to assessment decisions regarding *changing* that augmentative repertoire in some manner (e.g., the symbol/sign form; type of device).

To evaluate communication performance in this functional manner requires that the clinician conceptualize an idealized or optimal interaction between unimpaired speakers and users of augmentative techniques (at a particular developmental level and with or without a language disorder). This includes the levels of communication and language performance that might be expected given specific augmentative components and contexts, and the adaptive strategies that might be considered facilitory and successful for both partners. Augmentative communication teams and researchers are beginning to discuss what these competencies might encompass and how they might vary across aids, techniques, strategies, contexts, and language levels (Davis & Wilcox, 1985; Farrier et al., 1985; Kraat, 1985a; see chapter 9 for further discussion).  However, until such models of augmentative competency are developed, speech-language pathologists must rely on their collective experiences with clients, available research, and their own sense of what might be functionally possible and appropriate.

Clinicians may be interested in how augmentative interactions compare to the language and communication profiles that are outlined for persons using spoken language at various developmental levels.  This type of analysis may be useful in identifying specific aspects of a communication disorder (e.g., linguistic deficits in aphasia), or to more fully understand the differences that are present in using a specific augmentative repertoire.  However, this comparison should not be used as the sole basis of making judgments about performance of intervention planning.

2. *What are the strengths and weaknesses observed in the interactions?*  To identify the strengths and weaknesses within interactions, the clinician needs to consider observed communication behaviors, as well as those that are desirable but do not occur.  Both are important.  Strengths and weaknesses should be identified across contexts for both persons using augmentative components and for communication partners.  Partner behaviors of interest may include their performance as interactants in an exchange, and/or as a language and communication teacher or facilitator. Clinicians may find the case study presented in Light et al. (1986) useful in understanding how the strengths and weaknesses may be profiled.  In judging behaviors, it is also critical to acknowledge the effectiveness and efficiency of an interaction sequence.  For example, one dyad may finally negotiate a proposition after an unproductive series of yes/no questions, poor cueing from the person using augmentative techniques, and multiple communication breakdowns.  Another dyad may accomplish the communication task, but may use a yes/no question strategy quite effectively, along with the productive choice of available symbols, to quickly accomplish that exchange.  Both are successful, but one is more efficient than the other.

Strengths may be seen in multiple aspects of the client's behaviors, including frequent attempts at social interaction, the ability to shift speaking styles with a familiar or unfamiliar partner, the choice of language symbols used to accommodate a given communication situation, the beginning emergence of particular semantic relations or communicative functions, or the persistence displayed in gaining attention or pursuing a communication effort to its end.  A partner may display strengths in expecting participation from the client at the levels they are capable of, picking up on the client's leads, elaborating and guessing when provided with minimal cues, or providing models and feedback to the client.

Weaknesses can be observed in the unsuccessful or inefficient interaction sequences that occur. Problems areas can also be identified by outlining the communication levels and participation that are expected of individuals using a particular aid or technique but that do not occur. Weaknesses might include an adult's use of lengthy styles in situations where efficiency is needed; an overabundance of communication topics related to "self" in attempted social interactions; the lack of basic communicative functions, such as social greetings or requests for information; partners not expecting the client to participate in the conversation or not creating communication opportunities; inefficient guessing patterns of partners; or the need for partners to set up the aid for the client before linguistic communication can occur. The weaknesses that are determined to be most detrimental and critical to communicative interaction should be given priority in setting intervention goals.

3. *What are the causes of communication problems and weaknesses?* Communication difficulties can stem from many sources. Problems may be rooted in (a) a lack of novel experiences to talk about (Harris & Vanderheiden, 1980); (b) the extent of the language content available to the user; (c) the characteristics of the components themselves (e.g., language display size and layout, use of unconventional nonverbal signals, signs, and symbols); (d) the adaptive strategies employed by the user; (e) the adaptive strategies used by the communication partner; and (f) the cognitive, social, and language abilities of the clients or partners.

Consider the following examples. A client may experience communicative breakdowns because letter-by-letter spelling is not segmented into words (e.g., *ienjoyyourcompany*). This breakdown may occur because (a) a space indicator is not available for the client to use, or (b) the client is not using the available space indicator. The intervention objectives in these two instances are quite different. In the first case, a language item indicating *space* needs to be added to the vocabulary display; in the second, training strategies need to be directed toward appropriate use of this marker. In another example, a child may point to the symbol for *swing*, running his hand over the symbol slowly in contrast to his usual indication manner. He is attempting to make a comment about his favorite swing. His mother misinterprets the effort as a request to go to the swing, and replies "no." When the child again points to the symbol in an effort to repair the misunderstanding, his repeated efforts are seen as nudging and the child is scolded. In this example, several problems contribute to the misunderstanding: (a) the mother is not interpreting the child's communication behaviors and intentions appropriately; (b) vocabulary is not available for the child to express his intention in a clearer form (e.g., the words *love, like, fun*); (c) the child does not attempt to use available symbols to signal that a breakdown has occurred (e.g., *no* or *help*); and (d) the child has not been taught beginning strategies for signaling a breakdown. Multiple areas of training need to be targeted, including parent training, symbol additions, development of an understanding of signaling breakdowns, and training in when to use these new skills.

## SETTING INTERVENTION GOALS

### *Intervention Areas*

Table 5-3 outlines the general areas that frequently need intervention attention and planning for both the client and the communication partner.  Intervention may include training in augmentative components, speech and language acquisition or reacquisition, development of communicative interaction, and the development of skills for future and more advanced augmentative intervention.  Many areas outlined are unique to the clinical management of individuals using communication augmentation.  Others areas are also germane to the treatment of children and adults who are not using augmentative techniques.

Speech treatment is an integral part of the global intervention plan.  Placing an individual on an augmentative program does not mean that speech intervention is discontinued.  Long-term speech intervention, in conjunction with an augmentative program, is frequently quite appropriate.  Many individuals gain, or regain, sufficient speech or vocal abilities to produce some intelligible messages, and some go on to use spoken language as their primary means of communication.  Even limited vocal/speech abilities can provide meaningful ways of gaining attention, providing feedback to communication partners (e.g., giggle, "yeah"), indicating yes/no responses, or expressing specific meanings (e.g., excitement, distress).

For many clients, language acquisition or reacquisition is also an important focus of intervention planning (e.g., adults with aphasia or head injury; children with developmental disabilities or disorders).  In addition to speech and language needs, augmentative communication in itself requires extensive intervention.  All clients and partners need assistance in acquiring augmentative strategies to effectively communicate in everyday situations.  A communication aid may need to be constructed or purchased; symbols selected and acquired; clients instructed in coding or scanning techniques; partners trained in signs or other techniques and strategies.  Diagnostic questions may need to be answered (e.g., defining the communication needs in a work site; developing the nonverbal communication behaviors of an infant).  Individuals with developmental disabilities may also require additional experiences, attention to social development, or special training toward the development of independence (Warwick, 1986).  Given the severity of the disorders involved, the list of intervention needs within any one area may be extensive.  Goals should be prioritized, and those that appear to be most productive and urgent in each of the areas, should be outlined.

# TABLE 5-3. INTERVENTION PLANNING IN AUGMENTATIVE COMMUNICATION

## PERSONS IN THE ENVIRONMENT

Understanding of the physical operation, maintenance, and set-up of aided system components

Acquisition of the meaning of signs and symbols; nonverbal behaviors, vocalization/speech; how to participate in aided techniques; how to receive communication through these system components

Development of language and communication skills in persons using augmentation

- Providing social, cognitive, and language experiences
- Facilitating language and speech acquisition
- Providing models and experiences in use of augmentative components

Development of communicative interaction skills in communicating with persons using augmentation

- How to talk to persons using augmentation
- Strategies for expanding and elaborating incomplete utterances of nonspellers
- Awareness of conversational patterns that either facilitate or inhibit interaction
- Adaptive strategies to increase speed (prediction and verification)
- Strategies for handling and repairing communication breakdowns
- Development of general adaptive strategies for interacting with persons using augmentation

## PERSON USING AUGMENTATIVE COMMUNICATION

Individualizing communication system:

- Modes to be used
- Language content
- Construction/acquisition of aided boards and devices

Acquisition of nonspeech forms and techniques

Development of vocal/speech abilities

Development of language knowledge/reacquisition

- Language comprehension
- Language expression (content, form, use)
- Cognitive development
- General world experiences

Development of communicative interaction/use

- Development of general interaction/skills
- Social development/experiences
- Acquisition of adaptive strategies to accomplish various language and pragmatic tasks across partners and contexts
- Strategies to optimize speed and efficiency
- Attention to interfering nonverbal behaviors

Training abilities and skills for future augmentative systems (e.g., modes, techniques, language representation)

(Adapted from Kraat, 1982)

*Developing Intervention Goals*

The development of intervention goals is a continuous and on-going procedure throughout the clinical management process. It evolves out of formal evaluations or reevaluations, responses and behavioral changes in treatment, changes in speech and language abilities, or observations of daily interaction. Intervention goals are unique to a client, and are related to that person's language abilities, interaction patterns, learning abilities, environments, and the characteristics of the augmentative components being used.

Speech-language pathologists draw upon general language and intervention models in developing intervention goals. These include an understanding of the nature of language and communication, perspectives on language development, and assumptions about the underlying causes and remediation of various communication disorders. To this framework is added an understanding of the nature of augmentative communication, its multiple components, and the persons using them. These resources are collectively brought together in defining the specific intervention goals for each client and the client's partners.

The process of defining intervention goals is not an easy one, even given these resources. The jump from observations or assessment data to treatment goals is not always an obvious one, nor are the goals that need to be set following the completion of a goal always discernible. The process is further complicated by the multiple and extensive needs of the clients involved. Some guidelines for this difficult decision-making process are outlined below.

1. *Remember the purposes of intervention*. As one begins to formulate intervention plans, it is important to focus on the general purposes of intervention; that is, to facilitate a person's optimal communication functioning in everyday environments. The key words here are *communication, optimal,* and *everyday environments*. *Communication* does not imply how messages should be conveyed, but rather that they are effectively conveyed between two or more people. *Optimal* is a relative term suggesting that the maximal or best communication possible has occurred given the constraints inherent in augmentative components, the cognitive and developmental levels of the partners, and the physical and communicative contexts involved. The term *everyday environments* stresses that it is the performance in everyday situations (with multiple partners and communication contexts) that ultimately matters, not the ability to perform in a clinical situation or the mere possession of language knowledge. Remembering the purposes of intervention assists the clinician in integrating the multiple areas of need into an interconnecting structure with a functionally based direction. In this framework, intervention is not directed toward the acquisition of switch control, syntax, nonspeech forms, or vocabulary per se. These are not ends in themselves, but subgoals directed toward

achieving specific changes in communication levels or opportunities for the client in everyday environments. Thus, targeted goals that require a client to use a communication aid 80 percent of the time, to identify and produce five signs on command, or to label toys or colors would be incomplete and inappropriate. In the first example, intervention is directed toward increasing use of a device without attention to how, when, or why it is to be used, or for what interaction and communication purpose. In the other examples, vocabulary is being acquired with little concern for how it will be used in daily interactions. More functionally based goals would include use of the aid to accomplish an appropriate communication task and would target the use of referents in meaningful interactions (e.g., using signs to request a favorite snack from Mom; or using color attributes as a vocabulary expansion technique - "red toy").

2. *Select goals that have functional impact.* Given the enormity of the intervention needs in augmentative communication, clinicians should direct their attention toward those areas and behaviors that are likely to have the greatest functional impact on the individual's interaction experiences in everyday environments, or that modify the most urgent and critical problems. In this useage, functional impact refers to communication behavior that can noticeably change the daily communication and interactions of a client. Changes may be observed in: (a) increased communication clarity (e.g., intelligibility); (b) increased levels of communication or discourse that a client can successfully participate in; (c) expanded communication opportunities (e.g., new partners, contexts); or (d) increased effectiveness or efficiency during conversational exchanges. Functional goals might also include providing basic skills that are the underpinnings of future communication or interaction behaviors (e.g., developing prelinguistic communication behaviors prior to introducing symbolic communication (Goossens' & Crain, 1986). In formulating possible intervention goals, it is helpful for clincians to ask: (a) What changes in communication or language use will have the greatest impact on the everyday interactions of this client? (b) What targeted behaviors will actually change the communication level, intelligibility, interaction patterns, or opportunities for the client? and (c) Which communication needs are the most critical or urgent? For example, although it might be developmentally appropriate for a child to label clothing items (e.g., diapers, bib, shoe), language concepts and functions associated with *more, get down,* and *no* obviously will have a greater impact on daily interaction and might be addressed first. Likewise, expanded forms such as *when + swing, go + swing,* will likely have more functional impact than a more syntactically complete unit such as *the swing.* In some cases persons may be more significantly affected by goals that target increased eye contact, a yes/no response, eye-pointing to referents in the environment, or silences on the part of the caregiver.

3. *Identify communication goals before selecting vocabulary.* Clinicians frequently begin to plan an intervention by asking what vocabulary items should be selected.

Faced with a nonspeaker and a blank symbol board, or a person with two formal signs, this is understandable. However, this is not necessarily the first question that should be asked, nor the most productive. Vocabulary selection should follow the development and selection of client goals which, in turn, influence the language units that are chosen. For example, a general goal for a nonspeaking child mainstreamed into a regular first-grade classroom is to increase social interaction with his peers. This child is observed showing a nonverbal interest in interacting and competing with a peer who is seated nearby. Thus, this interest is capitalized on and a specific subgoal is set (i.e., initiation of challenging comments, such as "I'm going to get done first!"). The language unit evolves out of the goal set. In another example, an adult is observed having difficulties because his attendant frequently (and incorrectly) expands on a single word and does not ask for confirmation of those elaborations. The need to signal a breakdown and to repair it leads to the addition of language units (i.e., "That's not it, back up"). Again, this vocabulary selection evolved out of the communication goals established.

4. *Attempt to balance intervention needs in language development/reacquisition, communicative interaction, and skill development utilizing augmentative aids and techniques.* Often, intervention tends to focus on one area at the expense of others. An exclusive emphasis may be placed on: (a) developing language concepts and forms, with limited consideration given to on-going communicative interaction skills; (b) focusing on daily interaction, with little attention given to needed developments in language concepts and elements; or (c) emphasizing the acquisition of nonspeech signs, symbols, or device operations, with minimal attention given to either the communicative interactions that occur with those techniques or to on-going language development. All of these areas need attention during the course of augmentative interventions.

Clinicians need to develop unique approaches with children who use communicaiton aids to accommodate both language development and communicative interaction goals. If a child is using a restricted language set, those language elements must be carefully selected to provide the maximum degree of communication interaction possible. This size limit means that not all of the vocabulary and language understood by that child or being trained can necessarily be represented on the display. For persons using communication aids, the restriction may necessitate the use of multiple communication boards (e.g., a main interaction board, language/learning boards and activity-specific boards), the acquisition of language comprehension abilities that cannot be used productiveloy, and/or the use of a temporary segment of the language board for new but changing items. this situation does not occur with persons learning apoken language. With these individuals, language that is acquired is always available and can be used and practiced in any situation.

5. *Consider the client's motivations and interests in communicating*. Communication is a personal experience; that is, we communicate about what we are interested in and for reasons that we view as important. We are also generally more interested in communicating with some persons than we are with others. Clinicians should select language and communication goals that take into account what the client is interested in communicating about, with whom, and for what purpose. These motivations may become apparent through observations and interactions with the client, reports from persons who know the client, or by talking to an older child or adult. In discussions, the team may find that the client is more interested in acquiring skills related to participation in "social raps" than acquiring more complex syntactic or information-seeking skills in a classroom. A young child may be much more interested in seeking information about "What are we doing today?" or "Can I do it?" than asking *who* questions. Training goals and the selection of augmentative components need to reflect the user's motivations and interests in communication, as well as to expand their interests and communication opportunities.

6. *Incorporate both immediate and future needs into planning*. Intervention plans should address immediate needs as well as the development of skills necessary to fulfill future needs. As discussed in chapter 4, short-term goals are necessary to meet communication demands that are often immediate and critical. Long-term planning is needed in order to develop a cohesive direction for intervention and to identify preliminary skills that should be incorporated into current intervention programs. If intervention only addresses the present needs of an individual, future communication, social, language, and speech growth may be restricted or may occur more slowly. For example, if an individual who resides in a long-term care facility is taught only formal signs, then transfer to a group home in the community may be difficult because his communication repertoire will not be understood by those in the new home. Likewise, intervention goals directed only at the future may neglect current communication needs. If an augmentative team directs all of its attention toward the development of motor skills for the operation of a dial scanner, or the acquisition of six formal signs over a prolonged period of time, attention may not be given to helping this individual communicate and interact in the present.

## Reviewing Intervention Goals for Appropriateness and Scope

Once potential goals have been identified, they should be reviewed with regard to the following questions:

1. *Has developmental level been taken into account?* Conversational needs and capabilities differ along a developmental continuum, as do the form, content, and functions used. Clinicians may target behaviors that are beyond or below the developmental levels of their clients. Making developmentally appropriate judgments

is not an easy task because of the difficulties encountered when assessing clients with severe expressive communication disorders (see chapter 4).   These judgments are further complicated by the lack of information on developmental language stages for augmentative communication users.   Currently, clinicians need to use normative information on speaking children as a resource in determining the appropriateness of communication goals.

Clinicians should avoid selecting goals that an unimpaired speaker of a comparable developmental level would not yet be expected to accomplish, such as asking a speech-impaired child to use repair strategies or attention-getting devices that unimpaired children at a similar level are not capable of (Ervin-Tripp & Gordon, 1986); or asking an individual to spontaneously produce or respond to certain requests for information when he does not have the cognitive or pragmatic understanding to do so (Bloom & Lahey, 1978; Chapman, 1981; Schwabe, Olswang, & Kriegsmann, 1986). Similarly, intervention goals should not be directed at levels too low for an individual. For example, a child with a comprehension level of approximately 4 years of age without a formal sign or symbol system may not need to begin productive language training at the single word stage of normative development.

2. *Has chronological age and experience been taken into consideration*? Although developmental abilities dictate the general language and communication behaviors that are selected as intervention goals, the specific content and topics addressed in the intervention with older clients may be quite different from that of young language learners.   Differences in age, experience, and environments require adaptations to intervention planning.

3. *Have cognitive or language disorders been taken into account*? In providing an individual with a means of daily communication, underlying disorders must also be considered.   Clients often have language and cognitive disorders that will have an impact on their abilities to communicate using augmentative aids and techniques and that can change the focus of an intervention (e.g., creating the need to give more attention to the appropriate use of those forms in a child with autism) or the language and communication goals targeted.   Cognitive disorders might necessitate a reduced number of goals, changed expectancies, and/or smaller, more routinized subgoals. Clinicians must also appropriately shift intervention strategies when working with a client who has normal cognitive and language abilities.   For these individuals, several goals can be targeted at the same time, and the objectives necessary to achieve each goal may not need to be broken down into small, discrete steps.

4. *Have the differences associated with the use of augmentative communication aids and techniques been taken into consideration?*  In reviewing intervention goals, clinicians need to ask if they have targeted communication behaviors that are functionally appropriate for users of augmentative aids and techniques.   Have multiple modes of

communication been included in that plan? Have adaptive strategies that optimize the use of these expressive modes been considered? Have unique communication needs been taken into account (e.g., use of a limited language display space; need for vocabulary expansion strategies; use of special language items, such as *word is not on the board*; the need for partner participation)? Have the needs and communication behaviors of partners been addressed?

5. *Have the varied social contexts and environments of the client been taken into consideration*? Clinicians need to examine the pragmatic problems that confront the person using augmentative communication across multiple partners, different environments, and communication situations, and must address these problems in the intervention plan. The communication needs of a person in an intensive care unit may be quite different during interactions with medical personnel than with family members. The conversational content and communication rules that must be acquired in a classroom or vocational setting can be quite different from those needed at home or in social conversations with close friends. Partners, too, differ in their actions and reactions to an atypical communication mode and in their ability to guess or elaborate on communication efforts made. For the client to achieve higher levels of communication and interaction in daily environments, these differences need to be recognized and incorporated into the overall plan.

## THE INTERVENTION PROCESS

The intervention goals developed for a client or partner are often of a general nature. These goals need to be transformed into more specific intervention plans that specify training parameters, levels of performance, and procedures. In so doing, specific skills may be broken down into a series of subgoals or session objectives aimed at achieving that general goal.

There are several atypical aspects involved in further specifying discrete intervention goals. These may involve decisions about the form and content that might be used; how those language elements and notions should be represented in sign, gesture, or symbol; how signs or symbol associations are to be taught; what mode(s) of communication are best suited to a specific goal (e.g., nonverbal behaviors, vocalization, gesture, symbols); and how the necessary augmentative aids and techniques might be acquired. For clients with physical impairments, the intervention process is further complicated by the need to find appropriate contexts in which those skills can be taught and practiced. The typical play or conversational contexts used with speaking clients may be physically impossible or inappropriate for these clients.

Augmentative skills and adaptive communication strategies also need to be used, modeled, and responded to in everyday environments.  This requires special attention to creating opportunities to use these new skills in the environment and to intervention with multiple partners in that environment.

Four case examples are presented in this section to illustrate the process of further defining intervention goals when augmentative components are involved. Some of the concepts and parameters incorporated into those plans are discussed in the next sections as an introduction.

## Contextual Parameters

The ultimate goal of intervention is to increase a person's ability to communicate and interact in everyday environments.  Consequently, the contexts used for training should reflect situations that do or could occur in natural environments and incorporate the client's motivations for using a particular communication behavior.  The contexts selected may be everyday situations (e.g., a classroom; snack time at home) or contrived situations within a clinical setting.  Clients who are more cognitively able may have intervention plans that involve multiple partners and situations.  Those with more limited skills may initially be trained in one specific situation and environment, with new situations and uses gradually introduced.

In setting up contexts for training and practice, clinicians need to decide whether they are interested in the client's use of a particular behavior as a response, as a self-initiation, or both, as the prior events used to elicit these behaviors are quite different.  If the client is to use the behavior as a response, the behavior would be elicited by a direct question; if the behavior is to be used as an initiation, an eliciting event would be used.  Although both initiating and responding behaviors are ultimately of interest, initiation is frequently targeted during training, as this speaker role is particularly problematic to persons using augmentative components.  Eliciting events might include an internal need or state (e.g., wanting attention; hunger; boredom); an on-going activity or object of interest (e.g., a caregiver stops bouncing a child up and down; something new or interesting appears); the absence of an object or routine; or a prior utterance that does not obligate a response, but provokes a communication (e.g., "Let's put it away"; "The Mets are going to win tonight").

When targeting responsive behaviors, care must be taken to use eliciting questions that are functionally appropriate to the situation that the client is capable of comprehending, and that represent the types of questions that might occur in everyday communication.  While questions such as, "If you want the space ship to take off, what do you say?," or "What's this?" may elicit the language response desired, these questions rarely occur outside of a "teaching" situation. Questions such as, "What should we do?" or "What would you like?" may be more representative of real communication situations and use.

## Communication Parameters

The use of language encompasses multiple meanings, forms, and communicative functions. For example, the language symbol *open* may represent the notion of opening boxes, drawers, zippered bags, jars, windows, doors, and so on, with each experience being slightly different from the others (Goossens', 1983). The language unit *get*, in different combinations and situations, may refer to the act of physically obtaining an object in the environment, removing something ("get out"), getting to a place ("get home"), acquiring an illness ("get a cold"), or not understanding something ("I don't get it"). An utterance such as "I'm cold" may accomplish a variety of speech acts or communicative functions (e.g., to make a comment, give information answering a question, get someone to do something, to evoke empathy, to get out of going somewhere, and so on). Intervention planning for persons learning language and language use should specify the particular meaning(s) being developed or trained, the function(s) the language unit is to serve, and the modes and forms that are to represent the meaning(s) and function(s) involved. In so doing, the expectancies for use of language items are clarified, and untaught language behaviors needing future intervention are more clearly defined.

## Integrating Multiple Subgoals

Language and communication training may focus on acquiring a semantic notion, associating a symbol with a language concept, acquiring specific syntactic forms, developing the ability to use a specific technique or device, or learning how to use these skills during interactions with others. By focusing on how these skills will eventually be used in daily communication, these multiple areas of training can be integrated, rather than taught one at a time. For example, if one eventually would like a client to use *go + fast* to ask others to make play objects go fast or to get others to do things fast (e.g., pushing a wheelchair), this future goal can be made a part of early intervention. Initial training of the fast concept can include modeling of the forms (e.g., symbols, signs) and techniques that will be used (e.g., pointing to a language board). Although the child may not currently be expected to use those forms/techniques, the association is taught incidentally. The training contexts for teaching the concept of "fast" can also include situations where the child will later be expected to request that action. For example, for a child in a wheelchair, the symbol *fast* might be pointed to and the word spoken, followed by his being pushed fast to another partner, another modeling, and another consequence. Although the focus is on acquiring a notion of fastness, the intervention plan has included: (a) a form and mode of expression for that notion; (b) a specific function (that of making a request for an action); (c) use of the symbol as an initiation (rather than a response to a specific question); and (d) modeling symbol use and consequences in a variety of everyday activities of interest.

## *Case Examples*

The intervention examples that follow focus on the development of a single goal for each of four clients and the specification of the communication and contextual parameters involved. Obviously, several treatment goals can be addressed at one time. A single goal is used here for illustrative purposes. Although the case illustrations highlight individuals with severe physical disabilities who are acquiring language and communication behaviors, many aspects of the decision-making process are applicable to other clients as well. A summary of the decisions made is outlined in Table 5-4.

Case A. Marisol, a 4-year-old child with severe spastic cerebral palsy, has no independent means of mobility. She has had no prior speech, language, or augmentative services. During assessment, she could vocalize for attention and reach or eye-point toward objects of interest. While interacting with her mother, a smile was interpreted as a *yes* response, and the absence of a smile a *no* response. Following assessment, several speech, language, and interaction goals were outlined involving Marisol, her mother, and older brother. One of those general goals was to develop a more reliable *yes* response. This goal was selected because responses to yes/no questions were presently her primary communication avenue and communication breakdowns were occurring as a result of the lack of a reliable *yes* response form. It was targeted before the development of *no* response because of its additional importance as a response mode for scanning techniques.

*Yes* was initially targeted as an affirmation response to a specific situation. Marisol frequently reached or eye pointed toward an object or action of interest that was out of her reach. When she did this, her partner went to the object and asked her if that was what she wanted. This was usually followed by a smile or continued reaching and fussing when she did not get the object. This use of *yes* was selected for intervention training because of its functional impact because Marisol demonstrated beginning understanding of this affirmation (i.e., by smiling), and because partners were able to determine when she was trying to say *yes* in this context.

## TABLE 5-4. SPECIFYING INTERVENTION GOALS – CASE EXAMPLES

| CLIENT | GENERAL GOAL | MODE/FORM | FUNCTION | I/R* | CONTEXTS | PRIOR EVENT/UTTERANCE | CLIENT BEHAVIOR INITIALLY REQUIRED | CONSEQUENCE |
|---|---|---|---|---|---|---|---|---|
| Case A (Marisol) | Develop a reliable 'yes' response | Traditional headshake | Affirmation | R | Home: Snack, Pajamas, Play items; Clinic:Play Items | M. points, reaches, or eye points toward object/action of interest. Partner goes to, asks, 'You want ____? (touching it) | Head nod with physical assistance | Involvement with action or object |
| Case B (Victor) | Request to be taken along | 'take me' (take-symbol) (me-gesture) | Request for action | I | Home: going to laundry, mall box, getting Dad, going to work in the kitchen; Clinic: going to water fountain, down hall, copy machine, outside | Partner talks about going and begins to leave; V. fusses | | Taken along |
| Case C (Michael) | Understand that eye-pointing is communicative | Looking at object or action | Request for action (defined by partner's responses) | I | Feeding: favorite and undesirable | Two items present and in view | Incidental (looking at one item) | Fed small portion of that food |
| Case D (John) | Prevent communication breakdowns in use of 'name-calling' in language board communications | Use of "!!" following name-calling, | Teasing/challenging | I/R | Social conversation (home, school, clinic) | Topic or prior utterance that lends itself to name-calling | Being a receiver of utterances using name-calling without use of '!!' | Probable communication breakdown |

* I – Initiation
  R – Response

Both the eliciting question to be used by partners and the response form to be used by Marisol were further specified.  It was decided that partners should use the question, "You want (correct item)?", a form and meaning easily within Marisol's cognitive and comprehension abilities.  Several forms were considered for a *yes* symbol for Marisol, including looking at a *yes* symbol, looking upward, and a vertical headshake.  In consultation with physical and occupational therapy, it was determined that Marisol had sufficient head control to develop a consistent vertical headshake for yes.  In addition, situations and contexts were outlined at home and in the clinic in which this behavior could be prompted and elicited.  In the clinic this included strategic placement of objects (i.e., objects were not near each other and were out of her reach) that she would likely request during play.  At home, a snack activity (getting a bite of a donut), selecting her favorite pajamas over ones she did not like, and requesting specific play times in her room were identified as eliciting contexts in interactions with her mother.  Initially, Marisol was only required to nod her head (with physical assistance) in response to the questions of the clinician or her mother when she initiated a request through nonverbal behaviors.  That nodding was followed by involvement with the action or object that had caught her interest.

Case B.  Victor is a 6-year-old boy with severe athetoid cerebral palsy.  He has no independent means of mobility, and communicates primarily through direct selection on a 200-symbol word board.  He also uses vocalization, arm and eye-pointing, and a verbal "yeah" in his communicative interactions.  He is behind in language, social, and cognitive development, testing at about the 4-year-old level.  Several intervention goals have been targeted for Victor, including specific areas of language comprehension, looking at the person speaking to him, responding to the social greetings of others, development of index finger pointing, and multiple production goals.  Following observation of Victor's desire to accompany others during their activities (his attention-getting method was to fuss, whine, or cry), it was determined that one of his production goals would be to request, through linguistic means, to be taken along.

In planning an intervention program to teach this behavior, several decisions were required.  Victor needed to express his desire when people were in the process of leaving or talking about doing something.  In this context, it was unlikely that Victor would be asked if he wanted to accompany them, so the communication behavior needed to be targeted as an initiation; that is, Victor would have to learn to spontaneously make a request when a situation was occurring (e.g., Dad was going down to the mailbox).  That meaning and request could be expressed by several augmentative techniques and language forms, including (1) available symbols *I want go*, *me*, *Victor go please*; (2) pointing to himself; or (3) a distorted verbal approximation of *me*.  After evaluating these available modes and forms, it was decided to code the meaning and request with a new symbol *(take)* and  gesture *(me)*.  This decision was based on the fact that Victor was increasingly interested in "taking" behaviors (e.g., taking favorite objects to show others; telling on someone who took his possessions; taking a bath or ride; taking pictures with a camera), and that he would probably use this form enough to warrant its addition to his symbol board. These other meanings and uses of *take* were not included in his initial training. *Me* was initially coded by a natural gesture, so that the communication could be predicted by people out of physical range of his symbol board. In this case, the context, plus seeing Victor point to a symbol and gesturing *me*, would be likely to result in having the message understood.

Finally, contexts within the clinical and home setting were defined that had a high probability of eliciting this behavior, and in which Victor could in fact "come along." These included such home activities as going to the laundry room, getting the mail, picking up Daddy, and going into the kitchen during meal preparation. In-clinic activities involved going to places and activities of interest in that environment (e.g., going to the water fountain, copy machine, down the hall). As initiation of that request was of interest, training involved persons talking about and beginning to go to specified places without him. Initially, Victor was expected to imitate the form *take me* (modeled) following his fussing at not being included. This imitation was followed by the obvious consequences (i.e., being taken along).

Case C. Michael is a 2-year-old child with severe physical disability as a result of encephalitis at the age of 6 months. While his cognitive abilities appear to be nearly normal, his neuromuscular abilities are severely reduced. The prognosis for speech development in the near future is poor; therefore, augmentative intervention will be necessary. In the initial treatment plan, several goals were targeted, including continued speech treatment, assisting his parents and his sister in reading his nonverbal behaviors, training both parents to act as facilitators in developing appropriate cognitive and language experiences, and adapting toys. Goals also included the development of an augmentative technique (i.e., eye-pointing), as Michael's most controlled physical movement was eye movement. The intervention goal discussed here involves helping Michael to understand that "looking" can be communicative.

Michael, at this point, had no idea that he could make requests or get another person's attention by staring at an object or action in the immediate environment. He needed to learn this by experiencing the consequences that occur as a result of prolonged looking. A feeding context was used, as this activity was important to Michael and provided a repeated activity that could occur between Michael and his mother on a daily basis. Michael's looking, although not an intentional request on his part, was to be responded to as a request. The feeding activity selected provided Michael with two possible choices, his favorite food (cranberries) or an undesirable food (cold, unsalted oatmeal). These foods were placed in two distinctly different bowls and places. A simple picture symbol of cranberries was taped to that bowl so that Michael could incidentally begin to associate that symbol with that food and activity (a future goal). The initial behavior expected of Michael was any self-initiated looking at either bowl. The consequence of looking was being fed a small portion of that food.

<u>Case D</u>. John is a 13-year-old teenager who primarily uses a combination of spelling and whole word selection from a 300-item, direct-selection language board. His severe speech and writing disabilities are secondary to a traumatic brain injury sustained several years ago. Additional augmentative techniques used include arm-pointing, facial expression, and vocalization. John's intervention program includes language comprehension goals, learning how to alter his communication style when approached by or talking to strangers, improving writing and spelling abilities for communication purposes, and acquiring the interfacing skills needed to activate a computerized communication device. A specific area of communication breakdown was also targeted. In observing John's communication interactions with others, it was noted that he frequently attempted to tease others by calling them a name (e.g., *Big Ears*). These communications were frequently followed by confusion or a blank look on the partner's face. As the traditional paralinguistic features that would identify this behavior (e.g., pausing, stress, intonation) were missing in language board use, partners were interpreting these segments as the beginning of a sentence (e.g., Big ears are . . .) and not the teasing comments that were intended.

The general intervention goal established was to prevent the communicative breakdowns in the use of name-calling. Although the breakdown could have been prevented by having John drop this behavior from his interactions, it was felt to be an important part of his personality and interaction style. Consequently, several behaviors were explored to assist in preventing those breakdowns. These included: (1) the use of nonverbal facial expressions in conjunction with the board forms; (2) name-calling followed by the words *ha, ha*; *teasing*; or *joke*; or (3) the use of punctuation markers (*!!*) that would cue the listener. Nonverbal behaviors were ruled out, as it was observed that most partners did not notice his facial expressions while interpreting item-by-item messages on the language board. The use of punctuation was selected over joke markers, as it was felt that this sufficiently clarified his messages and intent without changing the nature of his teasing and humor. These punctuation markers were targeted for use for both initiations and responses.

Because name-calling was used by John primarily in general social conversation, this context was used in the intervention plan. In examining the aspects of the behavior that John needed to understand and acquire, several serial objectives were outlined. The first involved providing John with the experiences of his partners (i.e., confusion, difficulty in certain situations). The training context involved a social interaction with his therapist (also using a language board) in which name-calling without punctuation markers was used, resulting in breakdowns in John's understanding of those messages. Subsequent goals were directed at experiencing the difference when punctuation markers were used, being able to identify name-calling segments, and use of those punctuation markers in conversations with an increasing number of partners.

## SUMMARY

Intervention planning for persons using augmentative components shares many dimensions with the clinical management of other populations and disorders. That planning process also has many unique features, and requires an understanding of the capabilities and limitations of augmentative components, the special intervention needs of this population, and the adaptive strategies that are functional for these communicators and their partners. Several of these differences are discussed, and their relationship to the evaluation of communicative interaction and clinical management are outlined.

## STUDY QUESTIONS

1. Interact with a friend using spoken language, then using an augmentative aid (e.g., an alphabet board, 50-item word board, and/or an alphabet scan chart). Describe the differences that occurred when an augmentative technique was introduced. What was difficult for you or your partner? Easy? Frustrating? Did you observe any of the patterns reported in research on augmentative interactions? Others?

2. Outline some ways in which communication between natural speakers and individuals who use augmentative aids, symbols, and techniques may differ from spoken language conversations. For each difference, give an example of how this might affect an individual's ability to interact in daily communications. Outline one adaptive strategy that might be used by a partner and/or the person using augmentation to compensate for that difference.

3. Evaluation of communicative interaction requires an understanding of a person's communication repertoire, the pragmatic potentials of various augmentative components, and the adaptive strategies used.

What is meant by the preceding statement?    Illustrate your understanding by comparing and contrasting the communication behaviors that might be available to the following individuals:  (a) a 3-year-old child with athetoid cerebral palsy without any formal sign or symbol system; (b) a 12-year-old with severe verbal apraxia using 25 formal signs: (c) an adult with acquired quadriplegia and limited head, facial, and eye movements using an alphabet scan board.

4. What are some of the special considerations that need to be taken into account in obtaining and making judgments about communication samples involving individuals who use augmentative communication components.

5. Review the case examples given at the end of this chapter.  For each case, outline how the responses required of the child might change over subsequent sessions.    Develop a similar plan for (a) the development of a *no* response in Case A;  (b) the development of an initiated request for *taking off* a hand splint in Case B;  and (c) the subsequent steps that might be targeted in Case C.

## REFERENCES

Bedrosian, J. (1985).  An approach to developing conversational competence.  In D. N. Ripich & F. M. Spinelli (Eds.), School discourse problems.  San Diego:  College Hill Press.

Beukelman, D., & Yorkston, K.  (1977).  A communication system for the severely dysarthric speaker with an intact language system.  Journal of Speech and Hearing Disorders, 42, 265-270.

Beukelman, D., & Yorkston, K.  (1980).  Non-vocal communication:  Performance evaluation. Archives of Physical Medicine and Rehabilitation, 61, 272-275.

Beukelman, D., Yorkston, K., & Dowden, P. (1985).  Communication augmentation:  A casebook of clinical management.  San Diego: College Hill Press.

Blackstone, S., & Cassatt-James, E.  (1984).  Interaction skills in children who use communication aids.  Miniseminar given at American Speech-Language-Hearing Association, San Francisco.

Blank, M., & Franklin, E. (1980). Dialogue with preschoolers: A cognitively based system of assessment. Applied Psycholinguistics, 1, 329-352.

Blank, M., Gessner, M., & Esposito, A. (1979). Language without communication: A case study. Journal of Child Language, 6, 329-352.

Bloom, L., & Lahey, M. (1978). Language development and language disorders. New York: John Wiley & Sons.

Bolton, S., & Dashiell, S. (1984). INCH - INteraction CHecklist for augmentative communication. Huntington Beach, CA: INCH Associates.

Bonvillian, J., & Nelson, K. (1976). Sign language acquisition in a mute autistic boy. Journal of Speech and Hearing Disorders, 41, 339-347.

Bricker, D. (1972). Imitative sign training as a facilitator of word-object association with low-functioning children. American Journal of Mental Deficiency, 76(5), 509-516.

Bruno, J., & Bryen, D. (1985). The impact of modeling on language board users. Unpublished paper, Temple University and Children's Hospital, Philadelphia.

Buzolich, M. (1984). Interaction analysis of augmented and normal adult communication. Unpublished doctoral dissertation, University of California, San Francisco.

Calculator, S. (1985). Describing and treating discourse problems in mentally retarded children: The myth of mental retardese. In D. N. Ripich & F. M. Spinelli (Eds.), School discourse problems. San Diego: College Hill Press.

Calculator, S., & Dollaghan, C. (1982). The use of communication boards in a residential setting: An evaluation. Journal of Speech and Hearing Disorders, 47, 281-287.

Calculator, S., & Luchko, C. (1983). Evaluating the effectiveness of a communication board training program. Journal of Speech and Hearing Disorders, 48, 185-191.

Carlson, F. (1981). Alternate methods of communication. Danville, IL: Interstate Printers & Publishers.

Carrier, J. (1976). Application of non-speech language system with the severely language handicapped. In L. Lloyd (Ed.), <u>Communication assessment and intervention strategies</u>. Baltimore: University Park Press.

Chapman, R. (1981). Exploring children's communicative intents. In J. F. Miller (Ed.), <u>Assessing language production in children: Experimental procedures</u>. Baltimore: University Park Press.

Chapman, R., & Miller, J. (1980). Analyzing language and communication in the child. In R. L. Schiefelbusch (Ed.), <u>Nonspeech language and communication: Analysis and intervention</u>. Baltimore: University Park Press.

Coggins, T., & Carpenter, R. (1981). The communicative intentions inventory: A system for observing and coding children's early intentional communication. <u>Applied Psycholinguistics</u>, <u>2</u>, 235-251.

Colquhoun, A. (1982). <u>Augmentative communication systems: The interaction process</u>. Paper presented at the annual convention of the American Speech-Language-Hearing Association, Toronto, Canada.

Constable, C. (1983). Creating communicative context. In H. Winitz (Ed.), <u>Treating language disorders: For clinicians by clinicians</u>. Baltimore: University Park Press.

Craig, H., & Gallagher, T. (1982). Gaze and proximity as turn regulators within three-party and two-party child conversations. <u>Journal of Speech and Hearing Research</u>. <u>25</u>(1), 65-74.

Culp, D. (1982). <u>Communication Interactions--Nonspeaking children using augmentative systems and their mothers</u>. Paper presented at the annual convention of the American Speech-Language-Hearing Association, Toronto, Canada.

Culp, D., & Stahlecker, J. (1986). <u>Development and documentation of a communication facilitation program for nonspeaking children and their parents</u>. Paper presented at Fourth International Conference on Augmentative and Alternative Communication, Cardiff, Wales.

Davis, A., & Wilcox, J. (1985). <u>Adult aphasia rehabilitation - Applied pragmatics</u>. San Diego: College Hill Press.

DeVilliers, J., & Naughton, J. (1974). Teaching a symbol language to autistic children. Journal of Consultative Clinical Psychology, 42, 111-117.

Dollaghan, C., & Miller, J. (1986). Observational methods in the study of communicative competence. In R. L. Schiefelbusch (Ed.), Language competence: Assessment and intervention. San Diego: College Hill Press.

Duncan, S., & Fiske, D. (1977). Face to face interaction: Research methods and theory. Hillsdale, NJ: John Wiley & Sons.

Eddins, C., & McDowell-Fleming, M. (1984). Communicative behavior inventory. Paper presented at Third International Conference on Augmentative and Alternative Communication, Boston.

Ervin-Tripp, S., & Gordon, D. (1986). The development of requests. In R. L. Schiefelbusch (Ed.), Language competence: Assessment and intervention. San Diego: College Hill Press.

Farrier, L., Yorkston, K., Marriner, N., & Beukelman, D. (1985). Conversational control in nonimpaired speakers using an augmentative communication system. Augmentative and Alternative Communication, 1(2), 65-73.

Fishman, S., Timler, G., & Yoder, D. (1985). Strategies for the prevention and repair of communicative breakdowns in interactions with communication board users. Augmentative and Alternative Communication, 1(1), 38-51

Foulds, R. (1980). Communication rates for nonspeech expression as a function of manual tasks and linguistic constraints. Proceeding of International Conference on Rehabilitation Engineering. Toronto, Canada.

Fulwiler, R., & Fouts, R. (1976). Acquisition of American Sign Language by a noncommunicating autistic child. Journal of Autism and Childhood Schizophrenia, 6(1), 43-51.

Gallagher, T.M. (1983). Pre-assessment: A procedure for accommodating language use variability. In T. Gallagher & C. Prutting (Eds.), Pragmatic assessment and intervention issues in language. San Diego: College Hill Press.

Glass, A., Gazzaniga, M., & Premack, D. (1973). Artificial language training in global aphasia. Neuropsychologia, 11, 95-110.

Goossens', C. (1983). The use of gestural communication systems with non speakers. Workshop presented at Mayer Children's Institute, Omaha.

Goossens', C., & Crain, S. (1986). Augmentative communication intervention. Zurich, IL: Don Johnston Developmental Equipment.

Goossens', C., & Kraat, A. (1985). Technology as a tool for conversation and language learning for the physically disabled. Topics in Language Disorders, 6(11), 56-70.

Harris, D. (1978). Descriptive analysis of communication interaction processes involving non-vocal severely physically handicapped children. Doctoral dissertation, University of Wisconsin-Madison.

Harris, D. (1982). Communication interaction processes involving nonvocal physically handicapped children. Topics in Language Disorders, 2(2), 21-37.

Harris, D., & Vanderheiden, G. (1980). Enhancing the development of communicative interaction. In R. L. Schiefelbusch (Ed.), Nonspeech language and communication: Analysis and intervention. Baltimore: University Park Press.

Higginbotham, J., & Yoder, D. (1982). Communication within natural conversational interaction: Implications for severe communicatively impaired persons. Topics in Language Disorders, 2, 1-19.

Holland, A. (1982). Observing functional communication of aphasic adults. Journal of Speech and Hearing Disorders, 47, 50-56.

Huschle, M., & Staudenbaur, T. (1983). The occurrence of breakdown during the interaction between a familiar and unfamiliar listener and an augmentative system user. Unpublished manuscript, University of Wisconsin, Madison. (Abstracted in Kraat, 1985a)

Kraat, A. (1979). Augmentative communication system use in an institutional setting: A case study. Unpublished study reported in A. Kraat (Ed.), Communication interaction between aided and natural speakers: A state of the art report. Toronto: Canadian Rehabilitation Council for the Disabled.

Kraat, A. (1982). Training augmentative communication use: Clinical and research issues. In K. Galyas, M. Lundman, & U. Lagerman (Eds.), Communication for the severely handicapped. Bromma, Sweden: Swedish Institute for the Handicapped.

Kraat, A. (1984). Communication interaction between aid users and others: An international perspective. Proceedings of the 2nd International Conference on Rehabilitation Engineering, Ottawa, Canada.

Kraat, A. (1985a). Communication interaction between aided and natural speakers: A state of the art report. Toronto: Canadian Rehabilitation Council for the Disabled. (Also available from Trace Center, University of Wisconsin-Madison, 1500 Highland Avenue, Madison, WI 53705)

Kraat, A. (1985b). The jump from language boards to electronic/computerised devices: Some critical training issues. Proceedings of Fourth International Conference, Communication Through Technology for the Physically Disabled (pp. 58-63). Dublin: Central Remedial Clinic, Dublin.

Light, J. (1984). The communicative interaction patterns of young nonspeaking physically disabled children and their primary caregivers. Master's thesis, University of Toronto.

Light, J., Collier, B., & Parnes, P. (1985a). Communicative interaction patterns of young nonspeaking physically disabled children and their primary caregivers: Part 1 - Discourse patterns. Augmentative and Alternative Communication, 1(2), 74-83.

Light, J., Collier, B., & Parnes, P. (1985b). Communication interaction between young nonspeaking physically disabled children and their primary caregivers: Part 2 - Functions. Augmentative and Alternative Communication, 1(3), 98-107.

Light, J. Collier, B., & Parnes, P. (1985c). Communicative interaction between young nonspeaking physically disabled children and their primary caregivers: Part III - modes of communication. Augmentative and Alternative Communication, 1(4), 125-133.

Light, J., McNaughton, D., & Parnes, P. (1986). A protocol for the assessment of the communicative interaction skills of nonspeaking severely handicapped adults and their facilitators. Unpublished manuscript, Hugh MacMillan Medical Centre: Toronto, Ontario.

MacDonald, A. (1984). Blissymbolics and manual sign: A combined approach. Communicating Together, 2(4), 20-21.

Marriner, N., Yorkston, K., & Farrier, L. (1984). Transcribing and coding communication interaction between speaking and nonspeaking individuals. Working paper, University of Washington, Seattle.

Miller, J. (1981). Assessing language production in children: Experimental procedures. Baltimore: University Park Press.

Miller, A., & Miller, E. (1973). Cognitive-developmental training with elevated boards and sign language. Journal of Autism and Childhood Schizophrenia, 3, 65-85.

Morris, S. (1981). Communication/interaction development at mealtimes for the multiple handicapped child: Implications for the use of augmentative communication systems. Language, Speech, and Hearing Services in Schools, 12(4), 216-232.

Morris, S. E. (1982). Pre-speech assessment scale. Clifton, NJ: J.A. Preston Co.

Musselwhite, C., & St. Louis, K. (1982). Communication programming for the severely handicapped: Vocal and nonvocal strategies. San Diego: College Hill Press.

Potter, C., & Kraat, A. (1986). Look, big ear! A case study of the humor, attacks, and retreats of an augmentative speaker. Unpublished master's study.

Preisler, G. (1983). Deaf children in communication - A study of communicative strategies used by deaf children in social interaction. Stockholm: Trydells Trycheri.

Prutting, C., & Kirchner, D. (1983). Applied pragmatics. In T. Gallagher & C. Prutting (Eds.), Pragmatic assessment and intervention issues in language. San Diego: College Hill Press.

Reichle, J., & Ward, M. (1985). Teaching discriminative use of an encoding electronic communication device. Language, Speech and Hearing Services in the Schools, 6(1), 58-63.

Sachs, H., Schegloff, E., & Jefferson, G. (1974). A simple system for the organization of turn taking for conversation. Language, 50(4), 696-735.

Schaeffler, B. (1980). Spontaneous language through signed speech. In R. L. Schiefelbusch (Ed.), Nonspeech language and communication: Analysis and intervention. Baltimore: University Park Press.

Schwabe, A., Olswang, L., & Kriegsmann, E. (1986). Requests for information: Linguistic, cognitive, pragmatic, and environmental variables. <u>Language, Speech, and Hearing Services in Schools</u>, <u>17</u>, 38-55.

Shane, H., Lipshultz, S., & Shane, C. (1982). Facilitating the communication interaction of nonspeaking persons in large residential settings. <u>Topics in Language Disorders</u>, <u>2</u>(2), 73-84.

Shere, B., & Kastenbaum, R. (1966). Mother-child interaction in cerebral palsy: Environmental and psychological obstacles to cognitive growth. <u>Genetic Psychology Monographs</u>, <u>73</u>, 257-262, 286-302.

Skelly, M. (1979). <u>Amer-Ind gestural code</u>. New York: Elsevier Press.

Van Kleek, A., & Carpenter, R. (1980). The effects of children's language comprehension level on adults' child-directed talk. <u>Journal of Speech and Hearing Research</u>, <u>23</u>, 546-569.

Vicker, B. (1974). <u>Non-oral communication system project, 1964-1973</u>. Iowa City: University Campus Store.

Warwick, A. (1986). <u>Towards an understanding of the influence of self-esteem and independence on the communicative ability of physically disabled non-speaking children</u>. Unpublished manuscript, Hugh McMillian Center, Toronto.

Wexler, K., Blau, A., Leslie, S., & Dore, J. (1983). <u>Conversational interaction of nonspeaking cerebral palsied individuals and their speaking partners, with and without augmentative communication aids</u>. Unpublished final grant report.

Wiig, E. (1982). <u>Let's talk inventory for adolescents</u>. Columbus, OH: Charles Merrill.

Wilcox, J., & Campbell, P. (1985). Developing communication skills in young children with severe handicaps. Miniseminar given at the Annual Convention of the American Speech-Language-Hearing Association, Washington, DC.

Wilson, W. (1982). <u>An alternative communication system for the severely physically handicapped</u>. U.S. Dept. of Education grant report, University of Washington, Seattle.

Wollner, S., & Geller, E. (1982). Methods of assessing pragmatic abilities. In J. Irwin (Ed.), <u>Pragmatics: The role in language development</u>. LaVerne, CA: University of LaVerne Press.

Wood, B. (1981). <u>Children and communication: Verbal and nonverbal language development</u>. Englewood Cliffs, NJ: Prentice-Hall.

Yoder, D., & Calculator, S. (1981). Some perspectives of intervention strategies for persons with developmental disorders. <u>Journal of Autism and Developmental Disorders</u>, <u>11</u>(1), 107-124.

Yoder, D., & Kraat, A. (1983). Intervention issues in non-speech communication. In J. Miller, D. Yoder, & R. L. Schiefelbusch (Eds.), <u>Contemporary issues in language intervention</u>. <u>ASHA Reports</u>, 12, 27-51.

# CHAPTER 6

# TRAINING STRATEGIES

## OVERVIEW

SARAH W. BLACKSTONE

*American Speech-Language-Hearing Association*
*Rockville, Maryland*

## OBJECTIVES

● Review variables that may affect the successful training of clients in the implementation of augmentative interventions.

● Provide information about available resources to assist in training.

● Provide examples of a range of training strategies used by master clinicians in the augmentative communication area.

● Stimulate interest in research into the effectiveness of training strategies used in augmentative communication.

## INTRODUCTION

It is often tedious for partners to converse when a communication aid is the medium through which messages must flow. The rate of information exchange is slow, the speaker may fatigue, and the listener may become bored or distracted.  Likewise, it may be difficult or impossible for individuals to communicate using gesture or sign or to produce written communication symbols because of their physical, linguistic, and cognitive disabilities or because of the restricted number of partners capable of interpreting their messages.  Augmentative communication aids, symbols, and techniques are designed to enhance the interactive skills of persons who need them.  However, unless individuals are taught the skills and strategies that will enable them to use the aids and techniques effectively, interventions are not likely to be successful.

Intervention goals may include:  (a) enhancing a person's ability to participate in daily communication; (b) facilitating the development or return of speech, language, and communication skills; or (c) providing additional diagnostic information regarding the nature of an individual's communication problems.  Regardless of the goal, a training program for severely speech/language- and/or writing-impaired individuals should result in opportunities for more efficient and effective communication and more rewarding interactive experiences.  In general, training objectives for the individual using communication augmentation should include:

- increasing the rate and frequency of message exchanges;

- expanding the number of communication partners;

- providing new opportunities to communicate, such as computer access for vocational and/or educational purposes;

- increasing the number and type of messages expressed (i.e., telling secrets, joking, arguing, etc.); and

- improving the conversational skills of individuals who use augmentative techniques.

To accomplish these training goals and related objectives, speech-language pathologists and other professionals need to consider a multitude of variables in their augmentative communication intervention programs.  These variables will extend beyond the disabled individual and must include both the communication partners and the contexts within which communication occurs.  For example, if unimpaired speakers incorrectly believe that a physically handicapped person who uses a communication aid and produces telegraphic utterances (e.g., *go later store*) is cognitively disadvantaged (Creech & Viggiano, 1981), then they are unlikely to communicate appropriately with that person.

Training often means encouraging behaviors that would not have occurred without intervention (e.g., use of a language board or dedicated communication aid, utilization of a core vocabulary of manual signs to compensate for poor speech intelligibility, or production of written text using an eye gaze technique). Training strategies may also facilitate or increase the likelihood that existing behaviors occur on a more frequent basis and are maintained. For example, if parents are trained to recognize and to reinforce particular vocalizations of their physically handicapped child by responding to them as requests for attention, the child will probably begin to use these vocalizations communicatively.

In this chapter, general training guidelines and information about available training materials are presented, along with a collection of 13 strategies used by master clinicians in the augmentative communication area. By providing readers with examples of the training process, we hope to promote an awareness of procedures and materials that may be used to facilitate the development of language and communication competencies in augmentative interventions. We hope that the overview and examples of "how" clinicians with experience "do" what needs to be done will be helpful and will clarify the training process.

## EMPIRICAL BASIS FOR TRAINING

Good clinical practice dictates that solid theoretical constructs and empirical documentation should underlie all treatment approaches. Unfortunately, training strategies employed in the area of augmentative communication are rarely supported by empirical studies (Beukelman, 1985; Beukelman, Yorkston, & Dowden, 1985). Nevertheless, speech-language pathologists and others responsible for developing and implementing training strategies are required to make decisions and to provide necessary training in the absence of clear clinical guidelines. For example, nearly all communication necessitates the use of symbols, yet no definitive information is available about how the level of symbolic representation affects the initial learning and/or generalization of symbols (Kiernan, 1983; Tapajna & Blau, 1985). It is, therefore, possible that clinical assumptions regarding the ease with which particular groups or individuals learn certain symbols may be erroneous or shortsighted. Kiernan (1983), in a review of the use of sign language and other symbol systems with autistic children and adults, concluded that although there is ample evidence that autistic persons can learn to use symbols to communicate basic needs, most studies do not define subject characteristics and outcomes adequately. Similar methodological problems are cited in articles discussing the efficacy of using symbol sets and systems with other disabled groups (Lloyd & Karlan, 1984; Reichle, Williams, & Ryan, 1981). Although some empirical studies address the ease with which certain symbols are recognized and learned by unimpaired subjects (Clark, 1981; Doherty, Daniloff, & Lloyd, 1985; Luftig & Bersani, 1985), few conclusions can be drawn that can assist clinicians making decisions about their disabled clients.  In summary, few existing studies address specific questions about which features and characteristics of symbols, aids, and techniques most efficiently and effectively meet the communication needs of severely speech- and/or writing-impaired individuals (see chapters 7 & 9 for further discussion).

## APPROACHES TO TRAINING

Selecting and implementing training strategies that are likely to result in the achievement of intervention goals and objectives will require careful planning.  Such planning must take into consideration the individual client as well as physical factors and constraints related to the environment, communication partners, and task requirements of the communication situation.  In addition, characteristics, features, and constraints of augmentative communication symbols, aids, and techniques need to be taken into account because they will also affect the types of interventions possible.  As discussed in chapter 5, intervention programs in the augmentative communication area are often similar to those employed in other clinical areas of the communication sciences and disorders and special education.  However, in training clients who use communication augmentation, special considerations must be made.  For example, the adult patient with amyotrophic lateral sclerosis and the preschool child with cerebral palsy may require adaptive seating and positioning before they are able to use a communication aid, computer, or scanning selection technique.  In addition, clients and their primary communication partners may need to be instructed in the mechanics of the equipment (e.g., ways to turn on a computer, load a software program, edit text, use voice output, store and retrieve messages, and so on).

### General Training Approaches

Basic theoretical constructs in language, linguistics, psychology, and communication sciences and disorders provide clinicians with instructional models from which to begin training (Cole & Dale, 1986).  For example:

- Learning theory principles, such as elicited imitation and structured reinforcement paradigms, are effective in developing certain skills and are used in most clinical training programs. These are the principles that often underlie drill and practice teaching procedures. A major criticism of these procedures is that, in practice, they often fail to generalize behaviors that are taught (Harris, 1975; Stokes & Baer, 1977). Although the need to foster generalization is recognized and addressed in current behavior analysis literature, present clinical practices, particularly those conducted in one-on-one situations, may not adequately insure the generalization of functional communication skills across environments and partners.

- Language training principles and procedures (i.e., use of modeling techniques, semantic contingency, and symbol/referent pairings) are basic to communication training with children and adults. In practice, some but not all language teaching strategies provide ways to generalize trained behaviors to the environments within which a client lives, plays, and works. One example is the Environmental Language Intervention Program (MacDonald & Horstmeier, 1978) adapted for nonspeaking children by Lombardino, Willems, and MacDonald (1981).

- Incidental teaching (Hart & Risley, 1986), based on language learning principles, is a natural environmental training model and is increasingly recommended for use in augmentative communication training programs. Incidental teaching approaches reflect research in early language development (Bates 1976; Bruner, 1975; Snow, 1984) and attempt to teach language skills in a way that will generalize beyond circumscribed training settings. The effectiveness of incidental teaching has been shown to increase the variety and complexity of language in culturally disadvantaged children (Hart & Risley, 1974) and to be an effective strategy for teaching the functional use of manual signs to developmentally retarded children (Oliver & Halle, 1982).

- The application of metacognitive strategies to the communicatively impaired is a relatively new area of study. However, the approach is included here because it provides a structured approach to fostering improved conversational skills in higher functioning clients and to teaching communication skills and strategies to the partners of augmented communicators. The term *metacommunication* is used to describe an ability to consciously reflect on and manipulate different aspects of conversation. It involves two components: (a) an awareness of what strategies are needed in order to communicate effectively and (b) the ability to use self-regulatory mechanisms to secure successful execution of the discourse.  An intervention program aimed at developing metacommunication skills in individuals with severe expressive communication disorders might include strategies on how to secure a listener's attention, how to maintain one's conversational turn, and how to repair communication breakdowns.

Training conducted during discrete language sessions that constitute only a small portion of a client's daily or weekly schedule is less likely to be effective than instruction that occurs in context throughout the course of the client's day (Bonvillian, Nelson, & Rhyme, 1981; Snow, Midkiff-Borunda, Small, & Proctor, 1984).  However, the advantages (or disadvantages) of different procedures must be evaluated on a case-by-case basis (Cole & Dale, 1986).  For example, one-on-one drill and practice sessions may be the best way to train reliable switch activation and message storing procedures or to introduce a symbol system.  However, as a client progresses, the clinician may wish to conduct training sessions in an environment that stimulates interaction and approximates a more realistic communication task.  Therefore, an integrated approach that incorporates behavior modification techniques, language-based training approaches, incidental teaching, and metacognitive strategies, as appropriate, is preferable.  Training based on an eclectic approach can address the need for flexibility that is required in augmentative communication interventions.

## Augmentative Communication Training Approaches

Areas that require special consideration when teaching individuals who use augmentative communication are discussed below and include:  (a) setting up training contexts that accommodate physical, cognitive, and linguistic problems;  (b) incorporating the use of multiple communication modes;  (c) teaching augmentative symbols;  (d) developing conversational and discourse skills;  (e) systematically training primary communication partners to facilitate interaction; and  (f) using augmentative communication aids as tools that facilitate the development of communicative competence.

### *Setting Up an Appropriate Training Context*

Setting up a context appropriate to persons requiring augmentative interventions necessitates special consideration of environmental variables.  These individuals often have motor, cognitive, and/or language impairments as well as sensory or perceptual limitations and restricted social, academic, and vocational experiences. We are unlikely to change an individual's level of impairment (e.g., speech-motor dysfunction or ability to learn new information); however, we can provide compensatory ways of accomplishing tasks. Clinicians and educators structure training contexts so that they provide ample opportunities for practice, optimize learning, and account for relevant physical, cognitive, and social variables. Contextual variables include persons, objects, events, linguistic factors, communication aids, other equipment, time factors, and locations that can be manipulated during training.

*Physical considerations.* A properly thought out and constructed physical context is essential to persons with motor disabilities; otherwise, they may have no opportunity to interact directly with objects and people, to participate in activities, or to achieve independence. In constructing a training context that will accommodate a client's physical limitations, the clinician not only stabilizes and positions the client to optimize function, but also considers the location and arrangement of environmental variables (e.g., light and noise levels, the distance at which interaction occurs, availability of adaptive equipment, and degree of mobility). For example, Stuart (this chapter) describes ways to adapt a stage set designed to accommodate the needs of physically disabled "actors and actresses."

Setting up an appropriate context for physically handicapped individuals requires consideration of three areas: (a) stable positioning and seating; (b) access to the environment; and (c) physical comfort. Seating severely physically disabled clients in wheelchairs generally begins with stabilization and positioning of the pelvis and progresses to the trunk, head, neck, and lower extremities (Smith & Nwaobi, 1985). Occupational therapists, physical therapists, and rehabilitation engineers typically provide the necessary expertise on augmentative communication teams with regard to adaptive seating and postitioning (Beasley, 1977). For in-depth information on seating and positioning, the reader is referred to the following publications: Bergen and Colangelo, 1982; Finnie, 1975; Trefler and Taylor, 1984; and Ward, 1983. It is likely that various activities throughout the day will require different seating and positioning arrangements. For example, a child who uses a direct selection electronic communication aid that is mounted on a wheelchair may be unable to use this aid on the floor, while watching television, or at the dinner table or the beach. In these situations, the child will use other communication modes that may require alternative types of positioning and/or adaptive equipment. For example, Morris (1981) describes positioning considerations to facilitate interaction during mealtimes.

Once a client is properly seated and/or positioned, questions regarding access to communication and the environment (mobility, environmental controls, etc.) can be addressed. Adaptive equipment (e.g., head sticks, splints, dowels) are often required in order to use a communication aid (Goossens' & Crain, 1986a). For example, reliable control sites (e.g., finger, head movement, knee) need to be selected for access to communication aids and switches (Beasley, 1977; York, Nietupski, & Hamre-Nietupski,

1985). Access should permit interaction and enhance independence. For adults, this may require independent mobility, well-designed work stations and/or modifications of home/hospital environments to permit independent communication. For very young children, providing mobility (independent, if possible) and access to toys so they are able to play are often the first steps toward environmental and communication control. Available references to assist clinicians in fostering play skills with physically handicapped children include Burkhart (1980); Carlson; (1982); Coker (1984); Goossens' and Crain (1986b); Musselwhite (1985); and Wright and Nomura (1985).

In preparing training contexts, it is necessary to insure the client's comfort, keeping in mind that fatigue is an important factor. Considerable physical and mental effort may be required to operate certain communication aids or selection techniques. For example, visual scanning, which requires an individual to concentrate on and pay attention to the scanning array, can be physically and mentally fatiguing. While some clients with muscular weakness, such as those with amyotrophic lateral sclerosis, will fatigue very quickly, most individuals will fatigue somewhat after extended periods of physical exertion. Training contexts that minimize fatigue make the use of communication augmentation more rewarding.

The physical environment should also be taken into consideration when setting up a training context for the nonphysically handicapped client. For example, autistic individuals, hyperactive children, and individuals recovering from traumatic brain injuries may benefit from physical contexts that are free from complex stimuli and that are quiet and relaxed (see Kent-Udolf; Mirenda & Schuler in this chapter). Dowden (this chapter) reminds us that the physical context may be difficult or impossible to vary, as in the intensive care units of acute care hospitals.

*Cognitive considerations*. Constructing a context to optimize learning and minimize interfering behaviors requires that cognitive problems, such as attention and memory deficits, mental retardation, learning styles, modality preference, and behavioral disturbances, be considered. For example, in teaching mentally retarded individuals the meaning and use of symbols, it may be necessary to provide repeated exposure to and elicit the production of symbols over extended periods of time in order to establish symbol-referent pairings and the communicative use of symbols across contexts (Culatta & Blackstone, 1980).

Learning is more apt to occur if training activities and materials are appropriate to the clients' chronological age as well as their developmental level and interests. In addition, intervention programs that permit clinicians/teachers to respond to their clients' focus of attention, apparent desires and interest, and ability level from moment to moment and situation to situation are preferable. The use of everyday activities (see Higgins & Mills; Stuart; Van Tatenhove; Wasson) and structured play activities (see Bruno; Cassatt-James; Frumkin; Kent-Udolf; Light & Collier) provide training contexts designed to increase a client's opportunity to practice in "real" situations and emphasize the probability that generalized learning will occur. Training programs and materials that take into account cognitive variables are available. Some training programs provide ideas and strategies for integrating cognitive, linguistic, and play skills when training communication competencies (Goossens' & Crain, 1986b; Hanna, Lippert, & Harris, 1984).

*Linguistic considerations*. Creating an appropriate linguistic and social environment for children or adults with severe expressive communication problems is difficult for several reasons. First, it is difficult to ascertain the comprehension abilities of individuals with limited expressive output. As a result, teachers, clinicians, and families tend to "guesstimate" the linguistic knowledge and skills of severely speech-impaired individuals. Clinical experience suggests that overestimates of an individual's abilities and skills are just as likely to occur as underestimates. In either case, the linguistic competencies of children and adults with severe speech-impairments are often judged inaccurately. This creates particular problems for clients who are developing or relearning language. While unimpaired speakers can enhance their language comprehension through exposure to spoken-language models and the feedback they receive from their listeners, severely speech/language-impaired individuals are unable to make mistakes and, therefore, cannot receive appropriate feedback. Thus, any mistaken ideas on the part of the impaired individual about the meaning of words, the grammatical structure of spoken language or written text, and the use of language in social situations will remain unchallenged. A second problem is that individuals who use augmentative aids and techniques rarely, if ever, have contact with others who provide appropriate expressive communication models using similar augmentative symbols, aids, and/or techniques (see chapter 5 for further discussion). Yoder and Kraat (1983) conclude that severely speech-impaired persons are limited both by a lack of appropriate comprehension and expressive models.

Scripted and routinized contexts and role-playing activities (see Cassatt-James; Frumkin; Higgins & Mills; Stuart) can be used to control linguistic stimuli during training. In addition, elicitation techniques, modeling, expansion, prompting, and querying, can be used to encourage the expression of particular words, syntactic forms, and pragmatic functions. Many strategies in this chapter emphasize the need to develop expressive language skills in order to facilitate conversational competence (see Bruno; Frumkin; Light & Collier; Van Tatenhove; see also Goossens' & Crain, 1986a,b). In addition, one strategy (see Blau) discusses how to teach literacy skills in social contexts to children who use communication aids. Acquisition of good reading skills is of paramount importance because of its relationship to spelling and writing skills. Although the use of aids and techniques as educational and/or vocational tools is not the focus of this chapter, their importance for instruction, writing, computer access, and telecommunications should not be underestimated. Additional aspects of social contexts, including the number of communication partners, the communication modes utilized by actual and potential communication partners, the communication roles available to the client, and the amount and frequency of communication interaction, are discussed in the next sections.

### *A Multimodality Approach to Communication*

Effective and efficient communication requires the use of nonverbal and verbal modes (see chapters 1 & 5).  Although persons who use augmentative techniques and strategies always have reduced access to some modes, Harris (1982) and others have  concluded that all available modes should be used by impaired speakers and accepted by their partners.   In addition, the use of less ambiguous modes (e.g., communication aids) should be encouraged so that these individuals become active participants in the formulation and expression of messages.

The mode or modes best suited to meeting certain communication needs will vary.  In fact, Schuler (in press) suggests that the intent of a communication act may determine the most suitable communication mode.  Strategies in the chapter provide ideas for using various augmentative aids and techniques to address basic communication needs (see Dowden; Kent-Udolf; Mirenda & Schuler; Wasson) or more complex conversational (see Bruno; Cassatt-James; Goossens' & Crain; Higgins & Mills; Light & Collier) or writing (see Blau) requirements.

Training strategies designed to increase the use of several modes simultaneously should be introduced with some caution, and their effects on language, speech, and communication skills should be evaluated routinely.  For one thing, the effects on language comprehension and expression of teaching a client to use a combination of speech, standard, and special augmentative techniques is unknown.   While no controlled studies are available, Bonvillian et al. (1981) suggest that simultaneous signing and speaking does not exceed the processing limits of most children.  In some cases the use of one technique directly influences the use of others.  These effects may be positive (i.e., signing may facilitate the production of intelligible speech in hearing children), but the conditions under which this occurs are not well-defined (Schaeffer, 1977; Yamada, Kriendler, & Haimsohn, 1979).   In another example, the presentation of simultaneous modes (e.g., written words in conjunction with pictures and the use of shape and color cues) was successful with some, but not all, clients (Schuler, in press). In addition, the communication partners of motor-impaired individuals often require special training to recognize and respond appropriately to various modes.  Cassatt-James (this chapter) provides guidelines regarding how to train communication partners to recognize the communicative acts of physically handicapped individuals and to facilitate the use of multiple modes of expression.

## *Symbol Sets and Systems*

The use of static and dynamic symbols is unique to the area of augmentative communication (see chapter 3). Although orthographic codes are generally preferred for clients (and their partners) who read and spell because they provide access to novel messages (see Blau), physical and cognitive disabilities may make it difficult to use the alphabet or a word display. Special codes and techniques can provide this access (e.g., Morse Code, Braille, number encoding). For individuals who cannot spell and/or recognize words, graphic symbols (e.g., Blissymbols, rebuses, Picsyms, pictures), electronically produced speech (e.g., synthesized or digitized speech), and/or tactile symbols (e.g., objects, Blissymbols as adapted for the visually impaired) can be used to encode messages.

While many nonoral symbol sets and systems are available for individuals who cannot read, questions remain unanswered regarding how to teach them to individuals. How do young children learn to recognize and use Blissymbols (McNaughton, 1985)? What will facilitate an adult aphasic's ability to associate pictures with an object or event or as a means of requesting information (Helm-Estabrooks, Fitzpatrick, & Barres, 1982)? How can we teach a retarded child to use the manual sign *help* to request assistance (Culatta & Blackstone, 1980; Goossens', 1983)? The cognitive, sensory, perceptual, linguistic, and motor problems of individuals, as well as the nature of the symbols themselves, interact and confound our attempts to answer these quesions. Several years ago, Fristoe and Lloyd (1978) concluded that clinicians did not have enough information about, nor give sufficient attention to, symbol selection and training. More recently, clinicians and teachers have begun to teach nonoral symbols with somewhat more confidence. This may reflect their familiarity with language training programs and the augmentative communication area. In clinical practice, however, symbols tend to be "tested" rather than "taught." For example, clinicians may present a client with a new language board containing between 5 and 50 symbols and then provide instruction, such as "Here is the milk," "Look at the cookies," and so on. Then, the client is asked or tested (e.g., "Where's the milk?") or instructed to "Point to the cookies." This procedure merely teaches symbol recognition and/or assesses the client's recognition of specific symbols on a specific display. Symbol recognition is certainly not the end goal of augmentative interventions. Goals must be functionally based (i.e., the communicative use of symbols to accomplish certain communication tasks) (Culatta & Blackstone, 1980; Goodman & Kroc, 1981; Goossens' & Crain, 1986b; Helm-Estabrooks et al., 1982; Lombardino et al., 1981).

Symbol training may focus on teaching symbol/referent pairings (i.e., comprehension of symbols) or syntactic forms, or may emphasize the use of symbols to accomplish various communicative tasks. In most cases, training clients to use symbols communicatively requires teaching the use of symbol combinations to express complex ideas and to develop grammatical competencies and conversational strategies.

Unfortunately, vocabulary displays are restricted and contain a limited set of symbols that represent only a small proportion of a client's vocabulary (see chapter 5 for an in-depth discussion). In addition, many symbols on language boards are infrequently used. Clinicians should periodically evaluate the functional use of vocabulary items on displays and revise them, as appropriate. Initial vocabulary selection guidelines (see Mirenda & Schuler, this chapter) also can be used when revising symbol boards. Goossens' and Crain's and Van Tatenhove's strategies suggest ways of providing some flexibility for clients through the use of multiple communication displays that will enable them to communicate in different contexts about different topics. For additional suggestions in how to select vocabulary, see chapters 4 and 5 in this text, Brandenberg & Vanderheiden (in press), Carlson (1981, 1982), Fishman (in press), and Goossens' and Crain (1986 a,b).

## *Conversational and Communicative Competence*

Individuals who use augmentative aids and techniques typically play a passive role within communicative interactions, while unimpaired speakers initiate most topics and maintain control of conversational exchanges (Blackstone & Cassatt-James, 1984; Light, Collier, & Parnes, 1985; Light, Rothschild, & Parnes, 1985; Lossing, 1981; Wexler, Blau, Leslie, & Dore, 1983). As discussed in chapter 5, the characteristics of conversations between unimpaired speakers and individuals who use communication aids and techniques reflect the constraints of augmentative components, as well as to the disabilities of persons who require them and their communication partners (Bottorf & DePape, 1982; Calculator & Luchko, 1983; Harris, 1982; Yoder & Kratt, 1983). These characteristics are discussed throughout this text. To enhance conversational and communicative competencies, the following areas should be considered:

- features of augmentative aids and techniques (see chapters 3 & 5);

- altered conversational patterns (see chapters 4, 5, & 9);

- reduced speed of message transmission (see chapters 3, 4, 5, 7, & 9);

- laborious and tiring message formulation (see chapters 3, 4, & 5);

- neglect of multimodalities for expression (see chapter 1);

- limitations of nonoral symbols and vocabulary displays (see chapters 3, 4, & 5);

- the user's general experience and skill level (see chapters 2, 5, & 8);

- motivation level for communication (see chapters 2, 5, & 8);

- lack of conversational models (see chapters 5 & 9); and

- communication partners who are unfamiliar with communication aids, symbols, techniques, and strategies (see chapter 5 & 8).

Many strategies in this chapter address ways to develop conversational competencies. Initiation strategies (see Light & Collier; Higgins & Mills), turn-taking skills (see Cassatt-James; Frumkin; Higgins & Mills; Stuart; Wasson), requesting (see Dowden; Van Tatenhove) and commenting skills (see Wasson), timing (Stuart), and conversational repairs (see Cassatt-James), as well as general modeling (see Bruno) are discussed. In addition, establishing basic interactive routines is addressed by Kent-Udolf. Developing communication capabilities beyond conversation, specifically literacy skills, is discussed by Blau.

## Systematic Training of Communication Partners

Solving the communication problems of severely speech- and/or writing-impaired individuals requires that unimpaired speakers participate in ways that were not originally anticipated by sender-receiver models; this is due to the altered roles of participants discussed previously. For example, Light et al. (1985) demonstrated that facilitator training was effective in their clinical intervention with a 4-year-old physically handicapped boy who uses a nonelectronic communication aid. Whereas training the child alone had little effect on the initiation-response patterns of interactions with the mother, training the mother as well as the child had a significant effect on their interaction. Rosegrant (1984) reported that adult behaviors were strongly correlated with children's degree of progress in learning literacy skills. Similarly, training the caregivers of adults who use augmentative techniques in residential settings has resulted in increased use of the techniques (Shane, Lipschultz, & Shane, 1982). In a single case study of a 24-year-old nonspeaking adult with anarthria and spastic quadriplegia, Calculator and Luchko (1983) found that while client training alone had little effect on the subject's interaction patterns, partner training resulted in increased rates of client initiation.

Individuals, including those who use augmentative techniques, need to communicate with many partners (i.e., familiar and unfamiliar speaking persons of all ages, and those with and without a handicapping condition, including other nonspeaking individuals). Strategies designed to facilitate the interactive process by training a client's primary communication partners must take into account the individual needs and capabilities of partners. Partners may be taught to:

- understand the problems and processes involved in augmentative communication in general (multimodalities, listener role) and for the client in particular;

- become familiar with symbol sets and systems;

- understand the equipment (operation, mechanics, and maintenance);

- practice and demonstrate procedures employed in training;

- assist in evaluating the effectiveness of a training strategy; and

- demonstrate flexibility in carrying out the strategy.

In this chapter, all strategies involve some communication partner training. However, because most communication partners cannot be formally trained, the clinician should always provide written, pictured, or recorded directions to unfamiliar partners. Dowden's strategy points out that some contexts actually preclude extensive partner training. She points out that these constraints will affect the selection of aids and techniques.

## *Communication Aids as Tools*

The provision of a communication aid does not result in its ready integration or effective use by persons for whom it was intended. Tools of any kind are only useful when operated by skilled persons in order to accomplish some necessary task. Rodgers (1984) likens augmentative communication aids to musical instruments, since both are "mediums for communication" and require instruction before they can be used well.

Although most music teachers are competent musicians themselves, few teachers/clinicians are "master" communication aid users. Teacher and clinicians should not expect persons with severe expressive communication disorders (and other handicapping conditions) to do efficiently and effectively what they themselves cannot do and may not understand. To assist professionals, the manufacturers of dedicated communication aids and other materials provide an operations manual. Unfortunately, these manuals rarely include instructions or empirical data about how to utilize their product to enhance functional communication (i.e., human factors research is omitted). Therefore, strategies must be developed to teach all aspects of communication aid use, including how to:

- scan, encode, and use eye-gaze techniques (Blau, 1984; Fishman, in press; Goossens' & Crain, 1985);

- introduce electronics (Burkhart, 1980; Carlson, 1982; Coker, 1984, Goossens' & Crain, 1986b; Musselwhite, 1985; Wright & Nomura, 1985);

- program a dedicated communication aid (Goossens' & Crain, 1986b; see product manuals);

- increase speed of message transmission through the use of prediction, telegraphic utterances, and stored messages (Carlson, 1982; chapters 3, 5, 7, & 9);

- construct a communication aid (Carlson, 1982; Fishman, in press; Goossens' & Crain, 1986b; see Goossens' & Crane, Mirenda & Schuler, and Van Tatenhove, this chapter);

- organize a vocabulary display (Fishman, in press; chapters 4 & 5);

- teach skills for operation of a specific electronic communication aid (see operator manuals; Charlebois-Marois, 1985; Fishman, in press; Tapajna & Blau, 1985);

- program a text-to-speech synthesizer (see product manuals);

- set up a vocabulary on a discrete speech recognition system (Martin & Poock, 1985);

- customize computer hardware and software for clients; and

- use computers to serve multiple communication needs (Bowe, 1984; Fishman, in press).

## SUMMARY

This chapter, in addition to reviewing several theoretical approaches to training, discusses specific approaches that are applicable to augmentative interventions. The primary purpose of the chapter is to provide students and practicing clinicians with information and ideas about how to (a) set up a training context (taking into consideration pertinent physical, cognitive, and linguistic variables and social considerations), (b) develop a multi-component communication system by training speech/language-impaired individuals to use multiple communication modes, (c) teach symbol/referent pairings and teach strategies for using restricted vocabulary sets, (c) identify variables that may interfere with the development of conversational competencies, (d) delineate areas that require communication partner training, and (e) develop low- and high-tech aids as tools that actually enhance an individual's communication skills and options.

The remainder of this chapter presents 13 strategies that are designed to accomplish these objectives. These strategies, which are arranged alphabetically by author, do not represent a comprehensive collection of training approaches; rather, they provide the reader with samples of strategies presently employed by experienced clinicians in the augmentative communication area. By contributing to this chapter, these master clinicians are sharing their extensive clinical knowledge, experiences, and skills. The reader will note that the types of strategies presented are oriented toward children with congenitally based problems, thus reflecting the concerns of the U.S. Department of Education, which funded this project. The reader is referred to Beukelman, Yorkston, & Dowden (1985) for case studies that are oriented more toward an adult population. Clinicians may find these resources useful as they begin to provide augmentative communication training to individuals with severe expressive communication disorders.

## STUDY QUESTIONS

Following the format outlined in the next section of this chapter, develop a training strategy for one or more of the individuals described below. These study questions may also be useful in providing structure to small group or class discussions, particularly for those with limited clinical experiences.

1. A. is an 18-year-old, severely speech-impaired adult with a diagnosis of severe mental retardation and speech-motor dysfunction. He is ambulatory and has receptive language abilities approximating the 5- to 7-year-old level. To communicate, he uses gestures, vocalizations (yes/no; hi; drink); a communication book (with 100 rebus symbols); and a direct-selection technique (index-finger pointing). He interacts minimally with his peers in the sheltered workshop he attends as part of his educational program. In his group home, the staff reports that he responds to requests. His primary communication partners are two

professionals.    One provides his daily care and the other is a recreational therapist who takes him on a weekly outing in the community.

Develop a strategy to increase the number of appropriate initiations that this individual produces during daily activities. The reader may find the following strategies helpful in developing this training strategy:    Bruno; Cassatt-James; Frumkin; Goossens' and Crain; Higgins and Mills; Light and Collier; and Wasson.

2.  G. is a 7-year-old girl with normal intellectual abilities. She has athetoid cerebral palsy and a moderate dysarthria. She is mainstreamed for academics in a first-grade classroom at her local elementary school and has receptive language skills that approximate her chronological age. Speech intelligibility varies (according to the partner) from 20 to 40 percent. In addition to her speech, she uses a variety of augmentative components effectively, including gestures, vocalizations, and an LC-Etran (eye-gaze technique). Her symbols include a combination of 300 Blissymbols and words. Her linguistic expressions are often telegraphic. Recently, a voice output, portable communication aid with printed output was introduced, which she accesses using a head switch mounted to her wheelchair. G. has both normal and handicapped peers with whom she interacts. She relies most heavily on nonverbal mechanisms and residual speech to do so. At present, she has difficulty participating independently in activities.

Develop a strategy that will result in the development of more independent interaction skills with speaking peers during classroom and lunchtime activities. The reader may find the following strategies helpful:  Blau; Frumkin; Goossens' and Crain; Higgins and Mills; Stuart; Van Tatenhove; and Wasson.

3.  S. is a 4-year-old ambulatory child with autistic-like characteristics and diagnoses of moderate to severe mental retardation and a mild unilateral hearing impairment. He is enrolled in a self-contained class. Other children in the class are mentally and physically handicapped. S.'s receptive language capabilities can be measured at the 15-month level (i.e., he understands some single words). However, his response to language is inconsistent. Expressive communication skills are severely delayed, with speech and gestural behaviors approximating the 6-month level (i.e., vocalizations consist of reduplicative babbling with pitch variations; gestures that include reaching, pushing, and turning

away). S. has a very restricted communication repertoire. However, he is exposed regularly to basic signs, photographs of familiar objects, and people at home and at school. His family is very interested in improving communication skills and is available for training. His teachers are skilled, but busy. At the present time, his primary expressive acts consist of a whiny vocalization and reaching toward an object that he wants but is unable to procure.

The training goal is to develop appropriate requesting behaviors. The reader may find the following strategies helpful: Bruno; Cassatt-James; Kent-Udolf; Light and Collier; and Mirenda and Schuler.

4. D. is a 35-year-old adult with amyotrophic lateral sclerosis who is presently hospitalized with pneumonia, but will be released within one week. She is quadriplegic and has severe dysarthria and dysphagia. D. has only two reliable control sites left: her eyes and left thumb. She uses eye gaze to environmental objects/people for quick messages about basic needs, and employs a scanning technique (her partners scan the alphabet and she signals when the correct letter is reached) to produce elaborate messages. Communication partners include a devoted family and medical personnel.

Develop a strategy that will enable D. to ask questions. Consider why you would or would not suggest augmentative components that she is not presently using. The reader may find the following strategies helpful: Dowden; Higgins and Mills.

## REFERENCES

Bates, E. (1976). Pragmatics and sociolinguistics in child language. In M. Morehead & A. Morehead (Eds.), Language deficiency in children: Selected readings (pp. 411-465). Austin, TX: Pro-Ed.

Beasley, M. (1977). The role of the occupational therapist in interfacing communication aids. Proceedings of the Workshop on Communication Aids for the Handicapped (pp. 55-67). Ottawa, Ontario: University of Ottawa.

Bergen, A., & Colangelo, C. (1982). Positioning the client with CNS deficits: The wheelchair and other adapted equipment. New York: Valhalla Rehabilitation Publications.

Beukelman, D. (1985). The weakest link is better than the strongest memory. Augmentative and Alternative Communication, 1(2), 55-57.

Beukelman, D., Yorkston, K., & Dowden, P. (1985). Communication augmentation: A casebook of clinical management. San Diego: College Hill Press.

Blackstone, S., & Cassatt-James, E. (1984). Communicative competence in communication aid users and their partners. Paper presented at the Third International Conference on Augmentative and Alternative Communication, Boston.

Blau, A. (1984). Dial scan manual: Suggestions for training and use. Lake Zurich, IL: Don Johnston Developmental Equipment.

Bonvillian, J., Nelson, K., & Rhyme, J. (1981). Sign language and autism. Journal of Autism and Developmental Disorders, 11(1), 125-137.

Bottorf, L., & DePape, D. (1982). Initiating communication systems for severely speech-impaired persons. Topics in Language Disorders, 2(2), 55-71.

Bowe, F. (1984). Personal computers and special needs. Berkeley, CA: SYBEX.

Bruner, J. (1975). From communication to language--A psychological perspective. Cognition, 3, 255-287.

Burkhart, L. (1980). Homemade battery powered toys and educational devices for severely handicapped children. (Available from author, 8503 Rhode Island Avenue, College Park, MD 20740)

Calculator, S., & Luchko, C. (1983). The use of communication boards in a residential setting: An evaluation. Journal of Speech and Hearing Disorders, 47, 281-287.

Carlson, F. (1981). Alternate methods of communication. Danville, IL: Interstate Printers & Publishers.

Carlson, F. (1982). Prattle and play. (Available from Media Resource Center, MCRI, 444 S. 4th Street, Omaha, NE 68131)

Charlebois-Marois, C. (1985). Everybody's technology: A sharing of ideas in augmentative communication. Montreal, Canada: Charlecoms Enr.

Clark, C. (1981) Learning words using traditional orthography and the symbols of rebus, Bliss, and Carrier. Journal of Speech and Hearing Disorders, 46, 191-196.

Coker, W. (1984). Homemade switches and toy adaption for early training with nonspeaking persons. Language, Speech, and Hearing Services in Schools, 15, 32-35.

Cole, K., & Dale, P. (1986). Direct language instruction and interactive language instruction with language delayed preschool children: A comparison study. Journal of Speech and Hearing Research, 29, 206-217.

Creech, R., & Viggiano, J. (1981). Consumers speak out on the life of the non-speaker. Asha, 23(8), 550-555.

Culatta, B., & Blackstone, S. (1980). A program to teach non-oral communication symbols to multiply handicapped children. Journal of Childhood Communication Disorders, 4, 29-55.

Doherty, J., Daniloff, J., & Lloyd, L. (1985). The effect of categorical presentation on Amer-Ind transparency. Augmentative and Alternative Communication, 1(1), 10-16.

Finnie, N. (1985). Handling the young cerebral palsied child at home (2nd ed.). London: William Heinemann Medical Books.

Fishman, I. (in press). Electronic communication aids: Selection and use. San Diego: College Hill Press.

Fristoe, M., & Lloyd, L.L. (1978). A survey of the use of nonspeech communication systems with severely communication impaired. Mental Retardation, 16, 99-103.

Goodman, L., & Kroc, R. (1981). A classroom sign communication program for the severely handicapped. Language, Speech, and Hearing Services in School, 12, 233-239.

Goossens', C. (1983). The use of gestural communication systems with nonspeakers. (Available from MCRI, University of Nebraska Medical Center, 444 S. 44th Street, Omaha, NE 658131)

Goossens', C., & Crain, S. (1985). Eye-gaze communication systems: Assessment and intervention. (Available from authors, Sparks Center for Developmental and Learning Disorders, 1720 Seventh Avenue, South, Birmingham, Alabama 35233)

Goossens', C., & Crain, S. (Eds.). (1986a). Augmentative communication assessment resources. Lake Zurich, IL: Don Johnston Developmental Equipment.

Goossens', C., & Crain, S. (Eds.). (1986b). Augmentative communication intervention resources. Lake Zurich, Il: Don Johnston Developmental Equipment.

Hanna, R., Lippert, E., & Harris, A. (1982). Developmental communication curriculum. San Antonio, TX: Psychological Corporation.

Harris, D. (1982). Communication interaction processes involving nonvocal physically handicapped children. Topics in Language Disorders, 2, 21-37.

Harris, S. (1975). Teaching language to nonverbal children: With emphasis on problems of generalization. Psychological Bulletin, 82, 565-580.

Hart, B., & Risley, T. (1974). Using preschool materials to modify the language of disadvantaged children. Journal of Applied Behavior Analysis, 7, 243-256.

Hart, B., & Risley, T. (1975). Incidental teaching of language in the preschool. Journal of Applied Behavior Analysis, 8, 411-420.

Hart, B., & Risley, T. (1986). Incidental strategies. In R.L. Schiefelbusch (Ed.), Language competence assessment and intervention. San Diego: College-Hill Press.

Helm-Estabrooks, N., Fitzpatrick, P., & Barresi, B. (1982). Visual action therapy for global aphasia. Journal of Speech and Hearing Disorders, 47, 385-389.

Kiernan, C. (1983). The use of nonvocal communication techniques with autistic individuals. Journal of Child Psychology and Psychiatry, 24, 339-375.

Light, J., Collier, B., & Parnes, P. (1985). Communicative interaction between young nonspeaking physically disabled children and their primary caregivers: Part II-communicative functions. Augmentative and Alternative Communication, 1(3), 98-107.

Light, J., Rothschild, & Parnes, P. (1985). The effect of communication intervention with nonspeaking physicaly disabled children. Paper presented at the Annual

Convention of the American Speech-Language-Hearing Association, Washington, DC.

Lloyd, L., & Karlan, G. (1984). Non-speech communication symbols and systems: Where have we been and where are we going? Journal of Mental Deficiency Research, 28, 3-20.

Lombardino, L., Willems, S., & MacDonald, J. (1981). Critical considerations in total communication and an environmental intervention model for the developmentally delayed. Exceptional Children, 47(6), 455-461.

Lossing, C. (1981). A technique for the quantification of non-vocal communicative performance by listeners. Unpublished masters thesis, University of Washington, Seattle.

Luftig, R.B., & Bersani, H. (1985). An investigation of two variables influencing Blissymbol learnability with nonhandicapped adults. Augmentative and Alternative Communication, 1(1), 32-37.

MacDonald, J., & Horstmeier, D. (1978). Environmental language intervention program. Columbus: Charles E. Merrill.

Martin, B., & Poock, G. (1985). An initial applied look at stress and voice recognition. Journal of the American Voice Input/Output Society, 1(1), 24-33.

McNaughton, S. (Ed.) (1985). Communicating with Blissymbolics. Toronto: Blissymbolics Communication Institute.

Musselwhite, C. (1985). Adaptive play for special needs children: Strategies to enhance communication and learning. San Diego: College Hill Press.

Morris, S. (1981). Communication/interaction development at mealtimes for the multiply handicapped child: Implications for the use of augmentative communication systems. Language, Speech, and Hearing Services in the Schools, 12, 216-232.

Oliver, C., & Halle, J. (1982). Language training in the everyday environment: Teaching functional sign use to a retarded child. The Association for the Severely Handicapped, 8, 50-62.

Reichle, J., Williams, W., & Ryan, S. (1981). Selecting signs for the formulation of an augmentative communicative modality. The Association for the Severely Handicapped, 6, 48-56.

Rodgers, B. (1984). The holistic application of high technology for conversation, writing and computer access aid systems. In C. Smith (Ed.), Proceedings of Discovery 84: Technology for disabled persons. Menomine, WI: UW-Stout Vocational Rehabilitation Institute.

Rosegrant, T. (1984). Fostering progress in literacy development: Technology and social interaction. Seminars in Speech and Language, 5(1), 47-57.

Schaeffer, B. (1980). Spontaneous language through signed speech. In R. Schiefelbusch (Ed.), Nonspeech language and communication: Analysis and intervention. Austin, TX: Pro-Ed.

Schuler, A. (in press). Selecting augmentative communication systems on the basis of current communicative means and functions. Australian Journal of Human Communication Disorders.

Shane, H., Lipschultz, R., & Shane, C. (1982). Facilitating the communicative interaction of nonspeaking persons in large residential settings. Topics in Language Disorders, 2, 73-84.

Smith, P., & Nwaobi, O. (1985). Seating children who have cerebral palsy: Therapeutic and technical considerations. Alabama CEC Journal, 6, 20-29.

Snow, C. (1984). Parent-child interaction and the development of communicative ability. In R. Schiefelbusch & J. Pickar (Eds.), The acquisition of communicative competence. Austin, TX: Pro-Ed.

Snow, C., Midkiff-Borunda, S., Small, A., & Proctor, A. (1984). Therapy as social interaction: Analyzing the contexts for language remediation. Topics in Language Disorders, 4, 72-85.

Stokes, T., & Baer, D. (1977). An implicit technology of generalization. Journal of Applied Behavioral Analysis, 10, 349-67.

Tapajna, M., & Blau, A. (1985). The choice board: Perspectives on training and use. Lake Zurich, IL: Don Johnston Developmental Equipment.

Trefler, E., & Tayler, S. (1984).   Decision making guidelines for seating and
    positioning children with cerebral palsy.   In E. Trefler (Ed.), <u>Seating for
    children with cerebral palsy: A manual</u> (pp. 55-76).  Memphis, TN:  University
    of Tennessee Rehabilitation Engineering Program.

Vanderheiden, G. (in press).  Overview of basic selection techniques for augmentative
    communication:   Present and future.   In L. Bernstein (Ed.), <u>The vocally
    impaired: Clinical practice and research</u>.  New York:  Academic Press.

Ward, D. (1983). <u>Positioning the handicapped child for function:  A guide to evaluate
    and prescribe equipment for the child with central nervous system dysfunction</u>.
    St. Louis:   D. Ward.

Wexler, K., Blau, A., Leslie, S., & Dore, J.   (1983).  <u>Conversational interaction of
    nonspeaking cerebral palsied individuals and their speaking partners, with and
    without augmentative communication aids</u>.   Unpublished manuscript, Helen
    Hayes Hospital, New York.

Wright, C., & Nomura, M. (1985).  <u>From toys to computers:  Access for the physically
    disabled child</u>.  Lake Zurich, IL:  Don Johnston Developmental Equipment.

Yamada, J., Kriendler, J., & Haimsohn, M.   (1979).   The use of simultaneous
    communication in a language intervention program for an autistic child:   A
    case study. <u>UCLA Working Papers in Cognitive Linguistics</u>, <u>1</u>, 63-92.

Yoder, D., & Kraat, A. (1983).  Intervention issues in non-speech communication.  In J.
    Miller, D. Yoder, & R. Schiefelbusch (Eds.), <u>Contemporary issues in language
    intervention</u>. <u>ASHA Reports</u>, <u>12</u>, 27-51..

York, J., Nietupski, J., & Hamre-Nietupski, S.  (1985).  A decision-making process for
    using microswitches.  <u>Journal of the Association for Persons with Severe
    Handicaps</u>, <u>10</u>(4).

# SELECTED TRAINING STRATEGIES

# THE DEVELOPMENT OF LITERACY SKILLS FOR SEVERELY SPEECH- AND WRITING-IMPAIRED CHILDREN

*Andrea F. Blau*
*Consultant, Nonspeech Communication*
*New York, New York*

## INTRODUCTION

Recent research in literacy skills suggests two principal methods by which normal speaking adults identify printed words (traditional orthography). In the first method, termed the direct route, the individual identifies the visual form of the word. In the second method, termed the indirect route, the visual form is recoded into a phonological representation. Coltheart (1978) has suggested that these two routes operate in parallel, with the direct, visual route being the faster method for lexical access.

Developmental researchers (Jorm & Share, 1983) point out that skilled readers prefer the direct visual route, and use indirect phonological recoding only as a backup mechanism when access through the direct route fails. Phonological recoding, they suggest, plays a much more dominant role in reading acquisition. Young children who have had only limited experience with printed words have only limited visual representations of words in their mental lexicon. Jorm and Share (1983) and Mitchell (1982) have suggested that normal speaking children use phonological recoding as a self-teaching mechanism by which they ultimately learn to identify additional words by the direct visual route. A child's ultimate skill at word identification by the direct visual route, therefore, will depend in part upon his development of phonological recoding skills. Based upon their longitudinal studies of reading acquisition, Jorm, Share, Maclean, and Matthews (1984) suggest that competency in phonological recoding skills is predictive of later sight word vocabulary skill. They speculate that the two routes to the lexicon are developmentally intertwined and "do not represent independent abilities."

Nonspeaking children have not as yet been examined in terms of mental processes used for reading. Clinical debate has been ongoing for years as to whether persons with severe congenital speech impairments develop phonological skills in a manner similar to unimpaired speakers. Since phonological recoding demands that lexical entries be accessed as they would be for spoken words, questions have been raised regarding the psycholinguistic processes used by severely speech-impaired children. Concurrent with this debate has been the selection of methods for teaching reading skills to nonspeakers. Clinical experience supports the notion that severely speech-impaired children have a strong functional need for early acquisition of literacy skills, as their communicative and technological options increase once they have full use of the alphabet. Two distinct instructional methods are often used by educators, stressing either a sight word or phonic approach toward reading acquisition. Since literacy research suggests that both visual and phonological routes to lexical access are developmentally intertwined (and deficits in phonological awareness have been associated with poor reading acquistion), combining both sight word and phonic approaches toward reading instruction is preferred.

The following strategy takes advantage of the developmental lead available to severely speech-impaired children in terms of visual access to a large range of printed words (as paired with the symbols on their communication boards), while additionally facilitating the development of phonological recoding skills. Since many nonspeakers are also nonwriters because of physical limitations, the use of technical aids to facilitate writing and spelling skills, an integral part of literacy development, has also been included.

## PURPOSE OF STRATEGY

The purpose of this strategy is to teach literacy skills to severely speech- and writing-impaired children.

## UNDERLYING ASSUMPTIONS

1. *Client*. The child's cognitive and linguistic development ranges between 5 and 7 years of age, depending upon particular areas being assessed; chronological age varies between 5 and 8 years; diagnosis reflects a congenital nonspeaking condition, severe dysarthria, or developmental dyspraxia associated with a neurological disorder that has severely restricted the child's ability to speak and write; entry skill is at the kindergarten to first-grade level; social/emotional adjustment is at developmental age level.

**FIGURE 6-1. MINI-KEYBOARD.**

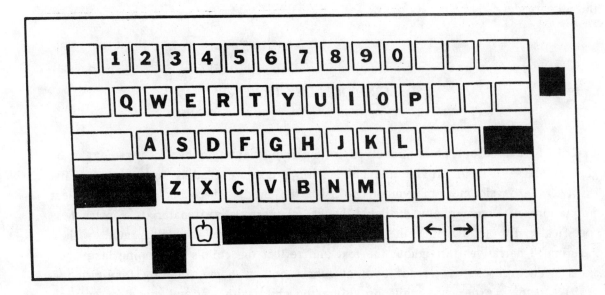

2. *Augmentative components*. The client's residual vocal and nonverbal skills are augmented by a direct select symbol/word communication board; symbols have been selected from a variety of picture-based symbol dictionaries, with several personalized symbols generated by the speech-language pathologist; child has had access previously to a range of communication boards; a large communication board is affixed under plexiglass to the child's desk/wheelchair and a range of mini boards are available in a portable communication attache; the Sharp Memowriter (Sharp Electronics Corporation, Paramus, NJ), Canon Typewriter (Telesensory Systems, Inc., Palo Alto, CA), and the Apple IIe or IIc computer (with speech synthesizer) (Apple Computer, Inc., Cupertino, CA) are used as educational aids.

3. *Environmental constraints*. The child comes from a supportive home environment and is in an educational program with speaking children; classroom staff are cooperative but may have limited experience with augmentative communication aids; development of adapted curriculum materials largely remains the responsibility of the speech-language pathologist; material preparation time is extensive; SRA reading series is used by classroom teacher (Rasmussen & Goldberg, 1976).

4. *Other basic assumptions*. Curriculum adaptations have been completed by the speech-language pathologist. These involve the preparation of a mini *keyboard* (Figure 6-1) located on the child's desktop communication board for phonics and spelling work and the augmentative communication adaptation of Part I of the SRA reading series. The symbols selected for the adapted SRA text match the symbols on the child's

communication boards, supplemented by illustrations of specific characters as used in the SRA reader.

## DESCRIPTION OF STRATEGY

There are four phases involved in the implementation of this strategy. The goal of Phase I is to provide the child with a positive reading experience. This involves the development of symbol books for the child. These books should reflect adaptations of commercially available books, or personalized materials constructed specifically for (and with) the child. Symbol sentences are illustrated within meaningful narratives throughout the text and reflect the child's developing language skills. These books are "read" both at school and at home, thereby facilitating a positive reading experience while providing the child with a visual model of symbol sentences and left to right sequencing within meaningful contexts.

The goal of Phase II is the development of a substantial sight word vocabulary. The symbols used within the adapted story books are systematically faded out while the printed words are highlighted. (For a developmental approach for moving from symbols to sight words, the Bridge Reading Kit (Dewsbury, Jennings, & Boyle, 1983) can be used as a guide.) A "reading" communication board is created that is similar in content and organization to the child's core communication board. Matching games are played in which the printed words are presented to the child while the child points to the corresponding symbol/word combination. Frequently used symbols are systematically faded out while the printed words remain on the child's board. As the child masters sight word recognition of each word, the symbol is replaced by the printed word on the core communication board.

Phase III involves the introduction of the phonic portion of the program. Using the keyboard and adapted SRA text (Blau, Valdes, & Quintas, 1985), letter/sound correspondences, sound blending, and phonic decoding skills are taught. The graphic symbol adaptations of the SRA text allow the child to point to symbols reflecting orthographic representations of words. Tasks are constructed in which the child must decode unfamiliar printed words (for which the segmented component parts have been mastered within previously learned word families) and select the symbols that reflect the identity of the new words. For example, having mastered the *an* family and the phonemes /d/, /m/, and /p/ in the initial position, the child is introduced to the *ad* family and asked to blend the aforementioned initial phonemes with the *ad* sound and then match these novel words to their corresponding symbols (i.e., *dad*, *mad*, and *pad*), giving evidence to the child's mastery of the sound-blending skill.

Since writing and spelling skills are part of literacy development, writing these words (both sight word and phonic targets) is done with the child's memowriter or typewriter. Additional experience with the alphabetic code and sound blending is facilitated through computer and speech synthesizer use. Software programs, such as Type and Speak, Keytalk, and Talking Textwriter, are selected to provide the speech-impaired person with auditory feedback for spelling and writing activities, while also providing the opportunity to explore a variety of consonant vowel combinations both graphically and auditorily.

Phase IV involves the development of sentence comprehension activities in which the speech-impaired person must access words through both the direct visual route and phonetic recoding. This involves creating meaningful contexts in which both sight word vocabulary and novel phonetic forms must be read for a given sentence to be understood.

## EFFECTIVENESS OF STRATEGY

Of the 6 children for whom this instructional approach has been used, all 6 have kept up with their speaking classmates in phonetic recoding skills (by successfully completing Part I of the SRA reader and other phonetic-based reading curricula), while exceeding their speaking peers in sight word recognition. Developing materials that reflected each child's emerging language skills contributed to the success of this approach.

## REFERENCES

Blau, A., Valdes, D., & Quintas, R. (1985). Nonspeech symbol adaptation: SRA basic reading series, Level A, Part I. Unpublished reading instruction material.

Coltheart, M. (1978). Lexical access in simple reading tasks. In G. Underwood (Ed.), Strategies of information processing. New York: Academic Press.

Dewsbury, A., Jennings, J., & Boyle, D.  (1983).  Bridge reading kit.  Toronto, Ontario: OISE Press.

Jorm, A., & Share, D.  (1983).  Phonological recoding and reading acquisition.  Applied Psycholinguistics, 4, 103-147.

Jorm, A., Share, D., Maclean, R., & Matthews, R.  (1984).  Phonological recoding skills and learning to read:  A longitudinal study.  Applied Psycholinguistics, 5, 201-207.

Mitchell, D.  (1982).  The process of reading:  A cognitive analysis of fluent reading and learning to read.  New York:  Wiley & Sons.

Rasmussen, D., & Goldberg, L.  (1976).  SRA basic reading series, Level A, Part I. Science Research Associates, Inc.

## *Talking Software for Literacy Development*

Computer Software for Remediation of Dyslexia (under development), available from B. Fox, Laureate Learning Systems, Inc., One Mill St., Burlington, VT  05401

Keytalk, available from Santa Monica, CA:  PEAL Software

Talking Textwriter, Apple II version available from Scholastic Inc., P.O. Box 7502, 2931 E. McCarty St., Jefferson City, MD  65102; IBM version entitled, "Listen to Learn," available at IBM product centers or authorized dealerships.

Type & Speak, available from H. Shane and A. Field, Institute on Technology in Education and Communication, Box 1155, Brookline, MA  02146.  Writing to Read, J.H. Martin, available at IBM product centers or authorized dealerships.

## ADDITIONAL READINGS

Rosegrant, T. (1984). Fostering progress in literacy development: Technology and social interaction. Seminars in Speech & Language, 5(1), 47-57.

Rosegrant, T. (1986). It doesn't sound right: The role of speech output as a primary form of feedback for beginning text revision. Paper presented at Annual Meeting of the American Educational Research Association, San Francisco. Available from Center for Learning and Technology, 217 Baldy Hall, State University of New York at Buffalo, Buffalo, NY 14260.

## MODELING PROCEDURES FOR INCREASED USE OF
## COMMUNICATIVE FUNCTIONS IN COMMUNICATION AID USERS

*Joan Bruno*
*Communication Technology Center*
*Children's Seashore House*
*Atlantic City, New Jersey*

## INTRODUCTION

The adult language model plays an important role in language acquisition for speaking children as well as children with severe speech impairments. There is limited yet positive evidence in the literature that supports the importance of modeling for language board users (Bottorf & DePape, 1982; Musselwhite & St. Louis, 1982). Successful modeling of a communication aid can be used to facilitate gains in syntactic development, semantic associations, and phonetic cueing. It also may increase the individuals's understanding and use of various communicative functions.

With modeling, performance of a task is the result of a demonstration, not an explanation. As a result, many populations, including motor, hearing, language, or cognitively impaired individuals who use communication aids can benefit from modeling techniques.

## PURPOSE OF THE STRATEGY

To facilitate an increase in the use of communication aids--electronic and nonelectronic--for a variety of communicative functions through modeling techniques.

## UNDERLYING ASSUMPTIONS

1. *Client*. This strategy can be used with children who are being introduced to a communication aid or who demonstrate limited use of their aid. These children

should be appropriately seated and positioned for using an aid and should have a reliable means of access. The children should not exhibit severe sensory impairments or social/emotional problems. It should be noted that the strategy may also be used with cognitively impaired adults.

2. *Augmentative components*. The clinician models either by pointing directly to the symbols on the client's aid, or by using the same technique as the individual (e.g., scanning on the person's electronic system to select appropriate symbols or eye pointing to encode a message). Appropriate symbols are available on the vocabulary display to encode the targeted communication functions.

3. *Environmental constraints*. The individual should have the communication aid available in multiple environments and for a variety of activities. Family/staff should be trained as facilitators to use appropriate vocabulary and to employ specific modeling techniques. Such training involves both the observation of treatment sessions and instruction in modeling techniques. During training, communication partners must be familiarized with the location of symbols on the communication board.

4. *Other basic assumptions*. Other basic assumptions include: (a) baseline data are available on the individuals's current use of various communication functions; and (b) data collected relative to the person's receptive language skills, memory capabilities, and syntactic abilities are utilized to determine the appropriate linguistic complexity to be modeled.

## DESCRIPTION OF STRATEGY

### Goal Setting

The speech-language pathologist selects the *target communicative function* (e.g., requesting information about the location of objects, commenting on an activity, telling a joke, responding to a question, etc.). Criteria are established regarding the complexity of targeted responses, such as single words, multiple symbol(s), and selection and sequencing of required lexical items (e.g., interrogative + noun). Then, with information from the family and educational staff, appropriate lexical items are targeted (e.g., Where + _____), and modeling contexts are selected (e.g., mealtimes). Speech-language pathologists and special educators should be sure that the client understands the symbol-meaning relationship. It is important to note that several communicative functions may be targeted simultaneously, if appropriate.

## *Facilitator Training*

During training, the speech-language pathologist describes the goals of the modeling program to the facilitator and demonstrates how the individual's symbols can be used to express the targeted message type. Facilitators can practice modeling on the client's display or on communication boards that are similar to the individual's communication board. This not only helps to sensitize them to the communicative constraints of the person's aid, but also increases their awareness of the content and location of the lexical items on the board.

The complexity of modeling is also demonstrated to the facilitator. Depending on the client's ability, the facilitator is instructed to use (e.g., point to, encode) complete sentences, telegraphic utterances, or single-word linguistic models. If necessary, the facilitator is taught the mechanics of the individual's augmentative aid and/or techniques. For example, in using a letter/number encoding aid, two options are given: (a) the facilitator can model by pointing directly to the lexical item(s) (e.g., *Where* is the *cookie*?); or (b) the facilitator can be taught and encouraged to model via the client's codes (e.g., *Where is the cookie?* may be entered as W2 C3).

As the facilitator models on the individual's board, continued use of spoken output should be stressed. Modeling may be telegraphic, but the facilitator should be instructed to use complete sentences, appropriate to the client's linguistic level, when speaking.

Training procedures are similar for modeling the use of a voice output communication aid. As part of the training procedure, the facilitator should not only be instructed to point to a symbol on the client's board, but to activate the voice as well. Again, while system modeling may be telegraphic, facilitators should reflect the intended meaning of the utterance and use mature sentence structure.

Training the facilitator increases the likelihood that modeling can and will occur outside the treatment environment. Modeling the "target function" can occur during role playing as well as in real-life situations.

## *Client Training*

Specific training strategies will depend largely on the targeted communicative function. For example, when teaching use of interrogative forms to request information, the clinician and facilitator may need to insure that needed objects are missing. They will model use of the communication aid to achieve the targeted function by selecting the appropriate lexical items from the client's aid. The facilitator will also model usage outside the treatment context, thereby increasing the client's exposure to the targeted function in the natural environment.  Obviously, use of the target function should be reinforced appropriately.  Partial responses from individuals should be accepted; however, the target form should be modeled again.

During initial training, modeling should be used all of the time.  Gradually, the use of modeling is decreased to determine whether the client is learning how to use the target function.  Frequent, spontaneous use of the function by an individual will indicate a reduction of the need for modeling by the speech-language pathologist and the facilitator.

If the client does not use the target function after considerable training, it may be necessary to utilize small group settings, with all members of the group working on the same function.  While it is not necessary for all group members to be severely speech-impaired, they should be required to use a communication board.  Thus, the frequency of modeling is increased and the severely speech-impaired individual can observe the consequences of correct use of the target form.  Failure to use the target function after repeated modeling of the function may indicate a need to reassess the appropriateness of the target.  Continued progress, however, indicates that the client is ready to be introduced to new functions and/or more complex forms.

## EFFECTIVENESS OF STRATEGY

Bruno and Bryen (1985) studied the frequency of modeling by speech-language pathologists in a therapy environment and its impact on physically handicapped children.  Subjects ranged in age from 5 years to 15 years 11 months.  Receptive language abilities ranged from 18 months to 15 years.  Results showed that among the clinicians who participated in the study, those trained in modeling procedures modeled significantly more than the untrained clinicians.  In addition, children exposed to modeling frequently generated statements that mirrored the facilitator's statements in both form and content.  Only rarely did a child generate a statement with fewer elements than modeled, and on no occasion did a child elaborate beyond what had been modeled by the clinician.  Modeling appeared to have a more significant impact on children with lower cognitive abilities.

While modeling is an important clinical tool, treatment activities and communicative context appeared to be equally important in influencing the type of statements that these children generated on a communication aid.  In this study, it was demonstrated that whether or not modeling was employed, the variety of communicative functions used by a child was largely dependent upon the type of therapeutic activity employed. In structured therapy sessions that utilized a stimulus-response format, the child only responded to the therapist's requests. However, in more activity-oriented sessions, opportunities arose that enabled the child to use a variety of communicative functions, including the target function.

## REFERENCES

Bottorf, L., & DePape, D. (1982). Initiating communication systems for severely speech impaired persons. Topics in Language Disorders, 2, 55-72.

Bruno, J., & Bryen, D. (1985). The impact of modeling on language board users. Unpublished paper, Temple University, Philadelphia, and Children's Seashore House, Atlantic City, NJ.

Musselwhite, C., & St. Louis, K. (1982). Communication programming for the severely handicapped: Vocal and non-vocal strategies. San Diego, CA: College Hill Press.

## ADDITIONAL READINGS

Calculator, S., & Luchko, C. (1983). Evaluating the effectiveness of a communication board training program. Journal of Speech and Hearing Disorders, 48, 185-191.

Conti-Ramsden, G., & Friel-Patti, S. (1983). Mothers discourse adjustments to language-impaired and non-language impaired children. Journal of Speech and Hearing Disorders, 48, 360-367.

Cross, T. (1984). Habilitating the language-impaired child: Ideas from studies of parent-child interaction. Topics in Language Disorders, 4, 1-14.

Harris, D. (1982). Communicative interaction processes involving non-vocal physically handicapped children. Topics in Language Disorders, 2, 21-38.

Lasky, E., & Klopp, K. (1982). Parent-child interactions in normal and language disordered children. Journal of Speech and Hearing Disorders, 47, 7-18.

Ratner, N. (1983).  How we talk to children:  Its theoretical and clinical implications. <u>Journal of the National Student Speech and Hearing Association</u>, <u>11</u>(1), 33-45.

Schodorf, J., & Edwards, H. (1983).  Comparative analysis of parent-child interactions with the language-disordered and linguistically normal children.  <u>Journal of Communication Disorders</u>, <u>16</u>, 71-83.

Yoder, D., & Kraat, A. (1983).  Intervention issues in non-speech communication.  In J. Miller, D. Yoder, & R. Schiefelbusch (Eds.), <u>Contemporary issues in language intervention</u>.  <u>ASHA Reports</u>, <u>12</u>, 27-51.

# ESTABLISHING THE USE OF MULTIMODALITIES USING THE COMMUNICATIVE INTERACTION ASSESSMENT PROCEDURE

*E. Lucinda Cassatt-James*
*American Speech-Language-Hearing Association*
*Rockville, Maryland*

## INTRODUCTION

Empirical studies have shown that many severely speech-impaired individuals who use augmentative aids and techniques are only passive participants in the social interaction process (Kratt, 1985). They rely very little on their formal communication systems when communicating with others, preferring instead those modes that are more rapid and less physically taxing such as gestures and vocalizations (Calculator & Dollaghan, 1982; Harris, 1982; Light, Collier, & Parnes, 1985b). These findings hold true regardless of whether clients communicate with electronic or nonelectronic aids. Research has also shown that the conversational skills of these persons are significantly affected by their communication partner because of the altered role of participants in natural-augmented speaker dyads (Kratt, 1985; Light et al., 1985b). The implication of such findings is that intervention programs for individuals who use augmentative aids and techniques must be dramatically altered. Focus must be shifted away from the provision of communication aids as a therapy goal and toward using them as a means of developing communicative competence. This strategy focuses on training conversational partners to identify and facilitate the use of multiple modes of communication in severely speech-impaired individuals. Communication via multiple modes, a philosophy which has received recent emphasis in the literature (Kratt, 1985; see also chapters 1, 3, & 5), enhances expression of the communicative intent of messages, permits more rapid communication, and reduces potential communication breakdowns by reducing message ambiguity.

## PURPOSE OF STRATEGY

The purposes of this strategy are to: (a) provide a structured procedure for studying the modes of communication employed by nonspeaking persons, and (b) systematically foster the use of multiple modes of communication by training the nonspeaking person's communication partners.

# UNDERLYING ASSUMPTIONS

1. *Client*.  This strategy can be used with children and adults who use various communication aids and techniques and who exhibit a wide range of developmental levels and handicapping conditions.

2. *Augmentative components*.  The strategy can be used to study and to foster the use of a variety of communication modes, including formal augmentative aids and techniques, vocalizations, verbalizations, gestures, signs, and eye gaze.

*3. Environmental constraints*.  The videotape analysis required for this strategy may limit its utility in some settings.  Individual clinicians, however, may find it beneficial to use the communicative interaction sampling technique to informally profile their clients' strengths and weaknesses even if they do not complete a formal analysis. On-line recording of interactional behaviors is possible; however, increased validity and reliability of the procedure occurs if the clinician works from a permanent recording of the interaction sample.

The clinical utility of this procedure depends on the active participation of the severely speech-impaired individual and the individual's communication partners. Partners must be willing to participate throughout the intervention phase of the treatment program.

# DESCRIPTION OF STRATEGY

This intervention strategy is organized into three phases:   (a) an evaluation phase, (b) a goal development phase, and (c) a training phase.

## Evaluation Phase

Determination of the types of communication modes employed by individuals with severe speech impairments necessitates systematic observation of their communicative behavior in a variety of contexts.  One formal method of studying interaction within nonspeaking/speaking dyads is the Communicative Interaction Assessment Procedure (CIAP).  This procedure is designed to:   (a) provide a comprehensive and indepth description of the dynamic interaction between persons who use augmentative communication techniques and their partners, and (b) allow the development of intervention goals based on this profile of strengths and weaknesses. The procedure can be used to study a variety of communication modes, including the use of augmentative aids, vocalizations, verbalizations, manual signs, informal gestures, and eye gaze. In addition, the CIAP enables the speech-language pathologist to determine the pragmatic variables that can affect communicative competence, including communicative functions of language and utilization of appropriate discourse maintenance strategies (see Table 6-1 for a listing of speech acts and discourse behaviors that can be assessed by the CIAP). A number of other extensive analysis systems are available for studying the interactional behavior of persons who use augmentative communication aids. The reader is referred to the work of Wexler, Blau, Leslie, and Dore (1983) and Light et al. (1985 a,b) for additional examples of indepth assessment protocols and to chapters 4 and 5 for further discussion.

## *Collecting the Data*

During the evaluation phase, data are systematically collected in two contexts: a naturalistic context and a contrived context.

*Naturalistic context*. The naturalistic context focuses on the "typical" communication produced by the participants during a familiar, unstructured event. The dyad is instructed to select and participate in a familiar, routine activity which is representative of a typical communication situation which the client experiences. Examples of selected activities include completing homework assignments, participating in games, and engaging in conversation. Although augmentative aids and techniques are always available during the observational period, partners are not asked to use them. Data from the observations provide information regarding the dyad's typical patterns of interaction. For example, it is possible to determine the severely speech-impaired person's favored communication modes, how communication aids are used during discourse, and what communication modes most frequently result in conversational failure. Information is also provided regarding the partner's recognition and acceptance of various communication avenues.

*Contrived context*. The contrived context involves utilization of a clinician-directed script that provides eliciting situations for each speech act and for topic initiation and maintenance strategies (see Figure 6-2 for an example of a script appropriate for a preschool child). This context attempts to ascertain the person's optimal communication behavior (e.g., whether the client has the capability to express

## TABLE 6-1. COMMUNICATIVE INTERACTION PROFILE CODING SCHEME

TURN

Intelligible turn
Unintelligible turn
No response
No opportunity to respond
Turn opportunity[a]

MODES OF COMMUNICATION

Verbalization
Vocalization
Gestures
Eyepointing
Head nod/shake
Idiosyncratic gesture
Communication aid
Laughs/smiles/cries

SPEECH ACTS[b]

Requests
  yes/no
  choice
  test
  closed
  open ended
  action

Responses
  confirmation/non
  process responses
  check
  reactive behavior

Statement
  labels
  explanations
  descriptions
  personal
  speaker action

Conventions
  exclamations
  calls
  social courtesies
  rhetorical questions
  game markers

Double scored
  speaker fill
  play

DISCOURSE

Main discourse
  topic continuity (new/old topic)
  discourse cohesion (forward/backward links)

Conversational breakdowns
  repaired
  unrepaired

Conversational repair strategies
  repetition request
  questioning
  suggestions
  prediction
  confirmation/non
  checks
  re-attempt (note mode used)
  third-person repair
  information
  miscellaneous

Composite speech act[c]
  questioning
  suggestion
  confirmation
  spelling
  letter/sound cueing
  information
  checks
  prediction
  guess
  miscellaneous

aAs defined by Light (1985a).

bDerived from Dore (1977).

cAs defined by Wexler et al. (1983).

**FIGURE 6-2. SNACK SCRIPT** *(CONTINUED ON NEXT PAGE).*

| CONTEXT | NARRATIVE |
|---|---|
| Child should be hungry. Teddy Bear & food are within view. | Hi (child's name.) |
| | Look at all this food. |
| | What should we do? |
| | I think somebody else is hungry! |
| Look to Teddy Bear | Call Teddy to come have a snack. |
| Bring out Teddy Bear. Let Teddy say "hi" to child. | Here's Teddy. He wants a snack. Teddy, say "hi!" |
| Put Teddy in chair and make food available. | Sit down, Teddy. It's time to eat. Who wants to eat? |
| | Teddy does. What do you want? |
| Pick up requested food. | What's this? |
| Give small amount of food to child. Pause for response. | |
| Direct attention away from child (up to 30 seconds). Wait for signal from child. | |
| (If no response) | Do you want some more? |
| | I wonder what you want? |
| Give child something other than what he/she asks for. | Here's the (requested food). |
| | Whoops, where is the (requested food). |
| Give child requested food. | I wish I had some! |
| If child indicates "yes"... If child indicates "no" ... If no response | Thank you Oh, well Can I have some? |

**FIGURE 6-2.  SNACK SCRIPT** *(CONTINUED)*.

| CONTEXT | NARRATIVE |
|---|---|
| Pretend you intend to eat all the food yourself.  Wait for response. | |
| (If no response) | Do you want some? |
| Present food so that child cannot eat it (e.g., no spoon, closed jar). | What's wrong? |
| | Oh dear.  What should I do? |
| Rectify problem and give child a few bites. | What is Teddy's favorite food? |
| | Well, let's be silly and give him some green beans instead. |
| Give Teddy green beans | Teddy says "yucky." |
| (Pause for response) (If no response) | Now what? |
| Comply with child's instructions. | |
| Have napkins, drink, cup in view. | I think Teddy wants a drink. What kind? |
| Give Teddy a drink, but spill some of it on child's table/tray.  Wait for a response. | What a mess. |
| If no response pick up napkin. (pause) | Who will clean it up? |
| Wipe up spill. | Who is still hungry? |
| Provide favorite food. | Time to clean up. |
| Pick up paper towel. | Who wants to clean the table? |
| | Does (caretaker) want to help? |
| If child responds "yes," | Call him/her |
| Clean the table. | Snack time is over. |
| Wave Teddy Bear's arm | Teddy says bye bye |

Revised from Blackstone, S., Cassatt, E. L., & Isaacson, R. (1983).  Snack script. in A. Kratt (Ed.), Communication interaction between aided and natural speakers:  An IPCAS study report.  Toronto:  Canadian Rehabilitation Council for the Disabled.

a greater range of speech act types, whether the client attempts to initiate communication if given the opportunity, and whether the client is skilled in repairing conversational breakdowns).

## Recording the Data

Because all modes of communication are being studied, as well as the behavior of both partners of the dyad, videotape recording is used to collect a sample of behavior. Overall, the entire procedure requires a minimum of 40 to 45 minutes. A brief warm-up period of 5 minutes is suggested prior to the formal data collection period.

## Goal Development Phase

## Using The Communicative Interaction Profile

Study of the communicative interaction profile provides information on a number of parameters, including: the number of modes used, whether specific modes are used to communicate specific speech acts, whether a partner responds to the use of various modes, and the roles of both partners in maintaining discourse. Speech acts used to initiate and maintain the discourse can be identified, and the balance of initiator versus responder roles can be evaluated. The profile also provides information on communication failures as well as data on each partner's attempts to repair conversational breakdowns. Just as important is information describing how the dyads maintain the discourse and how they circumvent possible communication failures. Validity and reliability of the data obtained from the evaluation phase can be strengthened if the clinician practices recording, transcribing, and analyzing several interactional samples. It is suggested that intermittent reliability checks be completed on a regular basis to insure accuracy of scoring.

## Targeting Intervention Goals

Selecting appropriate therapy goals requires identification of the communication skills of both partners. This will include identification of communication behaviors that facilitate or promote the maintenance of the conversation as well as behaviors that are absent from or which interfere with the successful completion of the discourse. This strategy demonstrates the use of the CIAP as a clinical tool for developing intervention goals in the area of multi-modal communication.

## *Considering Use of Multiple Communication Modes*

Before developing goals to foster a client's use of multiple communication modes, results of the assessment procedure must be considered from several perspectives. First, a similar pattern of mode use across the two assessment contexts may suggest that the range of communication avenues available to the client is related to client characteristics. For example, if a limited range of modes is recorded in both contexts, the clinician should determine whether the client's physical condition precludes use of a greater number of communication channels. Limitations in mode use could also be related to the client's lack of awareness of and/or experience with the different modes available for communicating. Also, restricted expression associated with some modes (e.g., the communication board) may simply be due to a lack of training in its interactional use.

In some instances, the clinician may find that the client utilizes a greater variety of communication channels in the contrived setting than in the naturalistic setting. This may be a direct result of the partner's behavior. Often, a partner's unresponsiveness to or lack of understanding of communication attempts via a particular mode results in restricted use of that mode. It may also be that partners are extremely successful at understanding messages produced via certain modes; therefore, the client prefers communicating via those modes to the exclusion of others.

In summary, evaluating multimodal communication is a complex process that requires the clinician to examine the performance of the nonspeaking person and the comunication partner in each of the assessment contexts. Observations reveal whether a nonspeaking client spontaneously uses a variety of communication modes. If limitations exist, the communication behaviors of both partners are studied in context to identify those variables that have a negative impact on the client's successful use of various modes of communication. Intervention goals may involve expanding the nonspeaking person's use of different modes and/or developing the partner's recognition and interpretation of communication via a variety of different modes.

## Training Phase

## *Employing Client-Centered Training*

In training, emphasis is placed on developing the skills of the client within a naturalistic setting. The task of developing the nonspeaking client's use of various communication modes will be influenced by a number of considerations, including developmental level and motoric skills. The developmental level of a client will influence the training approach. For example, older clients may benefit from didactic sessions that provide direct instruction on the use of specific modes to express specific communicative functions and from role play, interviewing, and dramatic play activities. Younger and less cognitively advanced clients will benefit from modeling, shaping, and contingent reinforcement of various behaviors during play routines or daily living activities. The impact of motor limitations on the use of various modes is obvious. Often, certain modes of expression are precluded due to a lack of volitional motor control. In some instances, use of other communication modes (e.g., reliable motor movement needed for switch activation) can be trained using systematic procedures and input from members of an interdisciplinary team.

## *Employing Partner-Centered Training*

Communication breakdowns may occur because the communication partner fails to recognize the various modes used by the client. In these instances, systematic partner training is required. To develop a communication partner's awareness and responsiveness to a client's use of various communication modes, a four-step procedure is employed. First, a didactic session is scheduled which focuses on the many modes of communication used by both unimpaired and impaired speakers during interaction. The ways in which various communication modes can be used to express similar communicative functions and the ways in which these various modes foster rapid and efficient communication are highlighted.

Second, videotapes of clinician-client interactions are reviewed. Initially, the clinician and the partner work together to identify each turn attempted by the client and to describe the communication mode employed. Using contextual information and background knowledge about the client, the clinician fosters the partner's ability to interpret the communicative intent and discourse function of the client's message. Gradually, the partner independently learns to identify the occurrence of turns, the communication mode used, and the general purpose of each of the client's communication attempts.

Third, videotapes of the partner-client interaction are presented. At this level, the client's behavior as well as the partner's responses are studied. This step provides the partner with more practice in recognizing various communication modes and their intent/discourse purpose. It also provides a means by which the partners can objectively study their style of interaction with the client.

Finally, after the partner reliably identifies the nonspeaking person's communication attempts using a variety of different modes, generalization practice is provided in the naturalistic setting. The purpose of this fourth step is to insure generalization of the principles identified using the videotapes. Using a functional context, the client and the client's communication partner are observed interacting during an activity of their choice. Throughout the activity, the partner labels the client's communication attempts, specifies the modes used, and responds appropriately depending upon the function of the message. The clinician observes but does not actively participate. The clinician's role is to provide support to the partner, reinforcing accurate responses and identifying the client's unrecognized communication attempts.

Maintenance sessions are provided on an intermittent basis. The partner's skill in recognizing and responding to various communication modes is monitored along with other treatment goals.


## EVALUATION OF EFFECTIVENESS:
## A CASE STUDY


To illustrate the use of the CIAP approach and multimodal training, data obtained from an analysis of the communication interaction between a 3-year-old, severely physically handicapped preschooler using a language board and her mother are presented. Observations regarding the use of multiple modes are described, and intervention goals derived from study of the findings are discussed.


*Observing the Client Using Multiple Modes of Communication in Two Contexts Revealed:*

1.  The intelligibility of the child's communication attempts varied depending upon the context. The number of unintelligible utterances was greater during the mother-child activity as compared to the clinician-child activity (24 percent and 12 percent unintelligible responses, respectively).

    The client used a full range of communication modes during both the mother-child and the clinician-child activities; therefore conversational breakdowns were not a result of the child's inability to express herself via a variety of different communication modes.

Both the parent and the clinician experienced difficulty understanding the child's communication produced via vocalizations/verbalizations. The mother, however, also experienced difficulty understanding eye pointing and informal gestures. The mother had difficulty interpreting her child's communication attempts via multiple communication modes. This resulted in the child's reduced intelligibility.

2. Study of the mother's behavior also revealed that she frequently did not recognize her child's communication. The mother responded most consistently to messages expressed via the communication board or to yes/no indications.

3. Further study of the mother-child interaction revealed that the preschooler frequently was given no opportunity to respond to contingent utterances. This caused significant asynchronism in the turntaking patterns of the two partners.

4. It was also observed that the child used her communication board less frequently when interacting with her mother than with the clinician (5 percent to 20 percent, respectively).

### *Fostering Successful Use of Multiple Modes of Communication*

During the goal development phase, the primary emphasis was on:

1. increasing the child's successful communication attempts via multiple communication modes; and

2. increasing the communication partner's recognition and acceptance of communication via a variety of channels.

During the training phase, objectives and training strategies for the partner included:

1. improving the parent's understanding of the child's communication. Strategy: The parent, under the clinician's supervision, practiced interpreting the intent of the child's messages (particularly those produced by eye pointing and gestures) by utilizing background knowledge of the child's interests and routines and by utilizing cues

available in the context. Conversational repair strategies (e.g., requesting repetition, requesting use of alternate modes) were also discussed and practiced. All activities were executed within the naturalistic environment.

2. developing an awareness on the part of the communication partner that the child was attempting to communicate. Strategy: The parent studied videotapes of the child interacting with various communication partners and identified when and how (i.e., with which modes) communication was attempted.

3. insuring that the child had ample time to initiate and/or respond. Strategy: The parent was taught to monitor her behavior and provide longer pauses between her turns.

4. encouraging use of the communication board. Strategy: The mother was taught to model use of the aid during all interactions. For example, if the client vocalized and gestured to a nearby object, the mother modeled the request using the formal communication aid and then provided the child with the desired object.

## REFERENCES

Blackstone, S., Cassatt, E., & Isaacson, R. (1983). Snack script. In A. Kraat (Ed.), Communication interaction between aided and natural speakers: An IPCAS study report. Toronto: Canadian Rehabilitation Council for the Disabled.

Calculator, S., & Dollaghan, C. (1982). The use of communication boards in a residential setting: An evaluation. Journal of Speech and Hearing Disorders, 47, 281-287.

Dore, J. (1977). "Oh them sheriff": A pragmatic analysis of children's responses to questions. In S. Ervin-Tripp & C. Mitchell-Kerman (Eds.,), Child discourse. New York: Academic Press.

Harris, D. (1982). Communication interaction processes involving nonvocal physically handicapped children. Topics in Language Disorders, 2, 21-37.

Kratt, A. (1985). <u>Communication interaction between aided and natural speakers: An IPCAS study report</u>. Toronto: Canadian Rehabilitation Council.

Light, J., Collier, B., & Parnes, P. (1985a). Communicative interaction between young nonspeaking physically disabled children and their primary caregivers: Part II - Communicative functions. <u>Augmentative and Alternative Communication</u>, <u>1</u>(3), 98-107.

Light, J., Collier, B., & Parnes, P. (1985b). Communicative interaction between young nonspeaking physically disabled children and their primary caregivers: Part I - Discourse patterns. <u>Augmentative and Alternative Communication</u>, <u>1</u>, 74-83.

Wexler, K., Blau, A., Leslie, S., & Dore, J. (1983). <u>Conversational interaction of nonspeaking cerebral palsied individuals and their speaking partners, with and without augmentative communication aids.</u> Unpublished manuscript, Helen Hayes Hospital, New York.

## AUGMENTATIVE INTERVENTIONS IN INTENSIVE CARE UNITS

*Patricia Dowden*
*Augmentative Communication Center*
*University Hospital*
*Seattle, Washington*

### INTRODUCTION

Serving severely speech-impaired patients in intensive care units (ICU) and emergency rooms (ER) differs in several respects from serving other individuals who require communication augmentation. These patients are medically unstable and unable to tolerate lengthy evaluations or training sessions. The daily schedule in intensive care is often full and unpredictable, necessitating rapid and flexible intervention procedures. In emergency rooms, the pace is even more rapid and unpredictable. This strategy focuses on intervention in the intensive care units of acute care hospitals.

### PURPOSE OF STRATEGY

The purpose of this strategy is to augment the communication of severely speech-impaired patients in intensive care units and emergency rooms.

### UNDERLYING ASSUMPTIONS

1. *Client*. The characteristics of patients in intensive care units (ICU) have been described thoroughly in a study at University of Washington Hospitals (Dowden, Beukelman, & Lossing, in press). According to this study, the majority of these patients have pulmonary insufficiency as either a primary or secondary diagnosis. This means that most of the patients are tracheostomized or intubated; the most common type of augmentative aid used to assist these patients is the electrolarynx or a modified airflow system available as part of specialized tracheostomy tubes. During

two years of data collection, these oral techniques accounted for 49 percent of all interventions. The majority of the adult patients studied had sufficient language abilities to use a variety of communication aids and techniques; therefore, a detailed language assessment was unnecessary in most cases. However, their cognition tended to fluctuate, often interfering with their use of a particular aid or technique. The patients also appeared to vary in their emotional response to augmentative communication. It is believed that approximately one-third of all failures were due to the patients' rejection of the communication aid or technique.

Emergency room (ER) patients are typically very different. Above all, communication is of secondary importance to any life-threatening medical condition; thus, the speech-language pathologist is called only when the patient's condition has been stabilized. In the case of traumatic injury, the patient is transferred to intensive care when stabilized, so the referral is made by ICU staff. There are, however, some patients in the ER who require our assistance. These patients are typically alert and not in a life-threatening condition. For example, speech-language pathologists are required when communication with the ER staff has failed because the patient does not speak English fluently or because the patient's speech is severely aphasic or dysarthric. Their role is to provide an interpreter or bilingual language boards for those who do not speak English. For language- or speech-impaired individuals, intervention varies, depending upon their capabilities and the needs of the ER staff at that moment. Often, speech-language pathologists assist by translating the most critical messages.

2. *Augmentative components and environmental constraints*. Environmental constraints in these settings are also unique. In most cases, the staff, the family, and the patient have no time or tolerance for training in the set-up, use, or maintenance of a communication aid or technique. An intervention must result in improved communication immediately with a minimum of effort (i.e., it must meet some of the communication needs of the patient that cannot be met by more conventional communication approaches). For example, it may not be an advantage to ICU personnel if a patient uses an aid to say *yes* or *no* instead of mouthing the words, since many people read lips very effectively. This is also true for mouthing some highly predictable words, such as *suction* and *air*, or for gestures of highly visual and predictable concepts, such as *hungry*. In addition, the use of any communication aid or technique in an ICU may be temporary due to changes in the patient's physical, cognitive, or emotional situation. It is essential that any intervention be reevaluated daily so that modifications can be made to reflect these changing capabilities or needs.

## DESCRIPTION OF STRATEGY

Evaluating patients for communication augmentation in any setting proceeds sequentially, beginning with a communication needs assessment and a capability assessment, and culminating in the selection of an augmentative approach. This is followed by training for the patient and significant partners. The effectiveness of this communication approach is then carefully evaluated. In emergency rooms and intensive care units, the entire process is severely truncated by the extreme time constraints. This discussion will focus on intervention in intensive care, where the time constraints are somewhat less severe. Since evaluation time is limited, however, the first two phases of the evaluation are conducted simultaneously rather than sequentially (see Dowden et al., 1986).

### *Needs Assessment*

The goal of this phase of the evaluation is to thoroughly assess the patient's communication needs. This information is obtained from the patient's chart or through interviews with the patient, the family, and the staff. Table 6-2 shows the major categories that are considered in the complete needs assessment, which includes over 70 questions about specific needs.

### *Capability Assessment and Selection of Augmentative Aids and Techniques*

Utilizing a hierarchy of assessment tasks, we try to determine during this phase of the evaluation whether the patient has the minimum abilities to utilize a given communication aid or technique. This phase of the assessment ends when we have sufficient information to arrange the potential augmentative communication techniques in a hierarchy from most to least desirable and to make recommendations. If it is determined that the patient has sufficient capabilities to use the most preferable communication technique and that this technique meets the patient's communication needs, the evaluation ends and trials with the technique are conducted. The hierarchy of communication techniques is shown in Table 6-3.

The various oral communication aids and techniques are considered simultaneously. The modified airflow devices are preferred, if possible, because of their similarity to natural speech. These devices include cuff deflation as well as use of the Pitt tube (National Catheter Company, Argyle, NY), the COMMUNItrach

## TABLE 6-2. NEEDS ASSESSMENT[a]

### 1. COMMUNICATION PARTNERS

- Perceptual abilities (hearing and vision)
- Proximity for communication
- Time constraints for communication
- Familiarity with the speech-impaired individual
- Familiarily with augmentative aids or techniques

### 2. ENVIRONMENT

- Locations
- Positions
- Physical constraints

### 3. MESSAGES AND MODALITIES

- Pragmatics of messages
- Output modalities
- Environmental control equipment

[a]From Beukelman, Yorkston, & Dowden, 1983.

## TABLE 6-3. COMMUNICATION AIDS AND TECHNIQUES

### 1. ORAL COMMUNICATION

- Modified airflow systems
- Electrolarynges

### 2. NONORAL COMMUNICATION

- Writing
- Direct Selection
- Limited Switch

(Implant Technologies, Inc., Minneapolis, MN), and other special types of tracheostomy tubes. The physician and the respiratory therapist are responsible for deciding which option to choose, although input from the speech-language pathologist may facilitate the decision.

If it is not possible to use the modified airflow techniques, then the electrolarynges are considered. These include the oral types, the neck types used at the neck or the cheek, and the nasal tube type, such as Venti-Voice (Bear Medical Systems, Inc., Riverside, CA). Frequently, the placement and the type of electrolarynx used are determined by medical considerations. These electrolarynges can be used independently, whether activated by hand or by a remote switch, or dependently, activated by the listener on cue from the speaker.

If it is an option, writing is the most preferable nonoral technique because it is the most conventional. Often, the speech-language pathologist or occupational therapist can make practical suggestions about the writing surface or utensil that will improve the efficiency of communication. For some patients, writing is useful for only part of the day (e.g., in a single position or only for brief periods). It can be supplemented by one of the direct-selection techniques.

The use of a direct-selection or limited-switch technique necessitates a longer evaluation than any approach described to this point. For these techniques the patient must be screened for motor, visual, and language capabilities. As mentioned above, screenings are conducted only until the patient's minimum capabilities to use the most desirable systems are ascertained. For example, if the patient can activate the keys on a Sharp Memowriter (Sharp Electronics Corporation, Paramus, NJ), trials with the system should begin immediately. If the patient can use this device with the staff to answer a few biographical questions, then the patient is presumed to have sufficient visual and language capabilities to use the aid.

More detailed assessments are required only if motor control precludes a direct-selection system. Before a limited-switch technique is tried, the patient's vision, language abilities in spelling and reading recognition, and motor control are screened by means of yes/no questions in switch trials. Using this information, the communication aids and techniques that are the best match between these capabilities and the patient's communication needs are selected for additional trials.

## Instructions for Patient and Partners

After the most appropriate augmentative components have been selected, it is essential to provide the patient, family, and ICU staff with sufficient information regarding the system, its use, and its maintenance. To some extent, this education is an on-going process that begins with regular in-services and presentations to ICU and critical-care unit (CCU) staff. These meetings are designed to familiarize the staff with communication augmentation in acute care, the techniques that are available for certain patients, and the operation and maintenance of the equipment. Then, when an augmentative approach has been recommended for an individual, we continue this training with more specific instructions and a demonstration for the patient and the primary nurse. Because hospital staff, families, friends and, above all, the patients have little time or tolerance for any training, the communication approach of choice should be as straightforward as possible, and the initial verbal instructions should be quite concise. These instructions are then followed by written instructions that are posted in the patient's room and inserted into the patient's chart with other daily care details for nursing. In most cases, we write both sets of instructions; in some ICUs, the chart information may be written by the primary nurse only.

The information that is provided in the patient's room and on the chart serves several purposes. Instructions must be provided that describe the set up of system components, including moving and repositioning the unit throughout the day, removing it in case of emergency, turning it on and off, and charging the batteries at night. There must also be instructions on how to interact with the patient, including where to stand for optimum communication, how to solve communication breakdowns, and how to maximize communication efficiency. In addition, there must be instructions relating to troubleshooting, including a list of potential problems and their solutions and whom to call if these solutions are ineffectual or if communication continues to be frustrating for whatever reason.

Although it is essential to make this information available, it is not sufficient to simply post it and expect everyone associated with the patient to be adequately informed. We often find staff, family, and the patient confused by equipment and extremely frustrated in their efforts to communicate, despite our careful instructions. Reasons for this failure vary. New staff or consulting staff often do not take the time to read the chart, or the information is removed from the chart in the patient's room. Family members and friends often do not read information posted in the patient's room because they believe it is personal information regarding the patient's medical condition. In addition, it is always possible that our instructions are insufficient and assume some familiarity with the aid or with communication augmentation in general. To counteract these factors, we take the following steps. First, we must determine that, at a minimum, the patient is completely familiar with system components and does not need additional instructions to operate it. Second, we provide the patient with a quick means of telling the staff, family, and friends to read the detailed instructions. One such method is simply to post the entire set of instructions (or a sign directing the reader to them) in a location convenient to the patient, so that the patient can point, gesture, or use eye gaze to draw the partner's attention to it. Third, we check back with the patient on a daily basis, often during both the day and evening shifts, to ascertain that everything is going smoothly. We use this opportunity to observe all kinds of partners in their interactions to determine whether the instructions we have provided require modification. We also use this oppportunity to evaluate the effectiveness of the communication approach, as described in the following section.

### *Evaluation of System Effectiveness*

The goal of the last phase of evaluation is to decide whether the augmentative system components recommended for a patient are appropriate. This can be determined by referring to the communication needs that were established previously. By consulting the patient, the staff, and the family, we determine the number of communication needs that are met. Whenever there are communication needs that were not met, we attempt to modify or change the aid and/or technique, or consider recommending additional ones to meet those needs.

## EFFECTIVENESS OF THE STRATEGY

In Dowden, Beukelman, and Lossing (in press), we describe the effectiveness of our intervention with ICU patients over a two-year period. We evaluated 50 patients, 48 of whom met our minimum-criteria on a cognitive screening task. Of these 48 patients, 3 were not served because they died or were transferred to another hospital. For the remaining 45 patients, we used 96 separate communication approaches, thus illustrating the instability of augmentative communication aids and techniques in the ICU.

Fifty-four percent of the interventions used during this 2-year period were successful, since the communication aids or techniques utilized met more than 50 percent of each patient's communication needs. In general, a combination of techniques was most successful in meeting the communication needs of these patients (e.g., an oral approach for speech and another aid to replace writing). We were least successful (i.e., met the fewest needs) with the patients who did most poorly on our cognitive screening task. In general, those patients who were unable to follow simple commands or to answer highly egocentric yes/no questions were not served well by the augmentative aids and techniques introduced. However, whether the patient was able to answer the questions relating to time or place appeared irrelevant to eventual success with a communication augmentation.

Approximately 39 percent of the patients used oral approaches, such as an electrolarynx or modified airway device. Forty-three percent of the patients used relatively inexpensive "light tech" aids, including plexiglass eye-gaze boards and various alphabet and word boards, despite the availability of high tech aids. Sixteen percent utilized the most common and inexpensive direct selection aids, such as the Sharp Memowriters (Sharp Electronics, Paramus, NJ) or the Canon (Telesensory Systems, Inc., Palo Alto, CA). Only one patient in this study used a more complicated aid. These findings suggest that speech-language pathologists can meet the communication needs of most patients typically seen in ICU with a few relatively inexpensive communication aids.

## REFERENCES

Beukelman, D., Yorkston, K., & Dowden, P. (1985). Communication augmentation: A casebook of clinical management. San Diego, CA: College Hill Press.

Dowden, P.A., Beukelman, D.R., & Lossing, C. (in press). Serving nonspeaking patients in acute care: Intervention outcomes. Augmentative and Alternative Communication.

## ADDITIONAL READINGS

Dowden, P.A., Honsinger, M.J., & Beukelman, D.R. (1986). Serving nonspeaking patients in acute care: An intervention approach. Augmentative and Alternative Communication, 2(1), 25-32.

Hammond, M., Cox, P., & Scarpelli, A. (1982). A remotely controlled neck-type electrolarynx for the tracheostomized quadriplegic. Paper presented at the Annual Convention of the American Speech-Language-Hearing Association.

Summers, J. (1973). The use of the electrolarynx in patients with temporary tracheostomies. Journal of Speech and Hearing Disorders, 38, 335-338.

## ENHANCING INTERACTION THROUGH ROLE PLAYING

*Judith R. Frumkin*
*Schneier Communication Unit*
*United Cerebral Palsy and*
  *Handicapped Children's Association*
*Syracuse, New York*

## INTRODUCTION

The successful use of an augmentative communication aid or technique is dependent upon the user's ability to interact effectively and efficiently within a communication environment. Persons who use communication aids must be able to initiate conversation, maintain topic relevancy, and adjust expressive output according to situations that may arise or cues that are given by a communication partner. Role-playing techniques using scripts that are written specifically for a client can be an effective intervention strategy that will encourage the development of pragmatic functions and conversational strategies for successful communication.

Lieven (1984) describes the creative skill of young language learners as they utilize routine utterances in unexpected but appropriate situations. Persons who use augmentative components also need to develop the ability to recognize situations where specific utterances can be utilized for maintenance of effective and efficient conversational pursuits. As the client becomes adept at role playing using the scripts, interaction in settings other than the originally selected environment will be facilitated.

## PURPOSE OF STRATEGY

The goal of this strategy is to facilitate the interactive competency of persons who use communication aids by utilizing role-playing techniques and scripted dialogues. Specific discourse functions, such as turntaking behaviors, repair and breakdown strategies, and maintenance of topic relevancy can be identified and developed through the use of structured role-playing activities. Guidelines and suggestions are provided for utilizing scripts in a variety of communication environments.   A communication environment is defined as a setting or situation where two or more individuals gather to exchange information of a communicative nature (Frumkin & Baker, in press).

## UNDERLYING ASSUMPTIONS

1. *Client*.   The age, diagnosis, or handicapping condition of persons using communication aids are irrelevant to the implementation of this strategy.   However, developmental level and cognitive abilities must be determined on an individual basis so that the selected activities and the linguistic content of the scripts are appropriately developed.

2. *Augmentative components*.   Any type of nonelectronic or electronic communication device with vocabulary and lexical entries that can be determined and programmed by the user and/or supportive personnel can be used.  Symbol selection, type of display, and access factors should not affect the decision to employ this strategy.

3. *Environmental constraints*.   The availability of staff, peers, and family (if possible) is considered an integral component for the success of this strategy. Individuals with whom the user can interact should be available throughout the training period.   Identification of communication environments and specific contexts where communication frequently takes place must be determined.   There are no time constraints that affect the training period; the strategy can be utilized as an integral part of the on-going process toward the development of interactive behaviors.

4. *Other basic assumptions*.   For training, several routine activities/communication environments have been selected, as well as vocabulary, lexical items, and dialogues that are appropriate to the client's participation in activities.

## DESCRIPTION OF STRATEGY

The steps that should be followed in implementing this strategy are outlined below.

*Selection of Communication Environments/Activities*

Factors that affect the selection of routine activities include the client's age, the various settings in which the client spends a majority of time, and the individuals with whom the client communicates in these settings. Examples of communication environments are illustrated in Table 6-4.

## TABLE 6-4. EXAMPLES OF COMMUNICATION ENVIRONMENTS

| Communication environment | Client | Primary partner | Discourse objective |
| --- | --- | --- | --- |
| 1. Playtime | Child | Caregiver (mother/father, etc.) | Topic Development/ turntaking |
| 2. Lunchtime | Child | Schoolmate | Initiation of conversation |
| 3. Recreation time | Adolescent | Rehabilitation counselor/aid | Conversation repair |
| 4. Work station | Adult | Manager | Topic relevancy/ clarification |

Considerations regarding the listener and the listener's role during conversation will depend upon the particular activity and the listener's familiarity with the client.

*Incorporating Communication Environments into a Role-Playing Activity*

After identifying and selecting a communication environment, the speech-language pathologist prepares a script to be used within that environment, presents it to the client for approval, and then prepares the vocabulary display and programs it into the communication aid, if necessary. For example, a child, age 9, using a Phonic Ear VOIS 135 (Phonic Ear, Inc., Mill Valley, CA), may have selected utterances related to a lunchtime routine programmed into the VOIS. The role-playing activity is presented as "Let's pretend it's (lunchtime). I'll be your (schoolmate) and this is what we might say." The dialogue for the listener's role is organized to prompt the production of the selected utterances by the aid user. In general, the vocabulary and dialogues will be personalized and the context specific, depending upon the client's situation and needs.

The following is an example of a scripted dialogue for playtime, which is an identified communication environment of a child, age 4. This child is using a picture communication board, with Picsym symbols and colored pictures, accessed directly with an index finger. The symbols placed on the board represent the entire utterance. For example, the sentence "I want to watch you make a necklace" is represented by the Picsym symbol *want* and a picture of a necklace incorporated into one picture (as illustrated in Figure 6-3). This enables the youngster to select messages efficiently using only one directed point. The burden of selecting more than one symbol for one utterance would interfere with the progression of conversation, thus impeding the effective interaction that is the objective of this strategy. The individual who trains the child to use this strategy reviews the picture symbols, identifying them as whole sentences during the initial training process. Complete sentences are used in the following example in order to facilitate the use of the script.

Communication Environment:  Playtime
  Materials suggested:  beads, string
  (key:  C = client;  P = partner)

P:      What shall we play with now?
C:      *I want to watch you make a necklace.  [want/necklace]*
P:      You will have to help me do it.  What should I do first?
C:      *Take a bead and put it on the string.  [bead/rope]*
P:      I have lots of beads here.  Tell me something about the beads that you would like.
C:      *I like big beads.  I want beads to wear on my neck.  [big/necklace]*
P:      You want a big necklace.  It will take some time.


(Partner deliberately does not tie a knot at the end of the string.)

P:      Oh no!  What happened?
C:      *The beads fell down.  There isn't a knot at the end.  You're silly! [down/silly]*
P:      You can help me.  Please hold the end and we'll see if we can make it work.
C:      *We did it.  Make another one.  [make]*
P:      I'll put these beads in the can and shake it up.  What a lot of noise.
C:      *That's loud music!  Put on the radio too.  I like that music.  [music/like]*

**FIGURE 6-3. "I WANT BEADS TO WEAR ON MY NECK"**

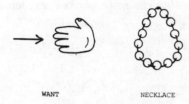

(Reprinted from F. Carlson (1985), Picsyms categorical dictionary, Lawrence, KS: Baggeboda Press.)

The following is a script for use with a 9-year-old child in a lunchtime communication environment. The augmentative communication device selected is a Light Talker with Minspeak software and spoken output (Prentke-Romich Co., Wooster, OH) that is accessed indirectly with a single switch (rocking lever in a row-column scanning mode). A combination of Minsymbols and Rebus symbols are utilized for utterance retrieval on the device's display. Whole utterances are programmmed into the Light Talker, requiring selection of an appropriate symbol sequence for expression. The utterances are reviewed during training with the user. Minspeak provides the user with a finite number of symbols that are used to represent concepts specific to the individual's situation and experience. The symbols are programmed in a sequence that is dependent upon utterances desired by the user. The selected utterances are summarized by the concepts or symbols most associated with their meaning. It is suggested that each script be designed according to a specific symbol theme, a feature that allows the user to categorize similar sentences with a concept grouping (e.g., sentences can be programmed under a theme of "dressing"; subsequent selection of symbols will recall programmed utterances related to that concept). For more detailed information regarding Minspeak, refer to the Minspeak application guide available through Prentke-Romich Co.

Communication Environment: Lunchtime
(key: C = client; P = partner)

C: *I'm hungry.*
P: Me too. Let's go eat.
C: *Will you help me carry my lunch?*
P: Sure.
C: *Thanks. What do you have to eat? I hope my food is good.*
P: My lunch looks okay.
C: *I wish we could go to Burger King instead.*

P:     Oh yeah.  Me too.  Their new Whoppers are great.

C:     *I think so too. I really like the milk shakes, especially chocolate.  Maybe we could go to a restaurant together sometime.*

P:     Okay.  Maybe.  Let's eat.

## *Expanding the Use of Dialogues*

Once the role-playing script is successful within the training context, the client is placed in "real" communication environment(s) (e.g., a 9-year-old child becomes involved in a lunchtime routine with another youngster).  Initially, personnel involved with the training should be present; the user can then be assisted, reinforced, and praised during the interactive situation.  Although a new partner's dialogue will vary from the script, the user will find the selected utterances available and useful within that setting.  Vocabulary selected for that activity can be enhanced and modified by other lexical items available on the communication aid.

As persons who use communication aids become more adept at utilizing practiced scripts and other vocabulary items, interaction in settings other than the original environment selected will be facilitated.  In this way, clients begin to establish a repertoire of utterances that nurture the development of appropriate pragmatic behaviors in various communication environments.

## EFFECTIVENESS

The use of role-playing techniques and scripts is described with a nonspeaking, 7-year-old child (J.) with spina bifida and complicating medical problems that include a permanent tracheostomy and oral-motor dysfunction.  Following an assessment of communication skills, treatment objectives were implemented, including training on symbol identification, use of symbols as representative language concepts, and initial communication aid usage.  The Phonic Ear VOIS 135 was selected as the most effective device for this child.  J. accessed the VOIS with a single digit, using Rebus symbols on the display for utterance retrieval.  Initial vocabulary selection programmed into the device included phrases and single words reflecting various semantic notions, such as requests ("I want _____," "I need _____"), significant persons, objects, and attributes.

Although J. understood how to activate the device, the VOIS 135 had limited conversational use.  Typically, J. would wait for an adult to ask a question and would then respond appropriately.  To enhance this child's interactive behaviors and successful use of the VOIS 135, a revision of utterances was suggested, along with modification of training and programming. Programmed utterances were changed to include scripts that reflected J.'s communication environments. Two environments were selected for use in role-playing activities (i.e., eating (snacktime) and going to the movies). The role-playing activities were introduced and trained at J.'s school by the speech-language pathologist who, following the guidelines for training role-playing skills, was able to integrate the role playing activities into J.'s routine during structured activities. To date, J. has attempted to utilize the selected utterances spontaneously, particularly during snacktime. An increase in initiation of conversation as well as an increase in J.'s willingness to participate more actively with peers and adults has been observed. Further training within other communication environments and investigation of ways to facilitate integration of scripts into J.'s spontaneous conversation with peers will continue as a primary emphasis of this child's therapy program.

## REFERENCES

Frumkin, J., & Baker, B. (in press). Minscripts. Syracuse, NY: Schneier Communication Unit.

Lieven, E. (1984). Interactional style and children's language learning. Topics in Language Disorders, 4, 15-23.

## ADDITIONAL READINGS

Constable, C. (1983). Creating communicative context. In H. Winitz (Ed.), Treating language disorders (pp. 97-120). Baltimore: University Park Press.

Friel-Patti, S., & Lougeay-Mottinger, J. (1985). Preschool language intervention: Some key concerns. Topics in Language Disorders, 5, 46-57.

Nelson, K., & Gruendal, J. (1979). At morning its lunchtime: A scriptal view of children's dialogue. Discourse Processes, 2, 73-94.

Snow, C., & Goldfield, B.A. (1983). Turn the page please: Situation specific language learning. Journal of Child Language, 10, 551-570.

**ESTABLISHING MULTIPLE COMMUNICATION DISPLAYS**

*Carol Goossens' and Sharon Crain*
*Sparks Center for Developmental and Learning Disorders*
*University of Alabama at Birmingham*

## INTRODUCTION

The productive vocabulary available to persons who use augmentative communication symbols, aids, techniques, and strategies is often severely restricted by lack of physical ability, visual limitations, and/or communication technique limitations (Yoder & Kraat, 1983). Augmentative communication clients are, therefore, frequently frustrated by their inability to accurately communicate thoughts and ideas.

Often, physically handicapped individuals are provided with a single communication display. Typically, this single display contains vocabulary items spanning a wide range of communication environments (e.g., home, school, church, Grandma's house, ballpark, McDonald's). The interaction potential of this single display for a given topic or activity is therefore diluted (i.e., the augmentative communication client can say a little about a lot of different topics, but is unable to say a lot about a given topic). In short, it is often very difficult for these individuals to be highly interactive with the diluted vocabulary set of a single display.

In an attempt to increase the number of vocabulary items available on a single display, many clinicians/teachers prematurely reduce symbol size. In so doing, they inadvertently increase the effort required to communicate. When effort to communicate outweighs desire to communicate, responding as opposed to initiating behavior tends to predominate in communicative interactions.

## PURPOSE OF STRATEGY

To provide the client with access to a larger productive vocabulary set, clinicians/teachers have begun to explore the concept of multiple communication displays. Multiple displays enable the clinician/teacher to provide:

1. a concentrated array of vocabulary that more adequately reflects the communication potential of a particular communication environment, and

2. the needed vocabulary for a particular communication environment without increasing the motor requirements involved in selecting vocabulary items.

## UNDERLYING ASSUMPTIONS

1. *Client*.    The clients may include individuals who use augmentative communication aids, have normal intelligence or are developmentally delayed, and have varying degrees of physical ability.

2. *Augmentative components*.    Direct selection, encoding, or scanning techniques can be used, as appropriate.  A variety of symbols may be used to make up the client's lexicon (vocabulary displays).

3. *Environmental constraints*.    The success of this strategy is highly dependent upon having the caregiver/teacher conscientiously change the various displays as needed by the client, and/or provide the client with a means of signaling a change of display.

4. *Other basic assumptions*.    The appropriate communication aid, response mode, and symbol set have been selected for the client.

## DESCRIPTION OF STRATEGY

The concept of multiple displays can be achieved in two ways:    (a) multiple independent displays, and (b) core display plus supplemental displays.

### *Multiple Independent Displays*

When using multiple independent displays, several displays are created to optimally serve a specific communication environment.  Displays may be accessed through direct selection, encoding, and scanning techniques.

*Direct selection*. For the nonambulatory client, multiple displays can be inserted into laptrays specifically designed to accommodate the concept of multiple displays. Communication displays can be stored in the laptray and can be routinely switched by the clinician/teacher/caregiver before proceeding to a new location or activity. With higher functioning clients, a symbol representation for each communication display should be located on the laptray, thereby allowing the client to independently request a change of display (e.g., pointing to a line drawing of a farm would indicate a desire to play with the toy farm during freetime; the teacher would then switch to the communication display for the toy farm).

Multiple independent displays can also be successfully used by placing semipermanent communication displays throughout the home, classroom, or institution (e.g., at the sink, on the wall beside the tub, at the toilet, beside the individual's plate at the table, at the headboard of the bed, at the sandbox, etc.). When establishing multiple independent displays throughout the home or classroom, clear plastic pouches and paste-on hooks can be used. Using plastic pouches, as opposed to clear plastic adhesive, allows flexibility in modifying the displays. In institutional settings a stronger, more permanent means of display is required; that is, one that cannot be easily destroyed. Displays designed for locations outside the home or classroom setting may be routinely kept in the car to insure that the appropriate display is always available for the client. Similarly, many parents have adopted a strategy of carrying a large bag, one side of which contains a transparent plastic pocket in which the multiple displays are housed. The caregiver routinely shifts the displays in the plastic pocket to expose the display that is unique to a particular activity.

The concept of multiple independent displays is equally applicable to direct-selection eye-gaze communication systems. When using a transparent eye-gaze frame/display, needed symbols may be temporarily displayed on the frame through the use of cup hooks, clear plastic pockets, and double-sided tape. To facilitate the process of quickly customizing the display for a given situation, pictures/symbols can be semantically organized and stored in a large three-ring binder containing plastic slide/photograph protectors. Equally amenable to the concept of multiple independent eye-gaze displays is a format described by Charlebois-Marois (1985). A clear sheet of mica containing several independent communication displays is suspended vertically between two window shade rollers. To change from one display to another, the caregiver merely advances the mica on its rollers. Message elements can be depicted using permanent overhead projector pens or, alternately, transparencies can be made of symbols that are not easily drawn. Transparent tape can be used to mount the symbols to the display.

When developing multiple independent displays within a direct-selection format, care should be taken to keep color coding consistent across different displays and, to the extent possible, to keep the locations of commonly used symbols roughly comparable across different displays.

*Encoding*.    The concept of multiple independent displays is crucial to maximizing the communication potential of area and color-encoded formats accessed through eye gaze (Carlson, 1982).   By way of example, four displays suitable for use on an eye gaze frame are depicted in Figure 6-4 (see also Van Tatenhove's strategy in this chapter).

*Scanning*.    Multiple independent displays reflecting various communication environments can also be developed for various electronic scanning formats.

Regardless of whether intervention is being conducted within a direct selection, encoding, or scanning format, each display should be planned in advance, taking into consideration the numerous interactions that can and do occur in a given communication environment.   Symbols may, however,  need to be introduced gradually. Various materials can be used to temporarily conceal vocabulary items that have not yet been introduced.    Figure 6-5 illustrates examples of materials that allow for gradual exposure of vocabulary items.

## Core Display Plus Supplemental Displays

Although the concept of multiple independent displays works well for many clients (especially during the early stages of intervention when display size is relatively small), the concept can be overwhelming for some.   An alternative concept that is frequently used is that of a core display plus supplemental displays.   A core display contains only those vocabulary items that are used with *high* frequency across a broad range of communication environments.   Additional vocabulary unique to a given communication environment is then provided in the form of a supplemental display.    Outlined in Figure 6-6 are examples of various core display plus supplemental display formats.

## FIGURE 6-4. FOUR EYE-GAZE ENCODED DISPLAYS REFLECTING THE USE OF MULTIPLE INDEPENDENT DISPLAYS

### Area & Color - Encoded Format

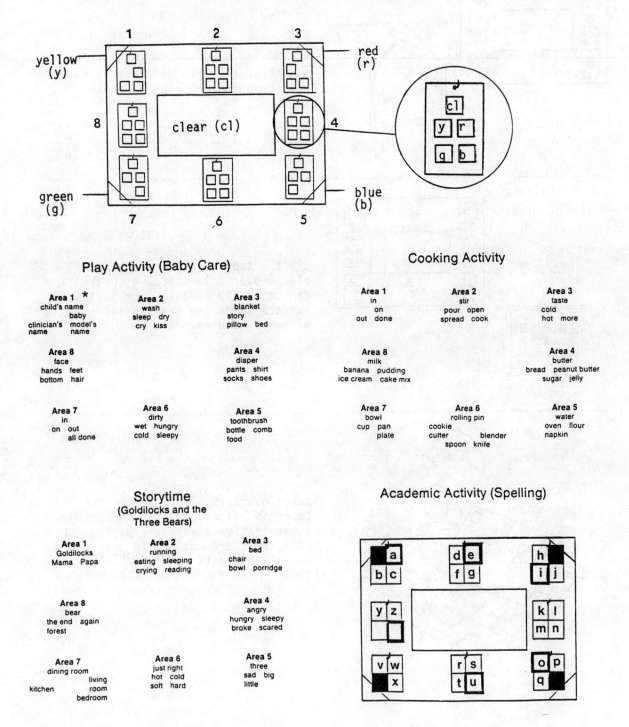

### Play Activity (Baby Care)

**Area 1** *
child's name
baby
clinician's model's
name name

**Area 2**
wash
sleep dry
cry kiss

**Area 3**
blanket
story
pillow bed

**Area 8**
face
hands feet
bottom hair

**Area 4**
diaper
pants shirt
socks shoes

**Area 7**
in
on out
all done

**Area 6**
dirty
wet hungry
cold sleepy

**Area 5**
toothbrush
bottle comb
food

### Cooking Activity

**Area 1**
in
on
out done

**Area 2**
stir
pour open
spread cook

**Area 3**
taste
cold
hot more

**Area 8**
milk
banana pudding
ice cream cake mix

**Area 4**
butter
bread peanut butter
sugar jelly

**Area 7**
bowl
cup pan
plate

**Area 6**
rolling pin
cookie
cutter blender
spoon knife

**Area 5**
water
oven flour
napkin

### Storytime
(Goldilocks and the Three Bears)

**Area 1**
Goldilocks
Mama Papa

**Area 2**
running
eating sleeping
crying reading

**Area 3**
bed
chair
bowl porridge

**Area 8**
bear
the end again
forest

**Area 4**
angry
hungry sleepy
broke scared

**Area 7**
dining room
living
kitchen room
bedroom

**Area 6**
just right
hot cold
soft hard

**Area 5**
three
sad big
little

### Academic Activity (Spelling)

*picture/symbols are organized according to conceptual groups.

## FIGURE 6-5.  MATERIALS ALLOWING GRADUAL EXPOSURE OF VOCABULARY ITEMS

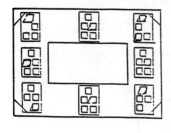
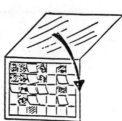

3-M "Post-Its" placed over "yet-to-be-introduced" message elements

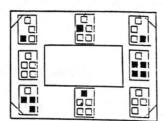

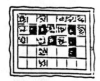

plastic tape (e.g., Scotch brand) placed over a laminated display (tape can be easily removed from laminated surface to expose the message elements when needed)

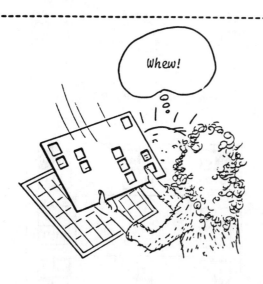

paper overlays, i.e., a sheet of paper is placed over the complete communication display. Portions of this sheet are cut out to expose the message elements beneath (Smith, 1983).

# FIGURE 6-6. EXAMPLES OF CORE DISPLAY PLUS SUPPLEMENTAL DISPLAY FORMATS

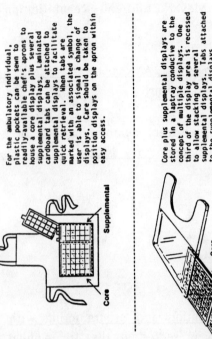

Core

Supplemental

The core display stays with the child at all times. For ambulatory children this can be achieved through the use of handle or a shoulder strap. Supplemental displays are then kept in their corresponding locations. For nonambulatory clients the core display is securely mounted on the individual's laptray. Supplemental displays are frequently kept in a pouch attached to the individual's wheelchair.

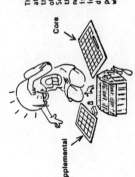

Supplemental

Core

The core display is securely mounted on the individual's laptray. Supplemental displays are vertically presented in a flip chart format. When supplemental displays assume a flip chart format, it is important to stress that vocabulary is arranged according to communication environments, not concept categories (e.g., one page for verbs, one page for adjectives, one page for prepositions, etc.). As much as possible, attempts should be made to reduce the need to flip through several pages to compile messages. Ideally, the core display and the supplemental display for a given communication environment should meet the majority of the required communications for that environment. The need to flip from page to page tends to slow down the communication process and considerably increases the level of effort required.

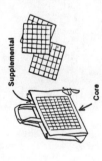

Supplemental

Core

The core display is mounted on the side of the parent's/caregiver's handbag. Supplemental displays are stored inside the bag and used as needed.

Core

Supplemental

For the ambulatory individual, plastic pockets can be sewn to readily-available chef's aprons to house a core display plus several supplemental displays. Laminated cardboard tabs can be attached to supplemental displays to facilitate quick retrieval. When tabs are marked with an associated symbol, the user is able to signal a change of displays. Care should be taken to position displays on the apron within easy access.

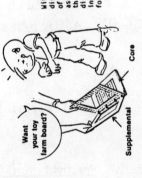

Core

Supplemental

Core plus supplemental displays are stored in a laptray conducive to the concept of multiple displays. One third of the display area is recessed to allow stacking of several supplemental displays. Tabs attached to the supplemental displays facilitate the exchange process.

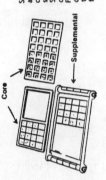

Want your toy /arm board?

Supplemental

Core

Within a notebook format, the core display is mounted on the final page of the book. Supplemental displays assume the shape of cardboard frames that form the perimeter of the core display. For the ambulatory individual, a strap can be attached for easy transport.

Core

Supplemental

Supplemental displays are mounted on a paper roll. An insert template containing the core display is then superimposed upon the roller base. Supplemental displays can be quickly changed by advancing the paper roll. For individuals with targeting difficulties, the core display template can assume a keyguard format (Charlebois-Marois, 1985).

# REFERENCES

Carlson, F.  (1982).  Prattle and play.  Omaha, NB:  Meyer Children's Rehabilitation Institute, Media Resource Center.

Charlebois-Marois, C.  (1985).  Everybody's technology:  A sharing of ideas in augmentative communication.  Montreal:  Charlecoms Enr.

Yoder, D., & Kraat, A. (1983).  Intervention issues in nonspeech communication.  In J. Miller, D. Yoder, & R. Schiefelbusch (Eds.), Contemporary issues in language intervention (pp. 27-51).  ASHA Reports, 12.

# ADDITIONAL READINGS

Smith, L.  (1983, October).  Practical hints for evaluation and programming with alternative communication systems.  Workshop presented at the 4th Annual Southeast Nonspeech Communication Conference, Birmingham, AL.

**COMMUNICATION TRAINING IN REAL ENVIRONMENTS**

*Jayne Higgins and Jane Mills*
*Encinitas, California*

## INTRODUCTION

Typically, during an augmentative communication assessment, a client's capabilities and skills are evaluated and matched with an augmentative communication technique. Very often, communication aids that seem perfectly matched during an assessment period are not successful over time in actual use. Sometimes the breakdown is caused by the device itself, but more often it is caused by environmental variables that were not considered.

To encourage an appropriate match between augmentative aids and techniques and a client, an environmental assessment of the client is recommended. An environmental assessment includes:

1. evaluation of the client in appropriate environments (home, store, school, work, leisure);

2. evaluation of augmentative communication symbols, aids, and techniques in appropriate environments (home, store, school, etc.); and

3. field testing of the use of recommended aids and augmentative techniques in various environments.

During this trial period or field testing phase, many questions should be considered for each environment within which the client needs to communicate, including:

1. What are the attitudes of the client and the family toward a communication aid and/or technique?

2. What is each environment like?

3. How accessible is it?

4. How efficient and functional is the aid/technique in meeting the communication needs of the client?

5. When comparing the cost of a communication aid to the change in the user's communication function, is the aid cost-efficient?

6. How tolerant to the use of the aid or technique are people in each environment (environmental tolerance)?

7. How adaptable is each environment to different augmentative communication techniques and strategies (environmental adaptability)?

8. How visually and auditorily understandable is the technique in each environment (comprehension in the environment)?

9. How familiar are people in the environment (environmental familiarity) with the severely speech-impaired person and with the augmentative communication components?

10. How many people need to interact with the client (environment number: one, a small group of three to five, or a large group of five or more)?

11. How necessary is each environment to the client (necessity of environment)?

12. What is the level of difficulty involved in communicating within each environment (ease of message completion)?

Figure 6-7 represents a sequence of environmental assessment variables. An important consideration during environmental trials is, "How successful is the link between equipment, client, and the receivers of information?" (Hagan, 1977). For example, in some environments, a computer-based system would lend prestige and credibility to the client (e.g., on a college campus), whereas in other environments, messages cannot be completed unless picture systems are used (e.g., in line in a fast-food restaurant). Therefore, it is important to determine how skills required by an environment relate to skills that have been acquired by the client. It is also important to note why and when communication breakdowns occur.

## FIGURE 6-7. ENVIRONMENTAL ASSESSMENT

PUPIL NAME _____
DATE _____
COMMUNICATION _____
ENVIRONMENT _____

1. N/A ___ N/I ___ Uses communication system in a one-to-one structured therapy session.

2. N/A ___ N/I ___ Uses communication system in a small group therapy session.

3. N/A ___ N/I ___ New environment is tolerant of system.

4. N/A ___ N/I ___ New environment adapts to system.

5. N/A ___ N/I ___ Supportive attitudes are present in the new environment.

6. N/A ___ N/I ___ New environment visually/auditorily understands the system.

7. N/A ___ N/I ___ New environment is familiar with the non-oral person.

8. N/A ___ N/I ___ New environment is familiar with the system.

9. N/A ___ N/I ___ New environment includes a single person or a small group for interaction.

10. N/A ___ N/I ___ New environment includes a large group for interaction.

11. N/A ___ N/I ___ New environment is necessary for the non-oral person.

12. N/A ___ N/I ___ Messages are completed in the new environment with the help of a buddy.

13. N/A ___ N/I ___ Messages are completed in the new environment independently.

14. N/A ___ N/I ___ Messages are completed quickly and efficiently and independently in the new environment.

15. N/A ___ N/I ___ Conversational interactions occur in the new environment.

16. N/A ___ N/I ___ Over time the communication system works in the new environment.

N/A—not appropriate
N/I—not interested

## PURPOSE OF THE STRATEGY

To insure optimal use of augmentative aids and techniques in the daily lives of persons who use augmentative components.

## UNDERLYING ASSUMPTIONS

1. *Client*.   This strategy is not restricted to a specific type of client; it is appropriate for any severely speech-impaired individual.   The training focuses on developing communicative competencies based on the daily requirements of the client.

2. *Augmentative components*.   Any augmentative aid or technique that the client uses.

3. *Environmental constraints*.   A "buddy," or back-up person, who is familiar with the client and the client's overall communication system must be available to handle any communication breakdowns during training in an unfamiliar environment.   When individuals in necessary environments demonstrate tolerance, comprehension, and an ability to interact with the client, and when the client is able to complete messages quickly, efficiently, and independently, a buddy is no longer mandatory.

The primary constraint of this training strategy is that a skilled professional (i.e., a speech-language pathologist) must train the client in the community.   This may be difficult because of time constraints and related cost factors.   In the initial stages of training, simulations of the actual environment may be used (i.e., setting up books, desk, table, and checkout area for a library; or a cash register, tray, and food for a fast-food restaurant).

## DESCRIPTION OF STRATEGY

Environmental training consists of four stages:   planning, initial training, environmental experience, and retraining.

## *Planning Stage*

During the planning stage, the speech-language pathologist and the client and/or caregiver brainstorm about the communication needs of a particular environment. For example, the following questions are posed:

1. What questions will the individual need to respond to or ask?

2. What will the individual do when misunderstood or unable to complete a message?

3. What components of the individual's communication system (i.e., gestures, electronic or nonelectronic aid) will be most functional for a particular environment?

4. How necessary is this environment to the individual?

5. How familiar is the environment with the individual and what effect might this have on communication?

## *Initial Training Stage*

The goal of the training stage is to initiate successful interaction between the client and the environment. This is accomplished through role playing in a simulated environment. The primary focus during this stage is to assist the client in acquiring functional communication skills. The training process includes "buddy training" to assist in facilitating successful communication. A buddy is a facilitator who can intervene when communication breakdowns occur and insure message completion. The process includes the following steps:

- The client and the speech-language pathologist model the interaction process for the buddy (e.g., the speech-language pathologist asks the client a question, and the client responds using selected augmentative components).

- The client and the buddy interact in the training session using augmentative aids and/or techniques (e.g., the buddy asks the client a question and observes the client's response).

- The client and the buddy role play in the simulated environment (e.g., client asks where a specific book is located in the library; the buddy responds; the client proceeds to check out the book).

- If appropriate, the client, the buddy, and the speech-language pathologist discuss the effectiveness of the augmentative components used and the environmental limitations.

An important consideration during the training stage, and one which should be considered when communication is unsuccessful, is the attitude of the client and significant others in the environment. Time must be spent discussing the importance of a supportive, positive attitude in the environment to insure long-term success of the communication augmentation (Hagan, 1977). Factors that must be considered include: the client's need to feel in control; the client's expectations for speech; the client's need to create or generate communication; the ability of particular augmentative techniques(s) to meet these needs; the client's need for independence; the client's need to communicate with many communication partners; and the inadequacies of the client's overall communication system.

## Environmental Experience Stage

The environmental experience stage will increase the communicative competence of the client and the buddy in the real environment:

- The client and the buddy interact within the desired environment and observe the success or failure of communication attempts (i.e., the client types out and hands the librarian a printed message; the buddy observes and/or intercedes if communication breakdown occurs).

- The speech-language pathologist is available for follow-up training and consultation.

Successful completion of a message generally results in an increase in client motivation and in the supportive attitudes of persons who are unfamiliar with the client in that environment. Failure to complete a message necessitates retraining.

## Retraining Stage

The retraining stage focuses on new goals or alternate procedures that are developed because of skill discrepancies observed during the environmental experience.

## EFFECTIVENESS OF STRATEGY

This strategy has been used with over 50 clients. As a result of the comprehensive design of the strategy, clients are learning to be independent communicators. One case study involves Martin, a 12-year-old male with a diagnosis of ataxic cerebral palsy. He is severely dysarthric and requires the use of several augmentative communication techniques to augment his speech. He is ambulatory, although he requires crutches for balance and support at all times. Academic performance level ranges between second and fourth grade. He is socially accepted by classmates within a physically handicapped school setting. During training, Martin used a lightweight, portable, electronic printout system, a communication book of approximately 200 words, and various mini books of selected vocabulary for specific communication situations (i.e., restaurant, morning circle, cooking).

Martin met with the speech-language pathologist to plan for his trip to the library with his buddy. A preferred augmentative technique was selected (i.e., a portable, lightweight, printout system). Martin practiced typing various questions for the librarian (i.e., "Where are books on lions?" "Where are books on gardens?" "Where is the restroom?" "How many books may I check out?"). Printing out the messages was practiced and demonstrated to the buddy by the therapist and Martin. Next, Martin typed a message and handed it to the buddy. They then practiced being at the library and asking the librarian (buddy) questions within a simulated setting. The effectiveness of the aid and possible limitations of the environment were discussed.

The following day, Martin and his buddy went to the library. The library was spacious, quiet, and unhurried. Martin located a librarian and typed his message. She waited patiently and then was handed the printed message. She took Martin to the two sections he was interested in and helped him locate his books successfully.

During the follow-up session with Martin's buddy and the speech-language therapist, it was noted that the librarian had to wait a long time for Martin's messages. Although the librarian allowed time for message completion, it was decided that a more expedient method could be used. Martin could either type out the most important messages prior to his visit and hand them to the librarian, or he could use a different communication aid that allowed for preprogrammed messages. It was determined that this environment was communicatively accessible in that the librarian tolerated, adopted, and understood the messages that Martin conveyed utilizing that particular augmentative aid.

# REFERENCES

Hagan, C.   (1977).   <u>Assistive communication systems:   A rationale for their use, selection and application</u>.  International Seminar on Non-Vocal Communication. Broma:  Swedish Institute for the Handicapped.

## ADDITIONAL READINGS

MacDonald, J.  (1978).  Language through conversation.  <u>Parent-child communication project</u>.  Columbus:  Nisonger Center, Ohio State University.

Mills, J., & Higgins, J.  (1983).  <u>Non-oral communication assessment and training guide</u>. Encinitas, CA.

# FACILITATING COMMUNICATION FOR SEVERELY SPEECH-IMPAIRED CHILDREN WITH ABNORMAL SOCIALIZATION PATTERNS

*Louise Kent-Udolf*
*Region II Education Center*
*Corpus Cristi, Texas*

## INTRODUCTION

Most behaviorally oriented language acquisition programs rely on discrete teaching formats. Procedures are described in minute detail and strict adherance is assumed. For children who display serious social-affective deficits, a different approach, called Intensive Play, is sometimes more successful. This approach is described by Bradtke, Kirkpatrick, and Rosenblatt (1972) and Kent-Udolf (1983, 1984). A similar strategy, called Intrusive Play, is set forth by Bell (1975) and is reflected in programming described by Lovaas (1981). These "play" strategies emphasize the importance of socialization to communication and language. The strategy described here is Bradtke's Intensive Play, a method designed to facilitate communication between severely speech impaired, affectively disordered children and their families. Because of their developmental status and history of minimal progress, these children usually receive only consultative speech and language services. Intensive Play is an alternative for clinicians who are able to provide direct services for these children.

Intensive Play is compatible with behavioral theoretical orientations and with current trends in the study of maternal interaction (Mahoney, Finger, & Powell, 1985). Intensive Play assumes that social-affective learning and communication can be facilitated through the application of principles of behavior analysis, that objectives can be stated in operational terms, and that improvement in communicative status can be measured reliably.

Intensive Play (IP) can be conducted by a parent, a speech-language pathologist, a teacher, or any person trained in the method; therefore, the term *teacher* is used to refer to an individual who works with the child and who makes teaching decisions during the IP sessions.

# PURPOSE OF THE STRATEGY

The goal of this strategy is to facilitate communication between the severely speech impaired, affectively disordered child and nurturing members of the child's environment. The long-range goals for the child include functional communication and language and the ability to learn in a small instructional group.

# UNDERLYING ASSUMPTIONS

1. *Client*. Intensive Play is a strategy for the child, under the age of 7, who relates poorly, or not at all, to nurturing adults. Because of the long-term nature of this strategy (12-24 months), children with certain degenerative conditions may not be appropriate candidates for IP since progress in communicating might be offset quickly by deterioration in the child's condition.

2. *Environmental conditions*. This strategy assumes that IP sessions will be held for at least 50 minutes daily, five days a week.

3. *Underlying assumptions*. The child's poor ability to generalize new behaviors necessitates the participation of family members and more than one teacher. Family participation includes observation of sessions, participation with the teacher in some sessions, and completion of assigned activities with the child at home. For this strategy to be successful, family members and teachers who work with the child need secure social-emotional support systems for themselves to minimize the effects of inadequate social reinforcement from their children. The adults must support each other until the children begin to provide them with an adequate level of support.

Preparation time is minimal once a plan for the child is designed and materials are assembled. Over time, the teacher collects a bank of audiotapes with music to suit different activities. A small audio cassette player/recorder is needed. Videotaping capability is helpful, but not essential, for evaluation and for communication among the teachers, including family members. A variety of edible reinforcers is also needed. Other needs include a large gym mat, a carpeted floor area, a large mirror mounted flush to the floor on one wall, open floor-to-ceiling shelves mounted on one wall, a rocking chair, a bean-bag chair, a soft blanket, small throw pillows, and a variety of play materials, such as pieces of cloth, facial tissues, toys, lotion, shaving cream, paper cups, and a plastic wash tub. A room that measures approximately 15 x 20 feet is desirable since too much space tends to prompt chasing (if the child can run) and makes "closeness" difficult, and too little space inhibits freedom of movement and makes group activities impossible.

## DESCRIPTION OF THE STRATEGY

The objectives and activities of Intensive Play are individualized for each child. No standard sequence of objectives is suitable for all children. There are six stages involved in Intensive Play; Table 6-5 lists sample objectives that have been developed by teachers for each of the six stages.

The procedures described below are used for each stage of Intensive Play:

1. The teacher talks and vocalizes to the child using child-oriented highlighting devices (see Table 6-6) to capture and maintain attention, to interest and amuse the child, and to create an aura of intimacy between the teacher and the child.

2. Tape-recorded music, prepared in advance, is used to complement the activities of each session. Listening to music with the teacher and responding to it through movement give IP a unique dimension.

3. The teacher comments on the child's or the teacher's own behavior with words and phrases that are common in early parent-child interactions. These words and phrases are uttered as the actions that they relate to occur. Table 6-7 lists examples of frequently used words and phrases.

4. Instruction includes the shaping of new behaviors needed to meet the criteria of each stage of IP. (Shaping is the systematic reinforcement of successive approximations to target behaviors.) For example, a target behavior might involve independently operating a jack-in-the-box toy or requesting that the teacher get a particular toy off the shelf. To strengthen newly shaped behaviors, edible reinforcers are paired with social reinforcers, such as praise, smiling, stroking, patting, hugging, and nuzzling. As target behaviors become stronger and are integrated into play routines, the teacher tries to maintain them with social reinforcers alone.

## TABLE 6-5. SAMPLE INTENSIVE PLAY OBJECTIVES

STAGE 1: ADAPTATION

- Child relaxes while being rocked in teacher's arms.
- Child relaxes while being held and stroked by teacher.
- Child tolerates manipulation of hands by teacher, such as, rubbing them or making them clap together.
- Child tolerates physical contact with no crying.

STAGE 2: ATTENDING

- Child is alert to teacher's voice and turns toward teacher.
- Child looks at foot when teacher removes child's sock.
- Child is alert to sound of mechanical toy and watches toy while it is moving.
- Child watches teacher polish mirror with spray and a cloth.

STAGE 3: TOUCHING

- Child touches teacher's hair, face, or throat.
- Child touches mirror.
- Child touches doll.
- Child touches mechanical puppy while still.

STAGE 4: ACTING ON OBJECTS

- Child opens box lid.
- Child shuts door.
- Child initiates play routine with doll.
- Child removes stocking cap pulled down over eyes.

STAGE 5: IMITATION

- Child imitates teacher's "making faces" in the mirror.
- Child imitates teacher's /m/ sound.
- Child imitates teacher's "putting doll to bed" and covering with a tissue.
- Child imitates teacher's swaying to music.

STAGE 6: COMMUNICATION

- Child greets teacher with eye contact and smile.
- Child turns teacher's face toward himself.
- Child communicates request to be put down during physical contact play.
- Child communicates request for toy during object play routine.

## TABLE 6-6. CHILD-ORIENTED HIGHLIGHTING DEVICES

- Exaggerating and varying voice inflection, pitch, stress, rate, and loudness

- Rhyming, repeating, and alliterating

- Using facial expressions, gestures, posture and movement

- Whispering

- Singing

- Dancing

- "Freezing" posture, facial expression, and voice

- Using nonspeech noises, such as animal noises, motor noises, silly smacking or popping noises

- Talking about what is happening

- Telling secrets

- Waiting silently for as long as 10 seconds for the child to respond

- Signing

- Using finger play

## TABLE 6-7.  EXPRESSIONS FREQUENTLY USED DURING INTENSIVE PLAY ROUTINES [a]

Hey!

Here.  Right here.  Here it is.  You got it!

There.  There it is.  Right there.

There you are!

This.  This one.

That.  That one.

Uh-oh.  You hurt yourself!

It fell.

It's broken.

Hi, there.  Hello!

Bye!  Bye-bye!

Whee!  This is fun!

Here we go!

You did it!

You like that!

Thank you!

You're welcome!

Ahhhh!  Oooooo!  Look at that!

Ooooo!  That's pretty!

Ooooo!  It's dark in here!

Yuck!  Dirty!  We don't like that!

Yuck!  Hands dirty!

Uh-oh.  I got it on my dress.

You're wet!

It's broken.

All done.  We're finished.

Oh, no.  Sorry.

Mmmm.  That's good.  I like that.

Look at that!

Wow!  New shoes!

Shhh. . .  Listen.  I hear something.

It's so quiet.  I like it.

You're happy now!

You want more!

Please!

Is that better?

You want to go, don't you.

Do you want this?

Again?  You want more?

You want to help.

You're tired of this, huh?

You want a little help there.

You want up!  You want to see?

You want down?

You want out of there!

Do you want more?  More?  Yes, you want more.

You don't want any more.  No.  No more for you!

Again?  You want me to....again?

No.  No more of that, huh.  No.

You want another one?  Another?  Yes, you want another . . .

Enough, huh?  Finished.

All gone.  You ate/drank it all gone.

It's gone!  (vanished)  Where is it?

Where is it?  Help me find it.

I'm looking.  I can't find it!

Here it is!

I'm finished!  All done.

Enough of this!  You want something else now.  Show me.  Tell me what you want.

You want me to stop!  Stop!

This is not the one you want!  No.  Look at that!  You're so pretty!

This one.  No.  This one.

That's mine!  Leave it alone!    Give it back!

It's my turn!  Your turn?

Let me see!

Too loud!  It hurts your ears!

Turn it off!  Make it quiet.

Thank you!

Let go of me!  Put me down!

I'll do it.  I can do it by myself!

Don't stop.  More.  Do it more.

Up!  Pick me up.

Help me.

Fix it.  It's broken?

Open this!

You're silly!

You're my honey!

Aaaaaaa . . . BOO!!

[a]No order or sequence is implied.

5. Family members are highly valued colleagues and are included in any
sessions they may attend. Eventually, family members view IP as a
method for themselves as well as for the child. IP encourages the
family and the child to enjoy their involvement with each other.

Children progress at their own rates through the six stages of Intensive Play.
While each stage has a different emphasis, they blend together with no abrupt
transitions. To progress from one stage to the next, the child must complete the
criteria of all previous stages (see Table 6-8). Each session, regardless of which stage
the child is in, is comprised of several common design elements: an opening, a warm-
up play routine, an intense physical contact play routine, a cool down, an object play
routine (either teacher- or child-led), and a closing.

## Stage One: Adaptation

The goal of Stage One is to make the child feel comfortable with the teacher,
the activities, and the setting. Activities might include rough-and-tumble mat play,
rocking in the rocking chair on the teacher's lap, dancing, singing, and clowning in
front of the mirror. Criteria for movement to Stage Two include absence of crying
during the session; absence of physical resistance when handled by the teacher; and
absence of escape attempts.

## Stage Two: Attending

The goals of Stage Two are to have the teacher identify a menu of positive
reinforcers for the child and to have the child attend to specific stimuli and stimulus
events. *Attending*, as used here, means that the child will physically and visually
orient or turn toward the stimuli. The teacher may choose activities that build on
those introduced in Stage One, or the teacher may introduce totally new activities.
Objectives might involve turning toward the tape recorder when the music begins or
stops, looking at a mirror when the teacher draws on it with shaving cream, looking at
a flash light when the light is turned on or off, gazing at a mechanical toy when the
toy begins to move or make noise, and looking at the teacher's face when the teacher
makes a "raspberry" sound. Suggested criteria for movement to the next stage include
maintenance of Stage One criteria plus attending to 80 percent of at least 20 stimuli or
stimulus events, with a latency of no more than 20 seconds, in each of three
consecutive sessions.

## TABLE 6-8.  SUGGESTED CRITERIA FOR STAGES OF INTENSIVE PLAY

### STAGE ONE:  ADAPTATION

- absence of crying during session,
- absence of physical resistance when handled by teacher,
- absence of escape attempts.

### STAGE TWO:  ATTENDING

- all of the above, plus,
- child attends to 80% of at least 20 stimuli or stimulus events with a latency of no more than 20 seconds for three consecutive sessions.

### STAGE THREE:  TOUCHING

- all of the above, plus,
- child indpendently touches at least 10 objects in each of three consecutive sessions.

### STAGE FOUR:  ACTING ON OBJECTS

- all of the above, plus,
- child independently acts on 20 different objects over no more than three consecutive sessions.

### STAGE FIVE:  IMITATION

- all of the above, plus,
- child imitates at least 10 actions modeled by teacher over three consecutive sessions.

### STAGE SIX:  COMMUNICATION

- all of the above, plus,
- child makes at least 20 responses in each of 10 consecutive sessions that can be described as communicative and pragmatically appropriate.

To compile a menu of reinforcers for the child, the teacher observes the child's preferences among edible reinforcers, such as ice cream, pudding, potato chips, crushed ice, frosting, banana, yogurt, popcorn, cookie crumbs, broken pretzel bits, sips of cola, and other foods and beverages. Family members can be helpful in suggesting foods and other reinforcers idiosyncratic to the child, such as scents, textures, and vibratory stimuli. The teacher also notes the musical selections that seem to calm, stimulate, and interest the child and the play routines that seem to amuse, comfort, and please.

## Stage Three: Touching

The goal of Stage Three is to have the child independently touch the stimulus materials. Again, the teacher may choose activities that build on those already used or introduce new ones to accomplish Stage Three objectives. The objectives pertain to reaching out and touching various objects. For example, the child may pat the mirror, touch a switch, touch the rocking chair, or touch the teacher's foot. *Touching*, as used here, refers to the child's attending to and touching an object with his or her hands. *Object* refers to any tangible stimulus in the setting, including the teacher. Suggested criteria for movement to the next stage include maintaining criteria from earlier stages plus independently touching at least 10 objects in each of three consecutive sessions.

Some children may already seem to touch "too much." When the child meets the criteria, with or without specific instruction, the child moves on to Stage Four.

## Stage Four: Acting on Objects

The goal of Stage Four is to have the child independently manipulate or handle objects to produce change, actions, or effects. The teacher may design activities based on the objects used in the previous stage or may introduce totally new activities using new objects. The child might learn to operate independently a jack-in-the-box, or climb into the rocking chair, or turn the light switch on or off, or activate a switch that operates a mechanical toy or the tape recorder. A second goal is to eliminate self-stimulating and self-injurious behaviors during the sessions. Suggested criteria for movement to the next stage include maintenance of earlier criteria and performance of at least 20 unprompted, appropriate actions over no more than three consecutive sessions.

## Stage Five:  Imitation

The goals of Stage Five are to have the child make eye contact with the teacher and to imitate behaviors modeled by the teacher.  A response qualifies as imitative when it occurs after a similar response is modeled by the teacher in the same session. The teacher may choose activities related to those used in Stage Three or may introduce new ones that encourage eye contact and the imitation of actions.  The actions to be imitated may include production of speech or nonspeech sounds or facial expressions, or they may be fine or gross motor movements.  Table 6-5 shows several sample objectives that might be included.  Edible reinforcers may be used to shape new responses; however, only social reinforcers are used to reinforce responses that meet criteria in this stage.  Suggested criteria for movement to Stage Six include maintenance of earlier criteria and imitation of at least 10 new actions modeled by the teacher over three successive sessions.

## Stage Six:  Communication

The goal of Stage Six is to have the child communicate with teachers and family members during familiar play routines.  Activities during this stage include the child's favorite play routines and the routines that the teacher thinks are especially productive for the child.  Table 6-9 shows a sample set of routines for Stage Six. Objectives pertain to the child's sending and responding to a variety of messages in a social context with the teacher.  Criteria for successful completion of this stage include the maintenance of criteria of earlier stages plus at least 20 responses in each of 10 consecutive sessions that can be described as communicative and pragmatically appropriate.

During this stage, if the room is large enough, more than one child/teacher team can work at the same time.  The advantages of doing this include the opportunity to observe and respond to changes in the child's behavior in the presence of others, the opportunity for the teachers to trade children without being completely separated from them, the opportunity to strengthen the child's attending behaviors in the presence of distractions, the opportunity to observe the child's tendency to attend to and imitate the actions of others, and the opportunity to observe the child's tendency to interact with others. Suggested criteria for successful completion of this stage include the maintenance of criteria of earlier stages plus at least 20 responses per session for 10 successive sessions that can be described with words and phrases in Table 6-7.

The stage is set for a child to learn language when:

**TABLE 6-9. SAMPLE ROUTINES FOR SIX INTENSIVE PLAY SESSIONS** *(CONTINUED ON NEXT PAGE)*

OPENING

- Child makes eye contact with teacher and smiles on entry.
- Child acknowledges greetings appropriately.
- Child separates easily from family member when necessary.
- Child exchanges farewell gestures.
- Child removes shoes and puts them away.
- Child turns on light.
- Child turns on music.
- Child looks at teacher.

WARM-UP PLAY ROUTINE

- Warm-up routines are gentle, physical contact activities. Background music should be toe-tapping, but not fast; folk music, peppy waltz, or march works well. There should be lots of animated talking and laughter to accompany this very intimate kind of play. Routines and music can be changed as appropriate.
- Teacher assists child in applying body lotion to arms and legs; child is encouraged to apply to self and teacher's arms; socks may be removed and child's feet massaged.
- Teacher may lead into finger play activity.
- Teacher may lead into peek-a-boo activity with blanket.
- Teacher may lead into mirror activity, playing with body lotion or shaving cream on mirror.

INTENSIVE, PHYSICAL CONTACT PLAY ROUTINE

- These are high energy activities with music to match. Vary the pace within but keep energy level high until music signals transition to cool down routine. Try some symphonic music. Take advantage of crescendos! End with a bang! Change routine and music as you like.
- Child notices change in music.
- Teacher leads into active movement routine; movements match the music; teacher may at first dance alone, focusing on the child, and may then pick up the child and continue dance routine holding child close.
- Teacher may lead into swinging the child out from teacher's body and lifting child up.
- Teacher may lead into mat play, moving away from and back to the child; teacher may tumble alone at first, focusing on the child, and then guide child through tumbling routine.
- Teacher may lead back into dance.

**TABLE 6-9.  SAMPLE ROUTINES FOR SIX INTENSIVE PLAY SESSIONS**
*(CONTINUED)*

COOL DOWN

- Music becomes calm and soothing, slow; may be hum-along or sing-along type music.
- Teacher may need to lead transition to cool down.
- Teacher engages child in finding the cushions, finding the blanket.
- Teacher and child move to the rocking chair.
- Child gets into teacher's lap in rocker.
- Teacher and child snuggle with blanket, rocking, cuddling, stroking child's hair and face.
- Humming, singing.
- Teacher responds to change in tempo of music in preparation for transition to Object Play Routine.

OBJECT PLAY ROUTINE

- Object Play Routines may be teacher- or child-led.  Teacher chooses one routine; if it seems to work, same routine is used for several sessions.  Teacher develops an order or sequence for the routine.  Routine will develop differently with different children.  New routine is introduced before old one gets boring. Each routine should have its own theme music.  By Stage Six, most children will have a preference for certain routines and will be eager to lead the routine.  Materials and toys are placed on shelves on the wall out of the child's reach.  Child must communicate preference to teacher by referring to items on shelves.

EXAMPLES OF OBJECT PLAY ROUTINES

- water play with plastic dishpan and assorted objects.
- comb/brush play beside mirror; child works on own and teacher's hair and vice versa; doll may be used.
- doll play routine: feeding, dressing, bathing, reading book, putting to sleep; choose no more than two per session.
- tea party routine: mixing "tea," or juice, stirring, setting table or spread on floor, pouring from pitcher, drinking from cups, using napkins.

CLOSING

- Closing is signaled when music stops.
- Child turns off tape player.
- Clean up time: Child helps teacher straighten room.
- Toileting or diaper change as needed.
- Child puts on shoes.
- Child puts on outer clothing.
- Child turns off light.
- Expressions of leave taking for everyone present: hugs, pats, kisses, waves as appropriate.

- the child, the family members, and the teachers discover and use mutually agreeable communicative modes;

- messages are sent and received with or without words;

- the child and family seem happier and more relaxed than before;

- the child's eye contact with family members and teachers is spontaneous and comfortably quick;

- smiling is reciprocal; and

- motor and vocal imitation are easily evoked in play.

With this quality of communication in place, language intervention strategies can be expected to facilitate the child's further development of functional communication and language.

Once the child meets the criteria for Stage Six, a comprehensive reassessment of the child's communicative status should be conducted. During the reassessment, the following questions should be addressed:

1. Does the child need an augmentative communication aid?

2. Does the child need a total communication approach that includes manual communication?

3. Does the child need a play group to nurture socialization and discourse or pragmatic development?

4. Does the child need intensive vocal imitation training to nurture phonological precision (Schaeffer, Musil, & Kollinzas, 1980)?

5. Does the child need 1:1 language therapy using a discrete trial format?

6. Does the child need 1:1 language therapy using a continuation of IP?

7. Is the child ready for trial group instruction with several other children?

## EFFECTIVENESS OF STRATEGY

Variations of Intensive Play have been used with speechless, affectively disordered children since the early 1970s. Bradtke, one of the original developers of this approach, reports (L.M. Bradtke, personal communication, 1986) that she knows of no systematic, longitudinal evaluation of the method. The need for this kind of evaluation is clear (Hersen & Barlow, 1976.) Gains reported anecdotally by parents and teachers emphasize positive changes in social behavior and communication.

There are no clear-cut reasons why this strategy is successful. Perhaps when the persistent intrusions of the adult on the child begin to bring some pleasure to the child, and when the child begins to reinforce the adult, communication has a chance to grow. Successful communication by the adults is strengthened by the child and vice versa (see Mahoney, Finger, & Powell, 1985). Having sampled success in nonverbal communication in an affective context, the child may respond more easily to the social reinforcers that encourage more functional communication and language. Having experienced success as teachers, the family members may deliver more reinforcers to the child than before. For whatever the reasons, IP offers a medium in which positive patterns of social interaction between child and nurturing adults can be learned.

## REFERENCES

Bell, V. (1975). A therapeutic approach through intrusive play. In M.P. Creedon (Ed.), Appropriate behavior through communication: A new program in simultaneous language for nonverbal children (pp. 30-44). Chicago: Michael Reese Medical Center.

Bradtke, L.M., Kirkpatrick, W.J., Jr., & Rosenblatt, K.P. (1972). Intensive play: A technique for building affective behaviors in profoundly mentally retarded yound children. Education and Training of the Mentally Retarded, 7, 8-13.

Hersen, M., & Barlow, D.H. (1976). Single case experimental designs: Strategies for studying behavior change. New York: Pergamon Press.

Kent-Udolf, L. (1983). Language deficits. In M. Hersen, V.B. Van Hasselt, & J.L. Matson (Eds.), Behavior therapy for the developmentally and physically disabled (pp. 81-108). New York: Academic Press.

Kent-Udolf, L. (1984). Programming language. In W.H. Perkins, (Ed.), <u>Language handicaps in children</u> (pp. 15-25). New York: Thieme-Stratton.

Lovaas, O.I. (1981). <u>Teaching developmentally disabled children</u>. Baltimore: University Park Press.

Mahoney, G., Finger, I., & Powell, A. (1985). Relationship of maternal behavioral style to the development of organically impaired mentally retarded infants. <u>American Journal of Mental Deficiency</u>, <u>90</u>, 296-302.

Schaeffer, B., Musil, A., & Kollinzas, G. (1980). <u>Total communication: A signed speech program for nonverbal children</u>. Champaign, IL: Research Press.

# FACILITATING THE DEVELOPMENT OF EFFECTIVE INITIATION STRATEGIES BY NONSPEAKING, PHYSICALLY DISABLED CHILDREN

*Janice Light and Barbara Collier*
*Augmentative Communication Service*
*Hugh Macmillan Medical Centre*
*Toronto, Ontario*

## INTRODUCTION

Clinical experience and research in the field of augmentative communication indicates that severely speech-impaired individuals typically occupy a respondent role within communicative interactions, while their speaking partners initiate most topics of conversation and control the development of the exchange (Calculator & Dollaghan, 1982; Calculator & Luchko, 1983; Colquhoun, 1982; Culp, 1985; Harris, 1982; Light, Collier, & Parnes, 1985; Light, Rothschild, & Parnes, 1985; Lossing, 1981; Wexler, Blau, Leslie, & Dore, 1983). Training strategies can be used to improve the interaction skills of physically disabled individuals with severe expressive communication disorders; however, these strategies should address not only the client's skills, but also those of the significant individuals within the client's environment.

## PURPOSE OF THE STRATEGY

To promote the development of effective initiation strategies by training nonspeaking, physically disabled children and their facilitators (e.g., parents, teachers, aides, residential counselors).

## UNDERLYING ASSUMPTIONS

1. *Client and augmentative components*. The implementation of this strategy is described with reference to the congenitally speech-impaired, physically disabled child who is nonambulatory and who has an established, graphic, augmentative

communication aid. With some modifications to account for the client's age, skill level, and interests as well as environmental factors, the strategy may also be appropriate for other age and disability groups. It is assumed that the client can effectively access a meaningful vocabulary display and that facilitators are familiar with and competent in interpreting the client's use of the augmentative aid(s).

2. *Environmental constraints*. Since communication is an ongoing process that occurs throughout the child's day, this strategy should be implemented during all aspects of the child's daily routine. In addition, since the communication process is strongly influenced by partner variables and contextual demands, the interaction strategies for a child may need to be adapted across various contexts. Initial training should begin with the child's primary facilitators within high frequency contexts or environments (e.g., with mother at mealtimes, with the teacher upon arrival at school). As the child becomes competent with familiar partners in routine contexts, training should be extended to include less familiar partners in nonroutinized contexts (e.g., with the waitress at a restaurant, with the secretary at the school office).

## DESCRIPTION OF THE STRATEGY

The goal of this strategy is to encourage the client's development of effective and appropriate initiation strategies. For the facilitator, training involves numerous strategies that include: (a) providing the time and opportunity for the child to initiate, (b) recognizing the initiation attempt, and (c) responding appropriately by establishing a shared focus in the interaction. For the client, initiating a topic is a two-step process involving: (a) securing a partner's attention, and (b) establishing the referent or topic.

### *Facilitator Strategies*

It is essential that facilitators who interact with children on a routine basis (e.g., parents, teachers, residential counselors, peers) are aware of the goals of the training strategy and are sensitized to respond appropriately to the child's initiation attempts. Therefore, training of facilitators should begin with a rationale for the implementation of the strategy, a clear delineation of the goals, and an explanation of the training steps involved. The facilitators should have opportunities to observe the clinician interacting, modeling, and demonstrating appropriate facilitator strategies with the client. The clinician should then observe the facilitators interacting with the client and using the targeted strategies and should provide them with appropriate feedback and encouragement throughout this process. The clinician may wish to use videotapes during the training period to clarify expectations and to illustrate appropriate strategies for the facilitators.

Specifically, facilitators should be trained in the following interaction strategies:

1. Providing opportunities for the child to initiate. Facilitators should be cautioned to avoid anticipating all of the child's needs and wants. They should be encouraged to observe the child's daily interactions and to identify situations in which the child is motivated to communicate (e.g., mealtime, playtime with favorite toys). They should then be instructed to use these opportunities to encourage the child to initiate.

2. Providing time for the child to initiate. Facilitators must insure that the child has sufficient time to initiate a topic. Recent research has shown that pauses in the interaction are highly likely to precipitate initiations from the child (Light, 1985; Light, Collier, & Parnes, 1985). Facilitators may initially require extensive modeling and observation time with a clinician to ascertain how much time the client requires in order to initiate.

3. Responding to the child's lead. To insure the child's success during attempts at initiating interaction, facilitators should be encouraged to carefully observe the child and to respond to the child's lead. Initially, this lead may be as subtle as the client looking in the direction of a desired object. Gradually, as the child's initiation attempts become more refined, facilitators should increase their expectations (e.g., client vocalizing and looking at the desired object).

## *Client Strategies*

Training the child to initiate effectively involves two strategies: (a) securing the partner's attention, and (b) establishing the referent or topic. Initially, familiar facilitators should be trained in the use of these strategies within supportive environments (e.g., facilitator within relatively close proximity to the client in a quiet context). Gradually, instruction in the use of these strategies should be in more demanding contexts (e.g., with an unfamiliar listener in a noisy room). Training of the client should take place in conjunction with facilitator training to incorporate carryover into the natural environment.

1. *Establishing attention*. With input from facilitators, a number of motivating contexts can be defined (e.g., mealtime, computer activities, play situations). The

clinician must then be sure that the client can effectively signal the facilitator's attention in these situations.  Possible modes for attention-getting within situations of such close proximity may include instructing the client to vocalize, use tongue clicks, hit the lap tray, or gesture to the facilitator.  The child may also use commercially available call bells and buzzers, operated by a single switch, or a loop tape with an appropriate phrase for initiating (e.g., "come here!"; "Mommy!"; "I want to tell you something").  Voice output communication aids with customized, preprogrammed, attention-calling phrases may also be used by the child.  In selecting an appropriate means for attention-getting, it is important to consider the preferences of the client and the facilitator, as well as the context.  If preprogrammed phrases are used for attention-getting, these phrases should be appropriate to the client's age, cognitive development, and personality.  Situations are then contrived within these contexts that require initiations from the client (e.g., at mealtimes the facilitator feeds another child and pretends to "forget" the client; during computer activities, the teacher gives an assignment and leaves the child, forgetting to boot the disk).  The clinician should model effective use of the targeted behaviors within a variety of meaningful contexts.  The client should then be given the time and opportunity to secure the facilitator's attention within the context.  Facilitators should be instructed to respond immediately to the child's attempts.  If no attempts are made to secure the facilitator's attention, despite sufficient time to do so, the clinician should prompt the child to initiate appropriately.  Prompts may include verbal cues, physical prompts, and/or models.  These prompts should then be faded until the child is spontaneously and successfully securing the facilitator's attention within a range of contexts.  Once the client is able to consistently secure the partner's attention as required, the clinician can then train the client in the next step of the initiation process.

2. *Establishing the referent*.  The focus of intervention at this stage is to establish the referent or topic of the interaction.  Again, facilitators should establish meaningful and motivating contexts in which the child is required to initiate (e.g., running an errand to the school office, taking a message home from school).  Initially, the task may be quite simple (e.g., asking the school secretary for a pen); later, as the child demonstrates the skills to establish a simple referent, the tasks may be made more complex (e.g., asking for assistance at the store, ordering lunch at a fast-food restaurant).

The clinician should first rehearse the entire initiation process with the child (i.e., securing the partner's attention and establishing the referent) through role playing.  The clinician should provide the child with appropriate feedback during the rehearsal process and should model more effective strategies for the client, as required.  During training, the child should be encouraged to identify the most salient referent in the interaction and to then choose an appropriate means of conveying this referent (e.g., communication board, gesture, pointing).

At this point, the clinician should unobtrusively observe the strategies employed by the client within the designated context. The clinician is only there to provide support for the child, to prompt or model strategies, if required, and to insure a successful interaction experience for the child.

If the child initiates appropriately by securing the partner's attention and clearly establishing a shared topic, the clinician should check to be sure that the partner responds appropriately. If the child does not use effective attention-getting strategies within the context, the clinician should retrain these strategies. If the child demonstrates effective attention-getting strategies, but has difficulty establishing the referent or topic, the clinician should determine the problem area (i.e., identify the salient referent, select an appropriate mode to convey that referent, or actually convey the referent intelligibly to the partner). The clinician should then provide the child with further training by modeling appropriate and effective strategies that are within the client's repertoire.

Again, the child will need opportunities to develop interaction skills within various contexts, with a wide range of partners, and around a variety of topics. Training should ultimately extend to multiple contexts within the client's natural environment, so that the initiation skills acquired are generalized and are truly functional.

## EFFECTIVENESS OF STRATEGY

Results of a single case study, involving a 4-year-old nonspeaking child and his mother (Light, Rothschild, & Parnes, 1985) lend support to the effectiveness of the training strategy described. This study examined the cumulative effect of the successive implementation of a two-phase intervention program involving direct client intervention and facilitator training. After training the child to request attention and to clearly establish his referent and training the mother to respond to the child's lead and to provide the time and opportunity for him to initiate, the child's initiations in a 10-minute segment of free-play interaction increased considerably. The child initiated nine times preintervention (14 percent of all initiations in the interaction) and initiated 21 times postintervention (55 percent of all initiations in the interaction).

# REFERENCES

Calculator, S., & Dollaghan, C.  (1982).  The use of communication boards in a residential setting:  An evaluation.  Journal of Speech and Hearing Disorders, 47, 281-87.

Calculator, S., & Luchko, C. (1983).  Evaluating the effectiveness of a communication board training program.  Journal of Speech and Hearing Disorders, 48, 185-91.

Colquhoun, A. (1982).  Augmentative communication systems:  The interaction process. Paper presented at the annual convention of the American Speech-Language-Hearing Association, Toronto.

Culp, D.  (1985).  Communication interactions - Nonspeaking children using augmentative systems.  In A.W. Kraat, Communication interaction between aided and natural speakers:  An IPCAS study report (pp. 190-191).  Toronto: Canadian Rehabilitation Council for the Disabled.

Harris, D. (1982).  Communicative interaction processes involving nonvocal physically handicapped children.  Topics in Language Disorders, 2(2), 21-37.

Keenan, E., & Schieffelin, B.  (1976).  Topic as a discourse notion:  A study of topic in the conversations of children and adults.  In C.N. Li (Ed.), Subject and topic (pp. 335-384).  New York:  Academic Press.

Kraat, A. (1985).  Communication interaction between aided and natural speakers:  An IPCAS study report.  Toronto:  Canadian Rehabilitation Council for the Disabled.

Light, J.  (1985).  The communicative interaction patterns of young nonspeaking physically disabled children and their primary caregivers.  Master's thesis, University of Toronto.  (Available from the Blissymbolics Communication Institute, 350 Rumsey Road, Toronto, Ontario, Canada, M4G 1R8.)

Light, J., Collier, B., & Parnes, P.  (1985).  Communicative interaction between young nonspeaking physically disabled children and their primary caregivers.  Part I: Discourse patterns.  Augmentative and Alternative Communication, 1(2), 74-83.

Light, J., Rothschild, N., & Parnes, P.  (1985).  The effect of communication intervention with nonspeaking physically disabled children.  Paper presented at the annual convention of the American Speech-Language-Hearing Association, Washington, DC.

Lossing, C.A. (1981). A technique for the quantification of non-vocal communication performance by listeners. Unpublished master's thesis, University of Washington, Seattle.

Mueller, E. (1972). The maintenance of verbal exchange between young children. Child Development, 43, 930-938.

Wexler, K., Blau, A., Leslie, S., & Dore, J. (1983). Conversational interaction of nonspeaking cerebral palsied individuals and their speaking partners, with and without augmentative communication aids. Unpublished manuscript, Helen Hayes Hospital, New York.

# TEACHING INDIVIDUALS WITH AUTISM AND RELATED DISORDERS TO USE VISUAL-SPATIAL SYMBOLS TO COMMUNICATE

*Pat Mirenda*
*University of Nebraska*
*Lincoln, Nebraska*


*Adriana L. Schuler*
*San Francisco State University*
*San Francisco, California*

## INTRODUCTION

Augmentative communication aids and techniques are currently being used to develop the communicative capabilities of individuals with autism and related handicaps. It has not yet been determined, however, when and how augmentative communication should be introduced, and which, if any, communication aids or augmentative techniques are best suited to this population.

Although decisions regarding the selection of augmentative components and effective ways of teaching clients to use them must be individualized, two generalizations about the application of communication aids with autistic individuals can be made. First, many individuals with autism seem to learn visual-spatial symbols more easily than spoken words. These individuals have been described as operating in a gestalt-like fashion; that is, stimulus input is analyzed as a whole rather than in terms of component parts (Prizant, 1983). This type of snapshot-like processing seems congruent with a mode of stimulus recognition that has been described as "simultaneous" (Das, 1984); that is, information is coded in a nonsequential manner. For example, entire spoken phrases may be echoed or reproduced in association with a specific person, context, and/or emotional overtone, rather than spoken communicatively in the right place at the right time. Because of these characteristics, individuals with autism may benefit from nontransient stimuli that remain visible over time. Thus, pictorial symbols can provide a suitable receptive and expressive language alternative to speech. These may include the use of written words (such as on a computer screen) or graphic symbols to augment an individual's understanding and use of speech and, to a lesser extent, sign language, gesture, and body language.

Not all individuals with autism will benefit from the use of graphic symbols; however, in many cases, they may constitute the best match between communication system requirements and a client's learning characteristics.

A second generalization is that communication skills should be taught in social contexts because generalization of appropriate symbol use is often a problem for individuals with autism.  Lack of speech is generally not the major roadblock to effective communication for individuals with autistic and related disorders, who are characterized by severe limitations in nonverbal as well as verbal communication behaviors.  Since the pragmatic and semantic aspects of communication are affected (Fay & Schuler, 1980; Tager-Flusberg, 1981), the mere introduction of an augmentative aid or technique will not result in improved communication.

If these individuals are to learn to use visual-spatial symbols to accomplish certain communication functions in daily situations, they must be taught to do so. Strategies have been developed specifically for the purpose of teaching clients with severe handicaps to use augmentative communication aids (e.g., Goetz, Gee, & Sailor, 1985; Keogh & Reichle, 1985; Reichle & Yoder, 1985).   Additionally, strategies developed specifically for other purposes, such as teaching verbal language, have been adapted for use with individuals who have severe communication disorders (e.g., Hart & Risley, 1975; Snell & Gast, 1981).  These approaches to training all incorporate the use of verbal cues on the part of the clincian as either a primary (e.g., Keogh & Reichle, 1985) or a "backup" instructional technique (e.g., Hart & Risley, 1975). Reliance on verbal cues to prompt a communicative response may be problematic for clients who tend to acquire new routines in a rather rigid, stimulus-specific manner, such as those with autistic-like characteristics who exhibit stimulus overselectivity. They may become overly dependent on instructional cues or prompts and have extreme difficulty in shifting and responding to more naturally occurring but less salient stimuli (Koegel, Russo, Rincover, & Schreibman, 1982).  This strategy provides an approach to training communication skills by accommodating to the learning styles of individuals with autism and related disorders.

## PURPOSE OF THE STRATEGY

The goal of this strategy is to develop a communication aid containing visual-spatial symbols that can be used by individuals with autism and related disorders, and to train these individuals to use the aid to communicate.

# UNDERLYING ASSUMPTIONS

1. *Client*.    This  strategy  is  appropriate  for  individuals  who  function communicatively at the late sensorimotor level or above.  Clients that may benefit from this strategy include those who exhibit one or more of the following:  (a) limited number  of  communicative  means  or  functions;  (b)  limited  understanding  of  causal relationships (means-ends); (c) limited knowledge of appropriate object use; and (d) limited symbolic ability.

2. *Augmentative Components*.  Any type of language board or book may be used. The  type  of  symbols  selected  will  depend  on  the  needs  and  capabilities  of  the individual.   While  the  needs  of  higher-functioning  and  verbal  individuals  are  not addressed in this strategy, it is suggested that use of nontransient symbols, such as written  words,  should  be  considered  to  augment  the  communication  skills  of  these individuals.

3. *Environmental Constraints.*  Communication  partners  should  be  willing  to implement this strategy.  No other environmental constraints exist.

# DESCRIPTION OF THE STRATEGY

## *Development of the Communication Aid*

*Symbols.*  The symbols selected for a client's communication system should be as small and as abstract as the client is able to consistently and accurately use to match objects/events to a referent.  For example, objects/events may be matched to:

- identical objects;

- identical miniature objects;

- large, identical, colored photographs;

- large, nonidentical, colored photographs;

- large, identical, black-and-white line drawings (e.g., Picture Communication Symbols, available from Mayer-Johnson Co., Box 56, Stillwater, MN 55082);

- abstract symbols (e.g., Blissymbols); and

- written words.

For some clients, selection of the most abstract level means that all of the pictures or symbols in the initial system will be at the same symbol level (e.g., objects or colored, nonidentical photographs). However, for many clients, pictures or symbols from two or more levels (e.g., some colored, nonidentical photographs, and some black-and-white line drawings) can be used. Such "mixed-symbol" sets should be encouraged, particularly for clients who exhibit a high degree of accuracy at one level and a lesser, but emerging degree of accuracy at the next level.

*Lexicon*. Several authors have described systematic procedures for selecting initial vocabulary items for an augmentative communication aid (Carlson, 1981; McDonald, 1980; Musselwhite & St. Louis, 1982; Yoder, 1980; see also chapters 4 & 5 in this text). An additional procedure that can be used effectively to determine vocabulary needs is derived from the ecological inventory strategy described by Brown and his colleagues (1980). Clinicians should consider selecting initial vocabulary items that correspond to communicative functions already expressed by the client using less formal communication modes (e.g., idiosyncratic gestures). For instance, pointing to a symbol that represents *more* to request the continuation of a favored routine may replace a more primitive, preintentional signal, such as motor agitation and proximity (for more examples, see Prizant & Schuler, in press; Schuler, 1985). In this procedure, the clinician uses highly motivating, nonabstract concepts, and gradually introduces additional functional vocabulary as the client begins to use some items spontaneously. This model emphasizes the use of nonabstract, meaningful vocabulary items in naturally occurring contexts (e.g., restaurants, grocery stores, etc.), with the gradual introduction of additional, functional vocabulary as the client begins to use the communication aid spontaneously.

*Vocabulary display*. Clients may have difficulty scanning complex visual arrangements. Assessment data should be collected by the augmentative communication team to determine the following:

- Is it easier for the client to look at symbols (objects, pictures, etc.) in a horizontal or a vertical array? For example, does the client's head or eyes move horizontally across a display containing several objects? Does the client scan objects placed in a vertical row at midline?

- Do error responses increase at the periphery of the display?

- Do error responses decrease when objects/pictures are placed closer together? farther apart?

- Do error responses decrease when the number of symbols in the display are decreased?

- Does the client tend to choose items on one side (right or left) of the anatomical midline? If so, does accuracy improve when all objects are aligned to that side?

Symbol displays should be developed taking these data into account. For example, the number and arrangement of pictures on each page or display should be confined to that which the learner can accurately and consistently scan. Some clients appear to be more successful at top-to-bottom (column) scanning than to the usual left-to-right (row) scanning, and pictures should be arranged in accordance with the preferred direction. Pictures should be arranged in both rows and columns only for clients with good visual scanning skills in both directions. The distance between pictures should also be individually adjusted. For some clients, the pictures may need to be displayed close together because of limited scanning abilities, while others may require a greater distance between pictures for accurate discrimination.

For clients with motor planning problems related to severe/profound developmental delays or a physical disability, it may be difficult to cross the anatomical midline with either one or both upper extremities. These clients may only be capable of pointing to pictures displayed on one side of the midline. If this occurs, the pictures should be arranged in a top-to-bottom array on the front (but not the back) of each page, and the pages should be bound together so that they can be turned in the opposite direction of the preferred hand. This eliminates the need to cross the midline, since all pictures are arranged on the client's dominant side at all times. Another solution is to arrange single pictures in the middle of each page and to bind the pages so that they turn upward. Such creative arrangements preclude the need to work on motor planning skills as "prerequisites" to communication book or board use.

The augmentative communication team should insure that the physical layout of the picture communication book/board accommodates the client's abilities and skill deficits and allows for maximum efficiency during use. For example, a client with a 25-page communication book may experience frustration and refuse to use the book because it takes so long to locate a desired picture. To facilitate more efficient use of the communication aid, pictures can be:

- grouped by color-coded categories (e.g., food pictures on blue pages, recreation/leisure pictures on yellow pages),

- divided using section dividers with large, protruding index tabs in colors that correspond to each section, or

- grouped by environmental category so that the book has school-related pictures in one section, home pictures in another, restaurant pictures in yet another, and so on. This approach often requires that some pictures (e.g., bathroom/toilet) appear in more than one section because their use is likely to occur across environments. This approach is often preferable for clients who receive frequent community-based instruction (Brown et al., 1980) as part of their school programs, or who are active in a variety of settings during nonschool hours.

*Construction*. Generally speaking, clients with autism will best be served by communication aids that are both portable and durable. Portability can be accomplished by compiling picture books that can be hand-carried, or by designing flip-charts or individual pages that can be worn on the belt, carried around the neck (for younger children), or attached to shoulder strap. Pictures can be preserved and made more durable if they are laminated, assembled in clear plastic pages such as Sturdi-Kleer or other products, assembled in clear photograph album pages with peel-back, self-adhesive covers, placed in the pockets of clear vinyl pages used to protect photographs or slides, or inserted in individual plastic covers such as those available with the Picture Communication Symbols (Mayer-Johnson Co.). The educator, clinician, and parent team responsible for designing the board or book will need to be creative and flexible in order to assemble the most portable and durable communication aid for each client (see Mirenda, 1985, for a more complete discussion).

## *Instructional Strategy*

This instructional strategy emphasizes the spontaneous use of the communication aid from the onset of training, thus avoiding the need for programming stimulus transfer from an instructional to a natural cue. The strategy consists of four general phases that can be adapted for individual clients. Phases 1 through 3 are conducted in structured training sessions, while Phase 4 is conducted in generalization environments (home, school, etc.).

*Phase 1: Establishing a Spontaneous Touch Response.*

1. Place a picture of a high-preference item on the table in front of the client so that it is "in the way." Place the corresponding high-preference item off to the side in view of the client.

2. Do not provide verbal cues or refer to either the picture or the item.

3. Engage in a simple activity during which the client is likely to touch the picture accidentally.

4. If the client touches the picture, either deliberately or accidentally, immediately provide the high-preference item for a brief period of time.

5. Once the client consistently touches the picture several times over several sessions, fade the high-preference item gradually until it is no longer visible.

Criterion for proceeding to Phase 2: The client will touch one symbol spontaneously in order to receive the referent (e.g., high-preference item.)

*Phase 2. Teaching Search and Locate Behavior*

1. Mask the picture used in Phase 1 with a translucent page (e.g., onionskin paper). The client must now lift the page and touch the picture. The clinician provides no verbal cues but does provide differential reinforcement (i.e., the high-preference item) for all attempts at page-lifting.

2. Once the client consistently lifts the translucent page and touches the picture, change to an opaque page and repeat the shaping procedure as necessary.

3. After mastery of Phase 2, mask the picture with two opaque pages and repeat the shaping procedure.

Criterion for proceeding to Phase 3: After lifting two opaque pages to find a picture, the client will then touch the picture to receive the referent (high-preference item).

*Phase 3. Increasing the Number of Symbols*

1. Place the original symbol and a blank "dummy" card of the same size and color on the table under two opaque pages.

2. Provide the high-preference item if the client touches the picture. Provide nothing if the dummy card is touched. Alternate positions of the picture and card randomly and continue to refrain from providing verbal cues.

3. Once the client consistently touches the picture and avoids the dummy card, provide the original picture and a second high-preference picture. Provide the item corresponding to the picture touched.

4. Gradually add pictures, one at a time, or as rapidly as possible without losing the search-locate-touch response. Be sure the pictures are added in accordance with the client's preferred visual scanning/motor response patterns.

5. Continue to provide the item corresponding to the picture touched and refrain from providing verbal cues.

Criterion for proceeding to Phase 4: The client will be able to choose one of several pictures arranged on one or more pages and should receive the item/event requested.

### Phase 4. Generalization

1. Provide instruction to family members, school staff, and all involved individuals regarding the purpose of the aid and how the learner can be expected to use it (i.e., to request items).

2. Provide the client with the aid across environments.

3. Continue to expand the picture vocabulary gradually, based on client interests, needs, and so on.

4. Gradually begin to establish practical parameters regarding affirmative responses to pictures touched. For example, begin to refrain from providing the item requested during inappropriate times. However, continue to respond affirmatively to the client's initiations as often as possible.

Phase 4 is ongoing and requires long-term monitoring on the part of those involved. During this phase, new vocabulary is identified and the symbol display is updated and maintained.

## EVALUATION OF EFFECTIVENESS

Use of a prompt-free instructional strategy to establish initial pictorial communication skills in individuals with limited communication skills may be preferable to strategies that employ a large number of external instructional cues because of the prompt dependence so commonly observed in autism. The effectiveness of this strategy was recently reported in a case study of a 9-year-old nonspeaking girl with "autistic-like" characteristics (Mirenda & Santogrossi, 1985).

## REFERENCES

Brown, L., Falvey, M., Vincent, L., Kaye, N., Johnson, F., Ferrara-Parrish, P., & Gruenewald, L. (1980). Strategies for generating comprehensive, longitudinal, and chronological age appropriate individual education programs for adolescent and young adult severely handicapped students. Journal of Special Education, 14, 199-215.

Carlson, F. (1981). A format for selecting vocabulary for the non-speaking child. Language, Speech, and Hearing Services in Schools, 12, 240-248.

Das, J.P. (1984). Simultaneous and successive processing in children with reading disability. Topics in Language Disorders, 4, 34-48.

Fay, W.H., & Schuler, A.L. (1980). Emerging language in autistic children. Austin, TX: Pro-Ed.

Goetz, L., Gee, K., & Sailor, W. (1985). Using a behavior chain interruption strategy to teach communicative skills to students with severe disabilities. Journal of the Association for Persons with Severe Handicaps, 10, 21-30.

Hart, B., & Risley, T.R. (1975). Incidental teaching of language in the preschool. Journal of Applied Behavior Analysis, 8, 411-420.

Keogh, W.J., & Reichle, J. (1985). Communication intervention for the "difficult-to-teach" severely handicapped. In S.F. Warren & A.K. Rogers-Warren (Eds.), Teaching functional language (pp. 157-194). Baltimore: University Park Press.

Koegel, R.L., Russo, D.C., Rincover, A., & Schreibman, L. (1982).   Assessing and training teachers.  In R. L. Koegel, A. Rincover, & A. L. Egel (Eds.), Educating and understanding autistic children (pp. 178-202).  San Diego:   College-Hill Press.

McDonald, E. T.  (1980).   Early identification and treatment of children at risk for speech development.  In R. L. Schiefelbusch (Ed.), Nonspeech language and communication: Analysis and intervention (pp. 49-79).  Austin, TX:  Pro-Ed.

Mirenda, P.  (1985).   Designing pictorial communication systems for physically able-bodied students with severe handicaps.   Augmentative and Alternative Communication, 1, 58-64.

Mirenda, P., & Santogrossi, J.  (1985).   A prompt-free strategy to teach pictorial communication system use.  Augmentative and Alternative Communication, 1, 143-150.

Musselwhite, C.R., & St. Louis, K.W.  (1982).  Communication programming for the severely handicapped: Vocal and non-vocal strategies. San Diego:  College-Hill Press.

Prizant, B. M.  (1983).   Language acquisition and communicative behavior in autism: Toward an understanding of the "whole" of it.  Journal of Speech and Hearing Disorders, 48, 296-307.

Prizant, B.M., & Schuler, A.L. (in press).   Facilitating communication:   Theoretical foundation.  In D. Cohen & A. Donnellan (Eds.), Handbook of autism and pervasive developmental disorders.  New York:  John Wiley & Sons.

Reichle, J., & Yoder, D.E. (1985).  Communication board use in severely handicapped learners. Language, Speech, and Hearing Services in Schools, 16, 146-167.

Schuler, A.L.  (1985).   Selecting augmentative communication systems on the basis of current communicative means and functions.  Australian Journal of Human Communication Disorders, 13, 99-116.

Schuler, A.L., & Prizant, B.M.  (in press).  Facilitating communication:  Prelanguage approaches.  In D. Cohen & A. Donnellan (Eds.), Handbook of autism and pervasive developmental disorders. New York:  John Wiley & Sons.

Snell, M., & Gast. D. (1981). Applying time delay procedures to the instruction of the severely handicapped. Journal of the Association for the Severely Handicapped, 6, 3-14.

Tager-Flusberg, H. (1981). On the nature of linguistic functioning in early infantile autism. Journal of Autism and Developmental Disorders, 2, 45-56.

Yoder, D.E. (1980). Communication system for nonspeech children. New Directions for Exceptional Children, 2, 63-78.

# EXPANDING SEQUENCING, TURNTAKING, AND TIMING SKILLS THROUGH PLAY ACTING

*Sheela Stuart*
*Crippled Children's Hospital and School*
*Sioux Falls, South Dakota*

## INTRODUCTION

When seeking experiences to foster any child's development and learning, the processes of drama are helpful (Cottrell, 1984). Personality growth in the areas of (a) imagination, (b) interaction, and (c) perception and response to aesthetic qualities are inherent goals within any drama experience. "Drama and speech are central to a language curriculum, not peripheral. . . . This thesis rests on the assumption that dramatic interaction--doing things verbally in situations with other people--is the primary vehicle for developing thought and language" (Siks, 1983, p. 11). These elements are recognized for verbal children who have vast numbers of other opportunities for learning.

Drama is a vehicle for children with severe expressive communication disorders as well. Nonspeaking individuals do not have the "ordinary" experiential opportunities of engaging in didactic communication. They have never had the opportunity to learn the processes involved in "talking Mom into letting us" or "talking our way out of a situation." Drama is used to facilitate personality growth and communicative competence by creating specific opportunities for such communication. An opportunity to role play with turntaking and episodic sequencing offers a mechanism to improve communication skills, provides elements for growth in creativity and imagery, and heightens self-confidence.

## PURPOSE OF STRATEGY

The purposes of this strategy are to enable persons who use communication aids to experience genuine didactic exchanges (i.e., you say this--then I say that--then you respond); to develop spontaneous problem-solving and conversational repair skills if something unexpected occurs; to emphasize sequential aspects of storytelling (i.e., beginning, middle, ending); to create opportunities for experience in fantasy and drama; and to develop personal awareness of expression through creative art.

Individual goals for nonspeaking persons for whom this strategy is employed will vary. Some goals may include:

1.  decreasing client's response time to five seconds or less using preprogrammed information within specific scenes;

2.  activating a communication aid appropriately five times during Act I and three times during Act II using accurate timing;

3.  maintaining attention and listening to the dialogue of other children and reacting appropriately throughout Acts I and II;

4.  using a variety of modes (e.g., saluting, searching, fist shaking, and device output) to enhance listener understanding in Acts I and II; and

5.  demonstrating the ability to entertain through communication.

## UNDERLYING ASSUMPTIONS

1. *Client*. The strategy is appropriate for most severely speech-impaired persons, regardless of age, developmental level, and educational placement. However, the type of "production" must be appropriate for the developmental, experiential, and disabling conditions of the clients. The strategy is not appropriate for individuals with cognitive abilities below a 3-year level and for those who do not use augmentative techniques consistently and meaningfully.

Higher functioning children should be encouraged to assume responsibilities for all aspects of the production, including:

a.  Writing the script for their own production following certain specifications. For example:

    1. It must be a total, well-sequenced story.

2. It must include dialogue and stage directions for each scene that tells the story.

3. It must include dialogue that conveys three different emotions and involves interaction between the characters.

b. Describing possible props and costuming needed for production.

c. Developing dialogue. Given the character's role, the children should make suggestions for actual lines.

2. *Augmentative components*. A variety of augmentative aids and techniques may be used in the "performance" (e.g., alternate display monitors, such as television screens and printers; electronic devices using synthesized speech output; laptrays with displays accessed by pointing; and eye-gaze displays that can be used together or grouped for specific scenes). The clinician must develop creative methods that will enable children to present the story and/or involve a narrator without intrusion.

For children with a limited vocabulary and/or who do not use electronic speech output devices, other alternatives are possible, as follows:

a. A portion of the play can feature use of an adapted toy, an eye gaze response, or use of some environmental control switch to turn on a radio, cassette player, or lamp, in conjunction with narration.

b. Individuals using signs can be easily included, making certain the narration or preceding dialogue cues the audience to their message.

c. Lines or limited communications can be written in symbols on large banner-type sheets. At the appropriate time, the client can lift the placard or "bring in" the banner to communicate their portion of the story.

3. *Clinician preparation*. The communication specialist and other staff members should:

a. Plan the production to insure that the action occurs smoothly and rapidly. This may require special music, narration, or older clients to cue younger children.

b. Balance the production so the children are all challenged while no one is overwhelmed or slighted.

c. Provide opportunities for clients to "act" within situations--being careful not to overdirect.  The clients' imagery and ability to pretend should be utilized.

4. *Environmental constraints*.  Employing this strategy requires additional use of space and materials, as well as additional staff attention and time.  Commitment from the administration to the project will help avoid difficulties.  Administrative permission should be obtained for committing time, space, and money to the project and for holding an actual performance.

Specific items to bear in mind include:

a. If everyone in the play is in a wheelchair, an auxiliary stage may be required.

b. Movement within scenes is constrained but possible with electric wheelchairs.

c. For children using speech output devices, auxiliary amplifiers may be necessary to enable the audience to hear.

d. "Spoken lines" that are stored in electronic devices must have recall codes that are remembered and accessed easily by device users.  Note: Many hours of staff time must be spent programming the speech output to be as "normal" as possible.

e. Practice sessions may take children out of other activities for dress rehearsals.

## DESCRIPTION OF STRATEGY

The greatest client development will result from the appropriate selection of clients for each production.  Successful mixing of clients with high and low functional abilities (according to role responsibility) provides more flexibility and allows for increased complexity of productions.  It is important to remember that the main purpose of this strategy is to encourage client communication within a dramatic structure, not to produce an award-winning extravaganza. The individual strengths and weaknesses, group size, and cognitive level of the majority will greatly influence all aspects of the production. The steps that should be followed in utilizing this strategy are discussed below.

## *Preparation for the Production*

*Select story theme*. When possible, the children should be involved in the selection process. For example, clinicians can encourage client suggestions by offering choices appropriate to the group (e.g., "What do people do on their birthday?") and then ask the group for their own ideas.

*Develop plot and characters*. In this step, the speech-language pathologist and other professionals outline the play (i.e., acts, scenes, and characters required to present the story). Careful consideration is given to the needs, the capabilities, and the communication, language, and speech goals of the nonspeaking and/or nonwriting participants.

*Develop dialogue*. The story outline is presented to the children and they become involved in the development of dialoque for each character. Young children can participate by suggesting, approving, or disapproving the script, while older children may actually write sections of the play. For example, the communication specialist may ask, "What do we say when we go to a birthday party?" or "Do you think Laura should say 'I hate birthday cake' when she gets to the party?"

## *Practicing the Production*

*Practice individual parts*. Each child is assigned a role and begins to practice the "part." The goals of this step are to:

1. Practice consistent use of preprogrammed information and/or actions within a constant environment.

2. Improve turntaking, which requires elements of attending, memory, and time.

3. Practice sequential communicative interactions through storytelling.

*Practice scenes and acts of play*. The children practice portions of the play together. The goals of this step are to initiate conversation; make clever, humorous, or directing interjections; and recover when communication breakdowns occur.  By participating in these predetermined interactions, the actors also gain personal experience using various augmentative techniques and strategies to consistently portray characters and to maintain a flow of conversational interactions.

## *Performing the Production*

A dress performance is recommended so that the children and the staff can anticipate some of the problems that might occur and the children can practice the entire production.  All performers should be congratulated for their efforts.

Performing for an audience offers an opportunity to experience collective efforts at peak performance.  The sense of self-trust and trust of others to achieve successful communication is fostered.  It also offers an opportunity for the children to experience drama and entertainment, giving of themselves through communicative efforts, and receiving praise and appreciation for their efforts.

## EFFECTIVENESS OF STRATEGY

The Communication Group at Crippled Children's Hospital and School in Sioux Falls, South Dakota, uses this strategy two to three times per year.  For example, in June 1984, the Crippled Children's Hospital and School Communication Group chose to write and produce a small play as a summer semester project.  Parts of that effort were videotaped for future reference and to share with families.  The total production was one act--riding on a bus going to a Halloween Party--that lasted about 10 to 12 minutes.

In May 1985, 20 nonspeaking children presented a three-act play entitled, *A Country Party*, based on a Laura Ingalls Wilder story (Wilder, 1937).  For this play, all group members used communication aids.  Eleven used electronic devices with printed and synthesized speech output.  The other children used a combination of "manual boards," (i.e., laptrays, eye gaze, notebooks, and adapted electronic toys).

In this production, we began by exploring several Laura Ingalls Wilder stories. The children expressed special interest in a vignette from *On the Banks of Plum Creek, Nellie Olsen's Birthday Party*.  The clinicians designed a basic outline of possible scenes. Activities for students focused on individual communication goals, which reflected the needs of children at a high linguistic level (writing lines for two characters in a scene depicting snobbery, jealousy, and embarrassment), through an intermediate level (requesting an object and an event during the play, on cue), and beginning level (use a communication aid with 90 percent accuracy to say, "Hello, my name is Heather," when requested). Individual tasks for each outlined step, such as script and dialogue development, were assigned according to functional levels and goals of the children participating. The group then met to "homogenize" the various individual products to meet the group goals of:

- writing a script, including each client's contribution;

- determining stage scenery, costumes, and so on;

- assuming individual roles;

- presenting a full scene; and

- performing a complete play.

As described earlier, many practice sessions are required. For example, in the May production of *A Country Party*, the group met for one hour weekly from January through March. In April, they practiced five days a week for one hour daily.

Special problems included staging, amplification, and maintaining pre-programmed information in aids due to some device breakdowns. The participants also found certain experiences frustrating, such as being asked to repeat a scene several times to assist one member to increase performance speed, waiting while a classmate tried to find the proper code to recall the appropriate line, and deciding what to do when the line was inappropriate.

Individual and group goals were met. However, this often required special practice during therapy sessions and individual assignments for homework. Carryover into other situations was noted in some areas, that is, more efficient device usage (faster code recall and timing) and increased ability to recover during and following a communication breakdown. Overall, group members seemed to communicate more frequently, creatively, and appropriately in social and academic situations. Best of all, they had fun and were proud of their performance.

# REFERENCES

Cottrell, J.  (1984).  <u>Teaching with creative dramatics</u>.  Lincolnwood, IL:  National Textbook Co.

Siks, B.  (1983).  <u>Drama with children</u>.  New York:  Harper & Row.

Wilder, L. (1937).  <u>On the banks of Plum Creek</u>.  New York:  Harper & Row.

## DEVELOPMENT OF A LOCATION, COLOR-CODED ETRAN

*Gail M. Van Tatenhove*
*Communication Systems Evaluation Center*
*Orlando, Florida*

## INTRODUCTION

An ETRAN is an eye point encoding system (see chapter 3 for a more complete description). It is an efficient augmentative or alternative communication technique, since eye encoding requires minimal physical effort and allows users to send messages quickly to familiar partners. An ETRAN can be designed in a variety of ways to match a user's cognitive and language abilities. This strategy describes a two-part encoding approach utilizing coding by location and color (LC-ETRAN). An LC-ETRAN can display up to 144 simultaneously presented messages. Additional groups of messages or entire displays can be interchanged, thus extending the message potential.

## PURPOSE OF STRATEGY

The purpose of this strategy is to develop an LC-ETRAN and to promote interactive use of the LC-ETRAN in multiple contexts.

## UNDERLYING ASSUMPTIONS

1. *Client*. The client must be properly supported through positioning for communication and must demonstrate a reliable and readable eye point, as well as an understanding of location/color encoding (i.e., the ability to scan a display in a left-to-right, top-to-bottom progression; discriminate between one-inch or smaller graphic displays (words, symbols, or pictures) placed 12 to 24 inches from his/her trunk; and match and discriminate among 12 colors). In addition, the client should have at least 100 to 144 messages to express. The LC-ETRAN must be acceptable to the client.

2. *Augmentative components*.  The symbols selected must be appropriate for the client and the client's partner, and messages selected should have interactive value to the client.  Symbols must accommodate a one-inch square target space.  Instructions for the use of an LC-ETRAN must be visible and understandable to potential communication partners and should include clear and concise directions, the location of additional displays, and information about the client and specific interaction strategies.

Materials required for constructing an LC-ETRAN and for making displays include:

1.  24 x 24 inch piece of 1/8 inch thick Lexan paneling

2.  wood for mount

3.  acetate sheets for displays

4.  color markers or acrylic paint to code locations

5.  bulldog clips to attach displays

6.  color pencils to code spaces

7.  velcro to attach displays

The equipment should be durable and portable (i.e., adequately mounted on the client's wheelchair laptray and easily transported between settings).  In addition, the displays must be protected by providing adequate storage (e.g., mailing tube or expandable file, transport tube, or bag on client's wheelchair).

3. *Environmental constraints*.  The communication partner must be available for a one-hour training session, must assume responsibility for providing feedback to the client and for exchanging displays, as needed, and must be willing to use the LC-ETRAN in multiple contexts.  The communication partner must understand the symbols and the encoding concept, and must be able to interpret the client's eye point.

## DESCRIPTION OF STRATEGY

### *Step 1.  Construction of the LC-ETRAN*

Cut an 8 x 8 inch window from the center of the Lexan panel (see Figure 6-8). Drill a hole into each corner of the potential window, insert saber saw, and carefully cut along grid lines.  Divide the remaining section of the Lexan panel into 12 4-inch squares by leaving 1 inch around the edge of the panel and 2 inches between potential locations.  Paint each of the 12 locations with acrylic paint.  Avoid placement of similar colors in close proximity.  After the panel has been color coded, construct a wooden mount that securely attaches to the student's wheelchair laptray.  Design the side supports of the mounts with a groove so that the Lexan panel will slide into it easily.

### *Step 2.  Construction of Displays*

*Twelve location displays.*  To make 12 location displays, cut a sheet of acetate to match the Lexan panel, round the corners, color code the spaces of each location using colors that correspond to each location, affix vocabulary to the display, and attach to the top of the panel with bulldog clips (see Figure 6-9).  Create as many displays as needed, storing extra displays in a mailing tube on the client's wheelchair.

*Individual location displays.*  To make individual location displays, cut and color code 1-inch square grid paper (4 x 4) with a 2-inch hole in the middle.  Place two loop sections of velcro dots, cut in half, on the upper rear corners of the location display square and place matching hook dots to the location on the Lexan panel (see Figure 6-10).  Store extra displays in an expandable file kept in a bag on the wheelchair.

### *Step 3.  Organization of Displays*

Compile a comprehensive vocabulary list for the display, including single words, phrases, and sentences.  From the list, select the best messages for initial use on the LC-ETRAN.  Analyze all messages selected and develop a master plan of locations needed, grouping vocabulary into 12 item classes.  Design placement of the locations on the LC-ETRAN as suggested in Figure 6-11.

# FIGURE 6-8.  SUGGESTED SPECIFICATION OF LC-ETRAN

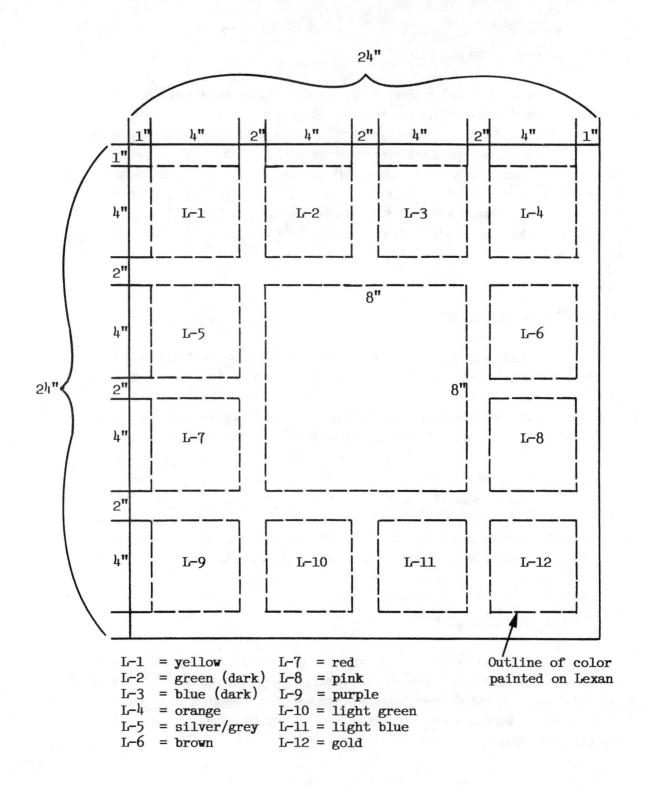

L-1  = yellow          L-7  = red
L-2  = green (dark)     L-8  = pink
L-3  = blue (dark)      L-9  = purple
L-4  = orange           L-10 = light green
L-5  = silver/grey      L-11 = light blue
L-6  = brown            L-12 = gold

**FIGURE 6-9. ACETATE DISPLAY**

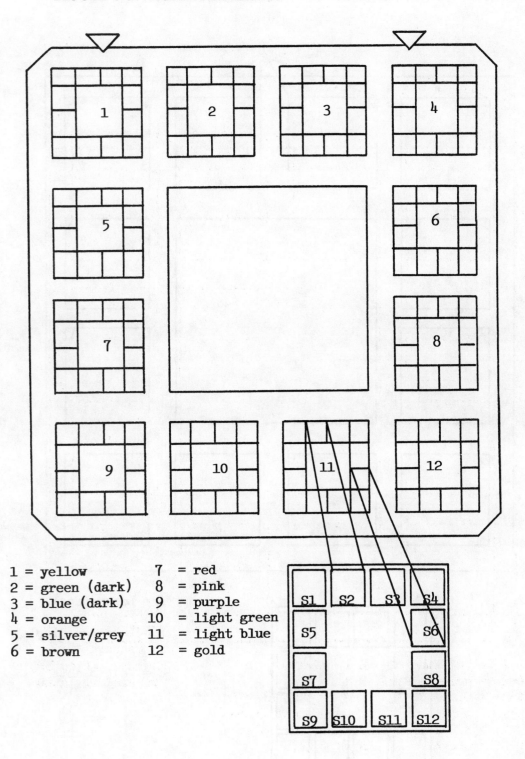

1 = yellow      7 = red
2 = green (dark)   8 = pink
3 = blue (dark)    9 = purple
4 = orange       10 = light green
5 = silver/grey    11 = light blue
6 = brown        12 = gold

**FIGURE 6-10.  INTERCHANGEABLE LOCATION OF DISPLAY SQUARES**

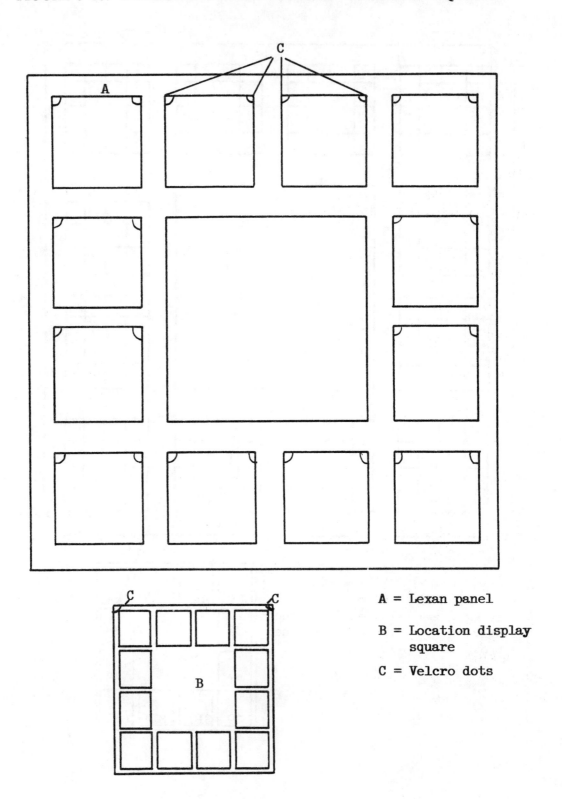

A = Lexan panel

B = Location display
    square

C = Velcro dots

**FIGURE 6-11. SUGGESTED DISPLAY ORGANIZATION FOR LC-ETRAN**

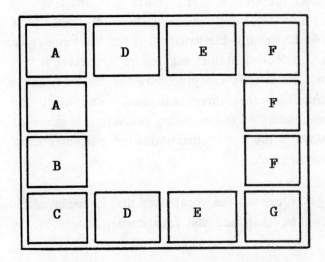

A – People
B – Places
C – Feelings
D – Actions
E – Modifiers
F – Objects
G – Phrases, sentences

*Step 4.  Understanding the Encoding Procedure*

The following is an example of a systematic method for teaching each step of the encoding process.

To teach the user that the panel is a significant whole made of distinct and important parts, say "Name (N), this is your communication board." Trace outline of the Lexan. "It is divided into 12 big squares. Here is one. Here is one." Touch each

location from left to right and top to bottom. "Each big square has a color. This one is red, this one is blue." Name each color, scanning left to right, top to bottom.

Once the user recognizes each of the locations, focus attention on the spaces. This teaches that each part of the whole is further divided into 12 additional subparts. Say "Look at this big square." Then point to each space and say "Each big square has many little squares. Here is one, here is one." To draw attention to the relationship of the colors of the locations and corresponding space, say "Each little square matches the color of a big square." Place one open hand behind a location. "Look at this little square. It is (color). It matches this big square." Point out the relationship of each of the 12 colors. Have the student match space and location colors to insure understanding of their relationship.

To teach the two-part sequence and coding needed to express a message, say "I am going to put a picture of X in this big square on the Y color." Place the picture in a corner location on a color corresponding to one of the three other corners. "If you want X, look at this big square." Place an open hand behind the quadrant to indicate the entire location. "Now look at the color the picture is on." Point with one finger to the color on the picture. "Find the same color big square." After N finds it, re-explain how it was done. "Good, you looked to this big square that has the same color. You told me you wanted X because you looked at this big square and then at this color." Point to the location and color. To solidify the procedure for the user, add a second, third, and fourth picture using the other three remaining locations in the corners of the Lexan. Adequate understanding of the encoding procedure is achieved when the student can indicate a message without the communication partner cueing selection of a location and the corresponding color.

*Note: Expansion of vocabulary.* To expand the vocabulary that is displayed, fill in the spaces of the four corner locations, then add the four corner spaces of the middle locations (see Figure 6-12).

Each time an item is added, emphasize the location and the corresponding color using variations of the given teaching script. Since the LC-ETRAN may be designed to allow individual locations to be exchanged, repeat the teaching procedure and review vocabulary when changing location displays. Once the four corner spaces of each location contain vocabulary, add the center spaces of the corner and center locations. This systematic addition of vocabulary is designed to insure client understanding and competence with the LC-ETRAN. Be sure that interactive activities are used in training and that the client understands the organization of the display.

## *Step 5: First Interactive Activity*

Choose and organize a fun, motivating activity that utilizes four to six vocabulary items or messages. This minimizes the demands placed on the client and prevents the client from becoming overwhelmed with the new augmentative communication technique. An example of an activity might be an excursion to a soda or candy machine. Place the pictures of money, soda, and candies, and so on, onto the display. To stimulate initiation of communication, model use of the device by saying, "I think I will have something from this big square and it is on the (color). It is a cola. What about you?" If the client fails to make a request, ask the client to indicate a preference. Expect the client to ask for money and to assist, if physically able, in purchasing the item of choice. Generalize use of the pictures displayed by intentionally meeting someone who is familiar with the LC-ETRAN and who will appropriately cue the client to relate what was bought, who purchased it, and how much it cost. Other excellent interactive activities include:

**FIGURE 6-12.  INTRODUCTION OF VOCABULARY**

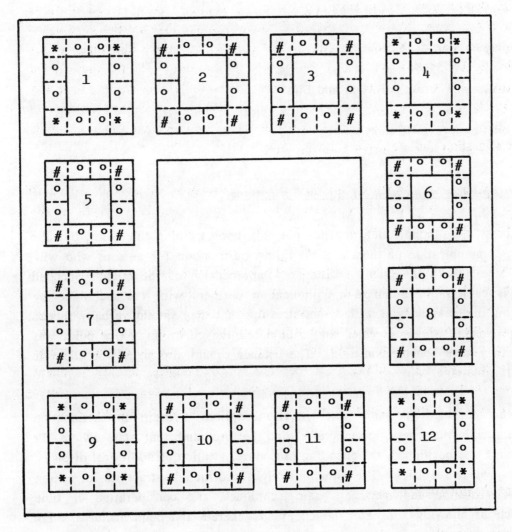

* = first priority to contain vocabulary; represents the corner
    spaces of the corner locations

# = second priority to contain vocabulary; represents the corner
    spaces of the middle locations

° = represents the remaining spaces of all locations; will contain
    vocabulary as needed, and no order is required when adding the
    vocabulary

1. asking directions

2. going to a restaurant or store

3. playing a favorite game

4. making a present for Mom and Dad

5. relating a favorite story

## Step 6:  Insuring Communication Success in Environment

Successful communication depends not only upon training the client, but also on training communication partners and providing information for persons who will randomly interact with the client.  Listener comprehension of the client's encoded procedure is critical.  Familiarize communication partners with the technique by demonstrating and reviewing it with them, stressing that they should verbally repeat the message they felt was expressed and should tell the client if an eye point was unclear or they have become confused.  The listener should also signal the client to repeat the last message.

Since untrained persons will require explicit written instructions to communicate with the client, directions should be provided that state where the listener needs to be positioned, the encoding procedure, location of additional displays, and how to provide feedback.  The directions might also include strategies for asking questions, clarification and message repair techniques, and consideration of time factors, such as allowing time for the client to generate independent ideas.  For example:

My name is X and I communicate by looking at messages on this Lexan panel, so stand in front of me and look through the window in my board.  I use a code to tell you what I want.  First I look at a big square. Please put your hand in the square you think I am looking at and I will know you are starting to understand my system.  You will see that each big square has 12 parts, so to tell you which part I want, I look at a second big square.  Put your other hand on the second square I look at. The message I want is in the first big square in the position or part that matches the location and color of the second big square.  Do you understand my system?  Good, let's communicate.  I'll start by looking at you, at the first big square, then the second big square and back to you. Please tell me what you thought I communicated and I will agree or disagree. I say yes/no by (describe client's method). I may need other displays that are on the back of my wheelchair. I'll tell you when I need one.

To enhance communication with untrained, nonreading persons, directions can be tape recorded and enhanced with pictorial explanations.

For successful communication, the client is responsible for signaling the receiver to study the directions. Selection and expression of messages that control and direct the interaction must also be taught to the client. Include messages such as "I need a new, big square/display," "It's not on my board," "I don't understand," or "Ask me good yes/no questions."

## EFFECTIVENESS OF STRATEGY

A case review of two clients evaluated at the Communication Systems Evaluation Center (CSEC), Orlando, Florida, indicates that this strategy results in effective interactive use of an LC-ETRAN and improved communication interaction. Client #1 is a 17-year-old male residing in a residential facility for the mentally handicapped. He is diagnosed as having athetoid cerebral palsy, persisting primitive reflexes, and increased muscle tone. Eye movements are his most reliable means of directly accessing messages. The client had an unsuccessful experience with an LC-ETRAN 6 months prior to the evaluation; however, no systematic teaching approach had been used. He was reintroduced to an LC-ETRAN using the procedures outlined in this strategy. After only 20 minutes of training, he completed each step without cueing. The persons accompanying the client were retrained, and follow-up information obtained 6 months later indicates continued ability to complete the encoding sequence independently.

Client #2 is a 6-year-old female with a diagnosis of athetoid cerebral palsy and mental retardation. She resides with her mother and extended family. She attends a program for physically impaired, educable, mentally handicapped students. Eye pointing is a more reliable means of access for her than the direct selection eye- and fist-pointing system that she had used during the previous year. She was taught a six-location, six-position LC-ETRAN system, learning the encoding procedures in 30 minutes. A reevaluation completed 18 months later indicated spontaneous use of her system, which she uses interactively with teachers and ambulatory peers. At the reevaluation, her system was expanded to 12 locations and 12 positions and she successfully generalized the encoding procedure following less than 10 minutes of explanation and modeling.

## ADDITIONAL READINGS

Ginsberg, H., & Opper, S.    (1969).    Piaget's theory of intellectual development. Englewood Cliffs, NJ:  Prentice-Hall.

McDonald, E.  (1980).   Teaching and using Blissymbolics.   Toronto:   Blissymbolics Communication Institute.

Musselwhite, C., & St. Louis, K.  (1980).  Communication programming for the severely handicapped.  San Diego:  College Hill Press.

Silverman, F.  (1980).   Communication for the speechless.   Englewood Cliffs, NJ: Prentice-Hall.

Vanderheiden, G., & Grilley, K.   (1975).   Non-vocal communication techniques and aids for the severely physically handicapped.  Baltimore:  University Park Press.

Van Tatenhove, G.   (1985).   Cognitive skills in consideration of an augmentative communication system.  Unpublished manuscript.

Vicker, B.  (1974).   Non-oral communication system project 1964/1973.   Iowa City: University of Iowa.

## APPENDIX A

The following materials for constructing an LC-ETRAN are available at local hardware stores:

1. Lexan (store personnel will cut to size)

2. wood

3. mounting brackets if needed

The following materials are available at local supply stores:

1. acetate sheets

2. color markers or paint

3. bulldog clips

Velcro is available from local fabric shops.

## MESSAGING AND REPORTING

*Patricia Wasson*
*Education Service Center*
*Region 20*
*San Antonio, Texas*

## INTRODUCTION

Notebooking is a method that is used to exchange information between persons at two locations through the use of spiral notebooks. In addition, notebooking:

- uses semantic contingency (the topics are user specific);

- gets the parents or principal caregivers actively involved and trained;

- provides feedback on out-of-school/clinic language usage and form;

- provides a vehicle for teaching certain linguistic forms; such as verb conjugation; and

- supplies an excellent data source.

Additional aims of notebooking are to:

- train listeners in communication techniques;

- provide additional information for the proper interpretation of unclear messages;

- provide a vehicle for practice in specific semantic, syntactic, morphologic, or pragmatic aspects of language; and

- provide opportunities for increasing performance in the use of augmentative aids and techniques.

## PURPOSE OF STRATEGY

The purpose of this strategy is to expand the use of augmentative communication techniques and strategies across audiences, situations, and topics by developing skills in messaging (the ability to accurately relay messages from one person or setting to another) and reporting (the ability to experience an event and report it to another person).

## UNDERLYING ASSUMPTIONS

1. *Client*. The type of disability or its severity is not important, provided the client is at least minimally functional in the operation of the augmentative technique and in the ability to respond. Notebooking would be inappropriate for clients who do not use augmentative techniques to respond. In addition, the client must spend time in at least two different settings.

2. *Augmentative components*. Any portable augmentative aid or technique is appropriate. Situational vocabulary selections must be available, as should the capacity for vocabulary additions.

3. *Environmental constraints*. Notebooking requires the availability and cooperation of individuals in the client's environment. This could include special teachers, mainstreamed teachers, speech-language pathologists, caregivers, vocational counselors, and significant others. A flow of information between at least two settings is necessary. A larger number of participants allows for faster generalization. Initial training time requires approximately 15 minutes. An additional 5 minutes daily is required for ongoing messaging.

4. *Other basic assumptions*. The participants in notebooking must understand the goals of the system and be familiar with the data recording system.

# DESCRIPTION OF THE STRATEGY

A spiral notebook for each separate setting is the only material required to start the procedure. Initial training time is minimal. A 15-minute visit or telephone call can get the process started. The goals of initial training are to delineate the purpose of notebooking, which is accurate message relaying and reporting, and to describe the process by which information is exchanged and data collected. Periodic 5-minute goal update sessions are suggested at least once a month. The estimated time needed daily for receiving the message, recording the data, and providing additional information is 5 minutes.

The time required of the primary facilitator, usually a teacher or speech-language pathologist, is 10 minutes daily. However, part of this time can be delegated if there is an aide or volunteer available. The responsibilities of the primary facilitator are to maintain the data sheets, prepare the notebook(s), and rehearse the targeted messages with the client.

The facilitator includes the following items in the notebook:

- the verbatim message as rehearsed;

- instructions on how to elicit the message;

- reminder of how to record the data;

- reinforcement statements;

- correction procedures; and

- additional information on events for verification of any spontaneous comments.

Example of these steps are detailed in the following section.

## Phase I

> *Goal*: The person using an augmentative technique will give a rehearsed message of specified length when asked questions about an event.

Criteria:      The daily message is repeated as rehearsed for five consecutive days.

The following is a sample notebook page, as prepared by the facilitator:

Ask:      What did you eat for lunch today?

Rehearsed phrase:      (Name) ate pizza lunch.

Directions:      Place the numbers 1-4 over the words in the order they are expressed by the client. Only number those words expressed, for example:

3      1      2

(Name) ate pizza lunch.

If correct, say:      (Name) ate pizza for lunch today. Was it good? (Continue the conversation, if possible, and record any additional comments [Name] makes.)

Additional comments:      _____

_____

If not correct say:      (Name) ate pizza lunch. (DO NOT ADD ANY OTHER WORDS, but check the response [Name] made after modeling).

_____Yes - repeated the phrase correctly after modeling
_____ No - did not repeat the phrase correctly
_____ No - made no response

Additional information:      We had a visit from the fire department today.

Record any spontaneous comments that (Name) makes.

Spontaneous comments:      _____

_____

*Phase II*

Goal: The person who uses an augmentative technique will give a rehearsed message of specified length when asked a nonspecific question.

Criteria: The rehearsed message is correctly given for five consecutive days with nonspecific questioning.

The following is a sample of a notebook page:

Ask: Tell me about school.

Rehearsed message: (Name) played bell music.

Instructions: Place numbers over the words reported in the order given.

If correct, say: (Name) played the bell in music. Was it fun? (Continue the conversation, if possible, and record any additional comments [Name] makes.)

Additional comments: _____

_____

_____

If not correct, say: (Name) played bell music. Say nothing else, but check the response [Name] makes after modeling.

_____Yes - repeated the phrase correctly after modeling

_____No - did not repeat the phrase correctly

_____No - made no response

Additional information: We had a fire drill at school.

Record any spontaneous comments that (Name) makes.

Spontaneous comments: _____

_____

_____

Phase III

Goal:  The person using an augmentative technique will relate a rehearsed event without cueing.

Criteria:  The person repeats a rehearsed event without cueing for five consecutive days.

The following is a sample of a notebook page:

Give social greetings.  Allow five minutes for (Name) to report.  Do not converse during this time.  If no message is delivered,

Ask:  What happened at school today?

Message:  Drew pictures today.

Instructions:  Place numbers over the words reported in the order given.

Check:  _____ spontaneous message given
_____ had to ask question

If correct, say:  (Name) drew a picture in art today.  How nice! What was the picture?

Record any additional comments made.

If not correct, say:  (Name) drew picture today.  (Check the response made after modeling.)

_____ Yes - repeated the phrase correctly after
modeling
_____ No  - did not repeat the phrase correctly
_____ No  - made no response

*Additional information*:  Nothing unusual today.

## Phase IV

*Goal*:  The person who uses an augmentative technique reports an unrehearsed event.

*Criteria*:  The person reports unrehearsed events for three consecutive days, both at school and at home.

The following is a sample of a notebook page:

Give social greetings.  Do not say anything else and allow time for spontaneous comments.  Write the comments as they are given in the notebook.

*Events*:  The following events happened at school:  (list events)

*If no response is given*:  Ask an unspecified question:  "What happened at school today?"  Record the responses as given.

The Goals of Phases I-IV are for messaging and reporting, but the rehearsed message can relate to other specific goals in terms of mean sentence length, syntax, semantics, or pragmatic objectives.  Goals to improve specific linguistic skills are appropriate for notebooking, as well.

The data sheets of the facilitator should reflect these additional goals, as illustrated in Table 6-10.  Additional data to be collected might include the effect of modeling on responding, spontaneous commenting, audiences with whom reporting occurred, and situations where commenting occurred.

### TABLE 6-10. MESSAGING AND REPORTING

### DATA SHEET

|  | *Date* *Assigned* | *Date* *Accomplished* |
|---|---|---|

Goal I   - relates rehearsed message with specific questioning

Goal II  - relates rehearsed message with nonspecific questioning

Goal III - spontaneously relates a rehearsed event

Goal IV  - spontaneously reports an unrehearsed event

*Behavior: Mean Sentence Length*

Goal I   - reports with two-word sequence

Goal II  - reports with three-word sequence

Goal III - reports with four-word sequence

Goal IV  - reports with five-word sequence

Goal V   - reports with five + word sequence

Future goals should include the use of messaging and reporting for different intentions, such as asking questions. The goal sequence would remain the same:

- a rehearsed question with specific cueing;

- a rehearsed question with nonspecific cueing;

- a rehearsed question with no cueing; and

- a nonrehearsed question with no cueing.

## EFFECTIVENESS OF STRATEGY

Preliminary data were collected from three teachers in self-contained classrooms, one school speech-language pathologist, and one clinical speech-language pathologist who used notebooking extensively with severely speech-impaired and physically handicapped children. Progress was noted for all students, as follows:

- Mean sentence length increased (one student went from two to seven words in less than a year).

- Spontaneous reporting was achieved when the goal sequence was followed.

- Reporting occurred in all settings where notebooking was used. This generalization seemed to occur simultaneously.

- No regression in reporting skills was seen over vacation time.

- Progress was noted in syntactic, morphologic, semantic, and pragmatic uses when these areas were addressed specifically.

Additional observations noted were:

1. When notebooking was first introduced without the data system, the initial response was enthusiastic, but the average number of messages received weekly from out-of-school sources quickly dropped to 1.5 per week. Use of the data system was effective in raising and maintaining a response ratio of four per week. Thus, it is

recommended that data collection responsibilities be given to the listener group.

2. Initial start-up time is demanding. The writing requirements on the facilitator decrease as participants learn the process. Therefore, note-booking should be introduced initially to one or two students in a class. Additional students can be added over time.

3. Responses may decrease periodically. If this occurs, several strategies may be used to increase the responses and to reestablish enthusiasm:

   • Ask for verification of information; for example, (Name) told me he went to the movies last night. Is this true? I could not make any specific comments since I did not have the verification of facts.

   • Introduce a change; for example, increase sentence length or add new vocabulary.

   • Make a telephone call to see if any unusual events have happened in the home that caused the decrease in note-booking.

## ADDITIONAL READINGS

Calculator, S., & Luchko, C. (1983). Evaluating the effectiveness of a communication board training program. Journal of Speech and Hearing Disorders, 48(2), 185-191.

Cross, T. (1984). Habilitating the language-impaired child: Ideas from studies of parent-child interaction. Topics in Language Disorders, 4(4), 1-15.

Fredericks, H., & Baldwin, V. (1975). A data based classroom for the moderately and severely handicapped. Monmouth, OR: Instructional Development Corp.

Grimm, J. (Ed.) (1974). Training parents to teach, four models, first chance for children. Technical Advisory Development System (TADS), 3, Chapel Hill, North Carolina.

Shearer, M. (1974). A home based parent training model. <u>Training Parents to Teach - Four Models</u>. First Chance for Children, <u>Technical Advisory Development System (TADS)</u>, <u>3</u>, Chapel Hill, North Carolina.

Shearer, M., & Shearer, D. (1972). The portage project: A model for early childhood education. <u>Exceptional Children</u>, <u>36</u>, 210-217.

# CHAPTER 7

# EVALUATING THE EFFECTIVENESS OF INTERVENTION PROGRAMS

DAVID R. BEUKELMAN

*Barkley Memorial Center*
*University of Nebraska-Lincoln*

## OBJECTIVES

- Present a model of communication disorder that can be used to evaluate the effectiveness of intervention programs.

- Review previous observations of impairment, disability, and handicap as a background to evaluate the effectiveness of intervention programs.

- Discuss measurement and procedural reliability and validity.

- Describe a structure to analyze intervention effectiveness and to modify intervention programs.

The preparation of this chapter was supported in part by Grant #G008200020 from the National Institute of Handicapped Research, Department of Education, Washington, DC, and the Barkley Trust of the University of Nebraska-Lincoln. The author wishes to thank Kathryn Yorkston for her helpful comments.

# INTRODUCTION

Human communication is a very complex activity that is reflected in numerous speaker and listener behaviors. The use of augmentative communication aids and techniques increases the complexity of human interaction. The impact of interventions that utilize augmentative aids, techniques, symbols, and strategies may be reflected in an almost unlimited number of behaviors. For example, use of a communication aid may improve spontaneous spelling, grammatical accuracy, and writing skills. In addition, use of the aid may be associated with increased motor control and improved posture. The user may also demonstrate improved interaction and social skills. In addition, having a functional way to communicate in school may improve academic performance.

Effectiveness evaluations are required to document whether the desired outcome of an intervention program has been achieved and, if not, what aspects of the program need to be modified. Evaluating the effectiveness of training also provides a basis for clinical research to identify and refine those strategies that are effective in meeting the communication needs of individuals with severe expressive communication disorders. Finally, there are a number of program management issues that can be addressed using outcome information. The issue of accountability is primary. Does the client achieve the desired improvement in communication function as a result of the time, effort, and money expended in an intervention? This question can be asked on an individual client basis, or on an agency or institutional basis, as the accountability of an augmentative communication program is assessed. In addition, evaluation procedures can be used to support quality assurance studies within a medical, therapeutic, or educational setting.

To evaluate the effectiveness of augmentative communication intervention, the clinician is faced with the difficult task of selecting those behaviors and measurement tools that will accurately reflect the impact of intervention activities. Without some model to guide these observations, evaluation of intervention effectiveness can become so difficult, so time-consuming, and therefore expensive, that it is eliminated from routine clinical practice. Although evaluation tools are limited and underdeveloped, intervention effectiveness in the augmentative communication area must continue to be evaluated.

# A MODEL OF COMMUNICATION DISORDER

A model of disorder has been adopted by the World Health Organization. This model, which can serve as a useful guide upon which to structure an evaluation of intervention effectiveness, has been discussed by Wood (1980) and Nagi (1977) and summarized by Frey (1984). The consequences of chronic injury, disease, or syndromes have been structured into a conceptual model and divided into three areas of disorder: impairment, disability, and handicap.

*Impairment* refers to "any loss or abnormality of psychological, physiological, or anatomical structure or function" (Wood, 1980, p. 4). For the severely communicatively disordered individual, the impairment may be reflected in the loss or abnormal function of those aspects of the body responsible for speech and/or language. For example, the individual with cerebral palsy experiences speech dysfunction (dysarthria) due to impairment in motor control known as spasticity, weakness, or dystonia. A careful assessment of many individuals with severe expressive communication disorders reveals an impairment that involves many of the subsystems of the body as well as those directly responsible for speech. In addition to severe dysarthria, the individual with cerebral palsy may also demonstrate impairment of posture and motor control of the hands, arms, and legs, such that control of augmentative techniques and aids is difficult. Impairment assessment involves the measurement of an individual's capability in terms of vision, cognition, language, and motor control.

*Disability* is that aspect of a communication disorder that refers to the reduced ability of an individual to meet the communication needs of daily living. The extent of disability is dependent on many factors, including the severity of the impairment, the communication life style of the individual, and the extent of an individual's compensation for the impairment through self-learning, specialized instruction, or prosthetic intervention, such as glasses, hearing aids, arm rests, and communication aids. Alterations in communication life style, such as changing jobs, beginning school, or retiring, have an important influence on disability level, even though the degree of impairment may not change. Assessment of disability includes a determination of the functional dimensions along which to judge the advantages of various augmentative techniques as they relate to an individual's efforts to communicate (see chapter 3).

*Handicap* refers to the societal disadvantage, due to an impairment and resulting disability, experienced by an individual with a communication disorder. Communication involves interaction among groups of individuals. The extent of a communication handicap depends upon the type of disability and the attitudes and biases of those who are in contact with the disabled individual. For example, the individual with a severe speech-impairment is often perceived as hard of hearing or mentally retarded. According to Frey (1984), the degree of handicap experienced by an individual or group can only be modified through education or legislation.

To thoroughly evaluate the effectiveness of intervention strategies, all aspects of a communication disorder that may be affected by interventions--impairment, disability, and handicap--must be considered. This can be accomplished by using the communication disorder model because it takes into account the variable relationships among the communication impairment of individuals with severe expressive communication disorders, their life styles, and society. For example, a change in impairment level may or may not influence a nonspeaking individual's ability to function in daily life. A person with Parkinson's disease may experience a reduction in motor control impairment (such as a reduction in stiffness) in response to medication. For some, the reduction in stiffness may allow improved speech intelligibility. Others will note the change in stiffness, but speech performance will not be changed enough to improve communicative interaction at home or work. However, if the reduction in impairment allows a critical change in the manner or efficiency with which an augmentative communication aid is controlled, a reduction in disability may be experienced.

A reduction in the level of handicap experienced by a nonspeaking individual may occur as a consequence of an intervention program and may even be the primary focus of an intervention program. However, the primary goal of an augmentative communication intervention program is to increase an individual's functional communication (i.e., ability to meet the communication needs of daily living), thereby decreasing the degree of disability. Therefore, evaluation of disability will be considered before the evaluation of impairment or handicap.

## EVALUATION OF DISABILITY

### Types of Communication Disabilities

Communication is particularly important to nonspeaking and nonwriting individuals in five different contexts: (a) social, (b) academic, (c) prevocational and vocational (d) recreational, and (e) self- and health-care.

*Social contexts*. Interpersonal communication is basic to our social participation and development. A comprehensive discussion of those characteristics of interpersonal communication that are particularly reflective of communication augmentation is found in previous chapters. Clinicians and researchers have focused on several characteristics of conversational interaction when quantifying the effectiveness of conversation between individuals using augmentative communication components and their unimpaired, speaking partners. Their work has suggested that individuals who use augmentative communication symbols, aids and techniques demonstrate minimal conversational control and that their speaking partners generally directed their interactions. These patterns existed even when nonspeakers demonstrated functional interaction skills during clinical training sessions (Calculator & Dollaghan; 1982; Calculator & Luchko, 1983). Farrier, Yorkston, Marriner, and Beukelman (1985) summarize research regarding communication interaction that involves the use of augmentative communication aids, symbols, techniques, and strategies by delineating variables affecting conversational control as follows:

> Conversational control may be defined as the manner and extent to which an individual directs and restrains communicative interaction. It represents a broad range of behaviors that occur in interaction . . . . Turn regulation, topic maintenance (including patterns of initiation and response), communicative functions/intents, grammatical forms, and communication modes used, and message transmission rates are among the variables that have been studied (Beukelman & Yorkston, 1980; Buzolich, 1983; Calculator & Dollaghan, 1982; Calculator & Luchko, 1983; Colquhoun, 1982; Culp, 1982; Harris, 1978; Kraat, 1985; Lossing, 1981; Morningstar, 1981; Wexler, Dore, & Blau, 1982). (pp. 65-66)

The subsequent research of Farrier et al. (1985) illustrated that unimpaired speakers (except for one dyad) who were required to communicate via an augmentative communication aid performed in a manner very similar to that reported for nonspeaking augmentative device users, thus illustrating the limiting effects of using augmentative aids during conversational interactions.

Several investigations have compared how the performance of nonspeaking persons was affected by the mode of communication they used. Wexler et al. (1982) reported that nonspeaking individuals with cerebral palsy produced 48 percent more initiations and 38 percent more complex conversational acts with the communication board than without it. Calculator and Luchko (1983) studied the cumulative effects of modifying a communication board and then instructing the "listeners" of an adult nonspeaking female to provide greater opportunities for her to communicate, particularly by situating the listeners in close proximity to the client and phrasing questions that encouraged elaborate responses from her. In this case study, the authors concluded that the client's ". . . new communication board was effective in overcoming some limitations posed by her former alphabet board in that she was more likely to respond to the initiations of others. However, the frequency of her own initiations did not increase."   In summary, the authors concluded that "each training phase contributed cumulatively to (the client's) overall communication effectiveness" (p. 190).

*Academic contexts*.  For most individuals, communicative behaviors exhibited in an educational setting appear to differ substantially from those exhibited during everyday conversational interaction. There has been little research in this area involving the communication behaviors of individuals who use augmentative communication aids in the classroom.  In most regular classrooms, a much greater emphasis is placed on written communication than on interpersonal communication. Academic communication also involves extensive stimulus-response interaction, which requires prompt, accurate responses.  In addition, academic communication involves group interaction, where interpersonal communication is much more didactic in nature. Finally, academic communication involves unusual formats, such as answer sheets and multiple-choice test forms.

*Prevocational and vocational contexts*.   Vocational communication can vary widely depending on the individual tasks and environments. There have been no reports of research on observations of severely speech- and/or writing-impaired persons in prevocational and vocational settings.  Clinical experience has shown that telephone skills, computer access, unusual writing formats, and environmental conditions involving special light and noise conditions are common in prevocational and vocational settings.

*Recreational contexts*.  The area of recreational communication is often ignored in communication intervention programs.  Most unimpaired speakers believe that communication during recreational activities is minimal.  For the nonspeaking individual, recreational communication involves words and messages, such as "Take two elephant steps" or "You forgot to discard" that are rarely used in daily communication.  Therefore, special provision must be made to facilitate and support recreational communication.  This type of communication often requires very specific messages that can be provided easily using a message retrieval strategy.

*Self- and health-care contexts*.  Although few unimpaired speakers consider self- and health-care communication to be different from other types of communication, many chronically disabled individuals do not share this view.  For them, numerous self- and health-care messages are communicated each day, involving some of the most repetitive forms of communication.  Yet, in analyzing the messages generated by five Canon Communicator (Canon USA, Canon Plaza, Lake Success, NY) users, Beukelman and Yorkston (1982) reported that 74 percent of the  messages classified as "requests for physical assistance" were uniquely different from one another, while 97 percent of the messages classified as "provisions of information" were uniquely different. Often, the self- or health-care requests are repeated again and again. Although the messages are very similar, they must frequently be well timed. An example of such a message would be, "Please put my feet on the footrests before you move the wheelchair."

## Measurement of Functional Communication

Communication is an extremely complex behavior. To measure the extent of each type of communication disability, dependent variables that best reflect patterns of communication interaction must be selected. Chapters 3, 4, and 5 contain discussions of the functional dimensions along which to judge the relative advantages of various augmentative techniques as they relate to the requirements of an individual's communication system.

A review of augmentative communication literature reveals that a number of approaches are frequently used to evaluate the communication performance of nonspeaking individuals. Yet, only a few of these procedures have been developed into tools that evaluate communication intervention effectiveness. These include an inventory of communication needs and direct observation of conversational interaction in natural environments.

### *Inventory of Communication Needs*

The assessment of communication needs is becoming a routine evaluation of disability. This functional assessment is utilized, in conjunction with the capability assessment, to guide augmentative communication intervention programs (see chapter 4 for a detailed discussion). Gradually, the needs assessment approach is also being used to document intervention effectiveness. For example, Dowden, Beukelman, and Lossing (1984) reported that nonspeaking patients in acute medical settings (intensive and cardiac care) had 95 to 100 percent of their communication needs met through a combined approach of augmented speech (electrolarynx) plus a scanning or direct selection technique. While those patients using only a scanning technique had 9 percent of their needs met, those with a speech-augmented technique (electrolarynx) had 64 percent of their needs met, and those with direct selection techniques had 61 percent of their needs met. In this research, the assessment of communication needs met was a useful measure of intervention effectiveness.

The validity of the "needs met" approach depends on the accurate development of a communication needs list. If the list is limited to a few aspects of the individual's communication life style, the information about intervention effectiveness will be similarly restricted.  Care must be taken to develop a needs list that is sensitive to the areas of functional communication and that takes into account any special needs as well.  In addition, it is important to determine which needs have been met as a result of a specific intervention.  Dowden et al. (1984) obtained this information by interviewing the nonspeaking individual, intensive care staff, and family members of each client.  If time and resources are available, it also may be useful to directly observe persons who use augmentative components to interact in order to document that communication needs are being met.

## *Direct Observation of Conversational Interaction in Natural Environments*

Observation in natural environments is necessary to collect actual performance data.  Several clinical and research groups have directly sampled and commented on patterns of communication interaction in the nonspeaking individual's environment in an attempt to measure intervention effectiveness.  They have relied on environmental observations that are recorded (e.g., on videotape or audiotape) and that require extensive review and analysis.  Few of the sampling procedures described below have found their way into regular clinical practice because they are time-consuming and, therefore, expensive.

*Videotape*.  Perhaps the earliest of these efforts was the doctoral dissertation of Harris (1978), during which she observed the communication interaction patterns of nonspeaking children in classroom settings.  Student-teacher interactions were recorded on videotape, and the tapes were analyzed in terms of participation by "senders and receivers," communication modes used, and communication functions expressed.  Calculator and Dollaghan (1982), using a design similar to that employed by Harris, video-recorded teacher-student interactions of mildly retarded individuals.  The communication samples were analyzed according to similar variables including "speaker role," "mode of student message," and "outcome of the message."  Finally, "successful" student initiations, defined as those that were followed by teacher acceptance, and "unsuccessful" student initiations, those resulting in teacher requests for clarifications, initiations of a new topic, or nonresponses were determined.

In a 1982 study, Culp investigated the communication interaction of nonspeaking children and their mothers in their home environments.  Twenty-five one-minute interactions were video-recorded.  The tapes were analyzed with respect to mode, mean length of utterance, communicative function performed, and initiator success.  In another study using video-recording techniques, Wexler et al. (1982) studied conversational functions between nonspeaking individuals with cerebral palsy and speaking adults.  Twenty one-minute conversations were recorded; for 10 minutes the communication board was used and for 10 minutes it was not used.  The severely speech-impaired persons were required to prepare several topics for conversation.

Using this approach, the nonspeaking individual, as the selector of the discussion topic, was given the opportunity for greater conversational control than in some of the other studies reported in this chapter.

*Audiotape and printed output*. In an effort to measure communication interaction without the constraints of cumbersome video equipment, several clinical research groups have reported alternative data collection techniques. Beukelman and Yorkston (1980) measured communicative performance in environmental settings using a method that involved analysis of dialogue that had been transcribed from audiotape operated by the listener and text that was printed by the user's communication aid. The recorded messages were categorized according to message type, such as greetings, requests for information, provisions of information, requests for assistance, and emotional expressions. The analysis was utilized to identify effective and ineffective communication partners based on the frequency of unresolved communication breakdowns.

*On-line observations*. In her master's thesis, Lossing (1981) developed a technique that would be less time-consuming and therefore less expensive than earlier data collection techniques. She asked communication partners to record data using a paper and pencil format. Lossing observed four different augmentative communication aid users during a total of 24 hours of communication interaction. The aid users and their communication partners were observed when the partners were tallying data and when they were not tallying data. She observed that:

> All partners consistently identified fewer communication exchanges than
> did the trained observer, the senior author who was active in developing
> the measurement tool. Further, the partners consistently underestimated
> the number of communication exchanges which had occurred during
> each session. . . . (Lossing, Yorkston, & Beukelman, 1985, p. 389).

These results reflect the caution that must be exercised when using minimally trained communication partners as data collectors.

*On-line observations with audiotape backup*. Calculator and Luchko (1983) employed a trained observer to tally the communication interactions of an adult communication aid user. The observer did not interact with the user or her partners. A concealed tape recorder was used to record interactions to confirm the observer's on-line recording of communication events. The dependent variables in this clinical study were partner type, proximity of partner, communication role in terms of initiator and responder, mode of nonspeech communication, communicative function, and form.

*Checklist*.  Recent efforts have been directed toward the development of more clinically applicable techniques for measuring the communication performance of severely speech-impaired persons.  In 1984, Bolton and Dashiell published *INCH: INteraction CHecklist for Augmentative Communication*.  The authors write:

> . . . (INCH) is not intended as a test.  Rather, the authors developed the checklist to describe the critical features of interaction between augmentative system users and their receivers.  The complete INCH program includes the checklist and a manual that contains theory, administrative procedures, and suggestions for intervention. Communication interactions are coded according to communication modes and strategies as described in the manual. (pp. 5-9)

## Direct Observation of Structured Interaction Tasks

Observation of structured interactions permits the control of several aspects of interaction in a way that is not possible during environmental observations.  For example, the content of the interaction can be controlled as well as the amount of information held by each of the participants.  Also, the familiarity and "helpfulness" of the listeners can be varied to determine how effectively the user can interact with differing types of listeners.  Finally, the structured interaction allows the user to assume different roles in an interaction.  The frequency of communication turns is usually quite high in the structured (as compared to the environmental) interaction. Therefore, the observation time is usually shorter for structured as compared to environmental interactions, making it more applicable in a clinical setting.  The presence of interaction patterns in structured settings does not necessarily mean that these patterns will occur in environmental settings.  However, if nonspeaking persons are unable to engage in interactional behaviors in the structured setting, they probably will be unable to do so in the environmental interactions.

Farrier et al. (1985) developed two structured interaction tasks for "in clinic" evaluation.  The first is a *direction-giving task* (see Figure 7-1 for an example of one of the 16 geometric designs used in this evaluation).  In this task, nonspeaking individuals are instructed to give their communication partners directions for reproducing a geometric design that is visible only to the nonspeaking person. Designs vary along five parameters, including color, shape, number of shapes, relative size of shapes, and position of the shapes on the card.  A plain, white index card is provided to the partner along with pens of different colors.  Partners are not allowed to observe the original card with the geometric design. No restrictions are placed on the interaction, which is video-recorded.

The second is a *decision-making task*. The general format of this task is a game in which cards are bought and sold to accumulate a specific number of points. Both the person using augmentative techniques and the communication partner are provided with a portion of the information needed to made decisions about buying and selling. The speech-impaired individual and the partner are not allowed to see each other's cards. They are instructed to share as equally as possible in the decision-making. There are no other restrictions on interactions, which are video-recorded.

**FIGURE 7-1. EXAMPLES OF GEOMETRIC DESIGNS USED IN THE DIRECTION-GIVING TASK**

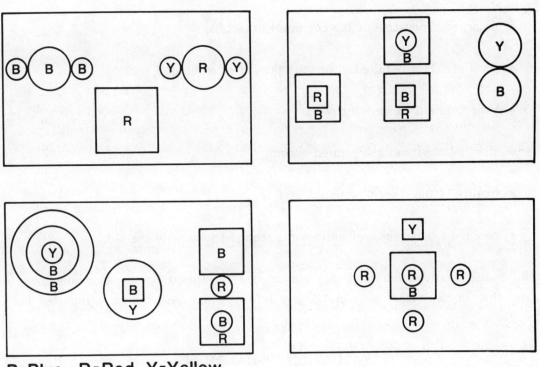

B=Blue, R=Red, Y=Yellow

*Note*: From "Conversational Control in Nonimpaired Speakers Using an Augmentative Communication System" by L. Farrier, K. Yorkston, N. Marriner, and D. Beukelman, May 1985, <u>Alternative and Augmentative Communication</u>, <u>1</u>(2), p. 66, Copyright 1985 by Williams & Wilkins. Reprinted by permission.

The interaction patterns resulting from direction-giving and decision-making tasks were analyzed to determine conversational control in terms of initiation-response and summoning power (McKirdy & Blank, 1982), total number of words, and duration of messages.

## *Assessment of User Satisfaction and Acceptance*

An important aspect of disability evaluation is the assessment of user satisfaction or acceptance.  Although an intervention technique or strategy may have the potential for meeting communication needs, the communication disability will not be reduced if the aid technique or strategy is unacceptable to the user.  At times, individuals find that characteristics of various augmentative components are unacceptable, such as:

- color, size, or shape of the communication aid,

- level of effort required to operate the aid or technique,

- time required to learn a strategy,

- size and clarity of the printed output,

- quality of the speech synthesis, and

- perceived bizarreness of movements required to control the aid.

Currently, user satisfaction and acceptance are measured using questionnaires; however, these measurement tools are largely informal and have not been reported in the literature.

## EVALUATION OF HANDICAP

Efforts to evaluate the presence and degree of handicap (i.e., societal disadvantages due to communication disorders) have been limited to questionnaires of listener satisfaction and acceptance. Although no standard approaches to elicit listener (communication partner) satisfaction or acceptance have been published, informal tools are used in several clinical centers.  These tools have not been evaluated at length as to their validity and reliability.  In 1984, Mathy-Laikko and Coxson presented a research report describing their initial efforts to quantify "listener reactions to augmentative communication system ouput mode."  Two groups of listeners were included in the study. The "sensitized group" included university students who had completed at least one course in special education or speech-language pathology. The "naive" group included university students who had completed no course work in special education or speech-language pathology. Both groups of listeners were instructed to rate their reactions to three modes of communication augmentation output: print, synthesized speech, and visual, nonretrievable symbol selection (alphabet and word communication board). Nine bipolar adjectives were rated on a seven-point gradient scale of acceptability (1 = best rating, 7 = worst rating), as follows:

1. practical - not practical

2. distinct - not distinct

3. fast - slow

4. clear - unclear

5. functional - nonfunctional

6. pleasant - unpleasant

7. positive - negative

8. approachable - not approachable

9. intelligible - unintelligible

Also included were the following interaction statements:

1. I would go out of my way to talk to a person using this system.

2. I would initiate conversation with a person using this system.

3. I would make additional conversation with a person using this system.

4. If I were having trouble understanding this system, I would continue trying.

The results of this study are too extensive to describe completely in this text. However, it is interesting to note that the "sensitized" group consistently rated all communication augmentation modes as more acceptable than did the "naive" group. Perhaps this study reflects how education may affect the attitudes of university students toward individuals with severe expressive communication disorders.

Development of tools to assess handicap will become increasingly necessary as more individuals who use augmentative communication aids and techniques are integrated into competitive secondary, post-secondary academic, and vocational settings. For example, disabled students often find some professors to be much more receptive of their disabilities than others. Some faculty members showed their lack of acceptance by "passing" disabled students with minimal effort, while at the other extreme, some called the Disabled Students' Center to complain about the presence of disabled students in the classes (C. Horn, personal communication, June 1, 1986). Evaluation of real or potential handicap will permit an analysis of those factors that contribute to intervention outcome.

## EVALUATION OF IMPAIRMENT

Capability evaluation is covered quite thoroughly in chapter 4 and will not be repeated here. The development of an augmentative communication aid, technique, or strategy can be viewed as an attempt to compensate for the impairments of a severely speech- and/or writing-impaired person. (Compensatory strategies may include an alternative language symbol system, specialized motor control interfaces, and many others.) Determining the level of compensated impairment should be considered in measuring the effect of an intervention program. For example, an improvement in written language skills is an expected consequence of using certain types of augmentative communication aids. If the effect of an intervention is to be assessed, the measurement of its impact on specific capabilities is necessary.

An illustration of the measurement of compensated impairment could involve the evaluation of a nonliterate person's knowledge of a specialized symbol system such as Blissymbols or Picsyms. Because a nonspeaking individual may not be literate, a specialized symbol system may be introduced through an intervention program. Measurement of the effectiveness of the intervention would involve the evaluation of the individual's knowledge of and ability to use a compensatory symbol system.

In another example, the accuracy and efficiency with which an augmentative communication aid user is able to transmit messages may be a measure of effectiveness for which the impairment has been compensated. Marriner and McDonald (1982) reported the accuracy with which 10 nonspeaking individuals, using a Morse Code-based augmentative communication technique, completed a dictation task. In addition to accuracy measures, they also measured the rate of message preparation. The accuracy and rate measures were combined and reported as a measure of message preparation efficiency in terms of "accurate characters per minute." A full discussion of their research results is beyond the scope of this chapter. However, the reader is referred to the Marriner and McDonald article as an excellent illustration of the evaluation of compensated impairment.

## PSYCHOMETRIC ISSUES

### *Measurement Validity and Reliability*

In 1972, Darley reviewed the aphasia treatment literature and urged renewed scientific rigor in investigations of aphasia. He wrote that treatment research required "more than an interested clinician's artistic and intuitive reporting of changes observed in his patients. Reliable quantitative data must be gathered with rigorous objectivity" (p. 11). Certainly, the study of intervention effectiveness in the area of augmentative communication should also be approached in a valid and reliable manner. Because augmentative communication is such a new area, most of the assessment tools are as yet informal and psychometrically incomplete. This is not unexpected. If studies in intervention effectiveness are to be completed in a scientifically rigorous manner, high quality assessment tools must be developed in the coming years. The Additional Readings section of this chapter includes several references that contain excellent discussions of evaluation tool development.

### *Procedural Validity and Reliability*

When evaluating the effectiveness of intervention, it is necessary to confirm that the intervention program actually occurred as planned. Due to the interdisciplinary nature of communication augmentation and the health status of some clients, several procedural validity and reliability problems occur frequently.

The potential for conflicting intervention goals exists among the various constituencies interested in the speech-impaired individual (e.g., team members, school personnel, health-care personnel, parents, and the nonspeaking individual). For example, a potential conflict can occur between the augmentative team and the professionals responsible for a child's physical development. Also, parents may not be convinced that augmentative communication equipment is appropriate for their child or they may be intimidated by the equipment.  If, as a result of this, they do not practice system usage with their child at home, the intervention program will not be delivered as expected.

A variety of other staff issues can result in modification of an augmentative communication program without the knowledge of the team leader/researcher.  Staff members may not have adequate training in the implementation of new types of interventions and the use of new equipment.  In situations where several staff members serve the same client (as often occurs in medical settings), some of the staff members may not be intimately familiar with the intervention program.  Of course, there is always the possibility that the intervention program has not been defined well enough so that staff members are able to follow it without error.

In general, an intervention program should be observed by the clinician/researcher at regular intervals to confirm that the plan is being implemented accurately.  In addition, the intervention staff should keep a log of intervention times and activities as a record that the intervention has occurred. The reader is referred to the Additional Readings section at the end of this chapter for references that contain excellent discussions of procedural validity and reliability issues.

### *Analysis of Intervention Effectiveness Results:* *Modification of Intervention Strategies and Programs*

The results of an intervention effectiveness evaluation are usually organized in response to  four basic questions:

1.  *Is change occurring?*  If the evaluation procedures have been completed properly, the question of whether change is occurring should not be difficult to answer.   Occasionally, the answer to this question will reflect problems in the evaluation process.  For example, the effectiveness evaluation may indicate no change, but the anecdotal comments of family and staff may report behavioral change. Conversely, family and staff members who have worked hard may find it difficult to admit that nothing has been accomplished unless objective methods are used  to guide their observations.   Measurement of change is not always easy.

Analysis of behavioral change is a general educational and rehabilitation issue that has frequently been discussed in detail by others (see Additional Readings).  One of the primary principles of measuring behavioral change is the establishment of a stable, or at least consistent, baseline performance prior to intervention.  A review of the intervention work in the augmentative communication area reveals that, for several reasons, this is rarely achieved.  First, the scope of the impairment of individuals with severe expressive communication disorders is so great that intervention teams struggle to complete the time-consuming capability assessments of impairment (e.g., cognition, speech, language, motor control, vision, perception, & others). Repetition of the assessment to establish stable baselines has been viewed as prohibitive. However, evaluation of intervention effectiveness requires that the principles of behavioral change measurement be respected. Care must be taken to select those dependent variables that will be sensitive to the impact of the intervention program and to measure them.

Documentation of change is useful for administrative and policy issues that extend beyond the needs of the individual client. From an administrative point of view, the development of an augmentative communication program is an expensive undertaking. Most service delivery programs undergo a regular performance review. Information confirming that the program's clients are achieving behavioral change and that this information is being documented is useful in sustaining and expanding service delivery capability. In addition, this information is effective in supporting the administrative performance studies that many medical and rehabilitation centers are required to complete. Nearly all of these uses of intervention outcome measures require more indepth analysis of results than simply an indication of rate of change. Other parameters of change that need to be measured include the nature of the behavioral change, the amount of change over a specified time period, the context in which the change is occurring, and the frequency of the behavior.

2. *Is the expected change occurring?* Intervention programs are designed to achieve a certain type of behavioral change. Almost without exception, there is a hypothesis about potential change that is shared by the treatment team. This expectation will guide and sometimes restrict the scope of the intervention effectiveness evaluation and lead the intervention team to inaccurate conclusions. One example of this involves a young woman who is currently an excellent user of a Morse Code-based augmentative communication device. One of her intervention staff members had previously reported concern about an earlier intervention program because this woman was unable to achieve an adequate level of motor control to use an Autocom communication device (Prentke-Romich Co., Wooster, OH) with a magnet mounted on a head wand. In retrospect, we are now aware that the Autocom experience contributed to this woman's spontaneous spelling skills, expressive writing skills, and head control, all of which have permitted the use of her current communication system. Therefore, it is important to measure pertinent areas of performance.

3. *Is change occurring at a different disorder level than anticipated?* As discussed previously in this chapter, the impairment, disability, and handicap aspects of a communication disorder may or may not be closely related in the case of a nonspeaking/nonwriting individual. In augmentative communication centers, we occasionally see parents and school personnel in conflict over the effectiveness of the

intervention program implemented by a school. School personnel will report improvement in performance, including reduction in impairment and improved motor control and language skills. However, the parents will report that their child's functional communication disability has not changed.

Both the parents and the school personnel are correct in their observations. Evaluation of the impact of an intervention must include measurement of all aspects of the communication disorder. This would include measures of the impairment (capability evaluation), measures of the disability (functional communication assessment), as well as measures of the handicap (attitude of those listeners who interact with the nonspeaking individual). A review of the augmentative communication literature reveals that this approach to evaluation of intervention effectiveness is not being reported in the literature.

In the case example presented above, behavioral change was occurring, but was not observed because the treatment team was observing at the functional communication (disability) level, while change was occurring at the capability (impairment) level. This example raises a difficult problem, that is, how does one decide which observations to make across the various levels of a disorder? There is obviously not enough time to measure all behaviors. To some extent, one can be guided by considering the changes in performance that will provide the building blocks for subsequent development.

4. *Is change occurring that will support future improvement in other levels of performance?* Because multiple capabilities (motor, visual, cognitive, linguistic, etc.) are required to communicate using augmentative aids and techniques, the development of skills in a variety of areas is needed to support the future use of advanced augmentative communication techniques. Evaluation of intervention effectiveness should be sensitive to capability changes that will support future multi-component communication systems. For example, in our clinical program, we are currently working with a local school district to serve the communication needs of an 8-year-old girl with cerebral palsy. Currently, she is using a two-switch scanning communication technique with one head switch and one hand switch. It has been difficult to individualize the system to allow the girl to control it accurately. At this time, she communicates very slowly with her aid. At her last progress evaluation, there was pressure from within the team to change the switch configuration "just one more time" in an attempt to enhance her communication speed slightly. However, evaluation results showed that since the aid has been operational, the girl has steadily improved her spontaneous spelling and written expression skills. Eventually, the decision was made to leave the augmentative components of her communication system alone for another 6 to 12 months, so that her language capability could continue to improve and not be interrupted by attempts to reduce her disability level in conversational interaction. In time, we intend to have her try a head-controlled Morse

Code-based communication system. For that system to be successful, spontaneous spelling skills at the third-grade level will be necessary. The current intervention program appears to have the potential of achieving that goal.

## CLOSING COMMENTS

The primary goal of a augmentative communication intervention is to provide individuals with severe expressive communication disorders with a means of reducing their communication disability. A review of the literature has shown that many intervention efforts have been successful, in that nonspeaking individuals have learned to operate selected augmentative communication aids and techniques. However, these studies also reveal some interventions that have resulted in minimal improvement in communication interaction ability. It is encouraging to observe that today, most augmentative programs are focusing on communication interaction training with an intensity that was not present two or three years ago. This change in emphasis is a direct result of the communication effectiveness research that has been completed.

A second area of impact has been the shift of intervention focus to the listener in addition to the nonspeaking individual. Previously, in many interventions, the listener had been totally ignored. However, the work of Calculator and Luchko (1983) resulted in specific intervention strategies that were directed toward the listener. The communication effectiveness study of Beukelman and Yorkston (1980) resulted in instruction to listeners about communication breakdown resolution strategies and interaction behaviors.

During the early years of the augmentative communication effort, the "demonstration of the possible" was adequate to justify formation of programs and to encourage workers in the area. Speech-impaired persons were able to communicate and that was good enough. However, early communication effectiveness measurement has begun to reveal that not all individuals who use augmentative communication aids and techniques experience a measurable reduction in their communication disability or handicap. Communication effectiveness evaluation results will become the primary base, for justifying and developing more appropriate interventions. In addition, the evaluations of effectiveness will play an increasingly important role in directing the modification and refinement of augmentative communication equipment. As augmentative communication practices mature, they will probably be guided to a greater and greater extent by our knowlege of the performance patterns of successful and unsuccessful users of augmentative aids, techniques, symbols, and strategies.

## SUMMARY

Evaluation of the effectiveness of augmentative communication interventions is completed for several purposes.  The service delivery needs of individuals with severe expressive communication disorders are assessed  to determine if intervention programs are to be maintained or modified.  In addition, effectiveness measures are used to determine if changes are necessary in the design and function of augmentative communication aids and techniques.   The performance measures obtained in effectiveness studies can also be used in the administrative assessment of agency or clinical performance.

A communication disorder has several aspects, including impairment (the loss or abnormality of structure or function), disability (reduced ability to meet communication needs of daily living), and handicap (societal disadvantage as a result of the disorder). To evaluate intervention effectiveness, each aspect of disorder must be determined.  While some intervention programs may affect each aspect similarly, other programs may have a positive effect on some aspects and a negative effect on others.

Numerous augmentative communication effectiveness studies have been reported in the literature.  Some have shown an important reduction in communication disability as a result of intervention, while others reveal a minimal reduction in disability.  Changes in training procedures have occurred as a result of communication effectiveness studies, thus producing a subsequent reduction in disability.

The analysis of intervention effectiveness can be structured using four questions:

1. Is change occurring?

2. Is the expected change occurring?

3. Is change occurring at a different level of disorder than was anticipated?

4. Is change occurring that will support future improvement in other levels of performance?

## STUDY QUESTIONS

1. Describe the relationships between the impairment and disability patterns of a severely speech-impaired individual.

2. Why are measures of procedural reliability so necessary in the evaluation of intervention effectiveness?

3. How can intervention effectiveness information be used to sustain or modify an intervention program?

4. What are the primary procedures used to collect intervention effectiveness information? What are their strengths and weaknesses?

## REFERENCES

Beukelman, D., & Yorkston, K. (1980). Nonvocal communication: Performance evaluation. Archives of Physical Medicine and Rehabilitation, 61, 272-275.

Beukelman, D., & Yorkston, K. (1982). Communication interaction of adult communication augmentation system use. Topics in Language Disorders, 2, 39-54.

Bolton, S., & Dashiell, S. (1984). INCH: INteraction CHecklist for augmentative communication. Huntington Beach, CA: INCH Associates.

Buzolich, M. (1983). Interaction analysis of augmented and normal communicators. Unpublished doctoral dissertation, University of Southern California, San Fransico.

Calculator, S., & Dollaghan, C. (1982). The use of communication boards in a residential setting: An evaluation. Journal of Speech and Hearing Disorders, 47, 281-287.

Calculator, S., & Luchko, C. (1983). Evaluating the effectiveness of a communication board training program. Journal of Speech and Hearing Disorders, 48, 185-191.

Colquhoun, A. (1982). Augmentative communication systems: The interaction process. Paper presented at the American Speech-Language-Hearing Convention, Toronto.

Culp, P. (1982). Communication interactions--Nonspeaking children using augmentative systems and their mothers. Paper presented at the American Speech-Language-Hearing Convention, Toronto.

Darley, F. (1972). The efficacy of language rehabilitation in aphasia. Journal of Speech and Hearing Disorders, 37, 3-21.

Dowden, P., Beukelman, D., & Lossing, C. (1984). Communication augmentation in intensive care units. Abstracts of the Third International Conference on Augmentative and Alternative Communication.

Farrier, L., Yorkston, K., Marriner, N., & Beukelman, D. (1985). Conversational control in nonimpaired speakers using an augmentative communication system. Alternative and Augmentative Communication, 1(2), 65-73.

Frey, W. (1984). Functional assessment in the '80s: A conceptual enigma, a technical challenge. In A. Halpern & M. Fuhrer (Eds.), Functional assessment in rehabilitation (pp. 11-44). Baltimore: Paul H. Brookes Publishing.

Harris, D. (1978). Descriptive analysis of communicative interaction processes involving non-vocal severely physically handicapped children. Unpublished doctoral dissertation, University of Wisconsin, Madison.

Kraat, A. (1985). Communication interaction between aided and natural speakers. A state of the art report. Toronto: Canadian Rehabilitation Council for the Disabled.

Lossing, C. (1981). A technique for the quantification of non-vocal communication performance by listeners. Unpublished master's thesis, University of Washington, Seattle.

Lossing, C., Yorkston, K., & Beukelman, D. (1985). Communication augmentation systems: Quantification in natural settings. Archives of Physical Medicine and Rehabilitation, 66, 380-384.

Marriner, N., & McDonald, J. (1982). Quantifying aspects of nonspeech communication. Short course at the Second International Conference on Nonspeech Communication, Toronto.

Mathy-Laikko, P., & Coxson, L. (1984). Listener reactions to augmentative communication system ouput mode. Paper presented at the American Speech-Language-Hearing Convention, San Francisco.

McKirdy, L., & Blank, M. (1982). Dialogue in deaf and hearing preschoolers. Journal of Speech and Hearing Research, 25, 487-499.

Morningstar, D. (1981). Blissymbol communication: Comparison of interaction with naive vs. experienced listeners. Unpublished manuscript, University of Toronto.

Nagi, S. (1977). The disabled and rehabilitation services: A national overview. American Rehabilitation, 5, 26-33.

Wexler, K., Dore, J., & Blau, A. (1982). Conversational functions of the nonvocal/vocal dyad. Short course presented at the American Speech-Language-Hearing Convention, Toronto.

Wood, P. (1980). Appreciating the consequences of disease: The classification of impairments, disabilities, and handicaps. The WHO classification of impairments, disabilities, and handicaps. The WHO Chronicle, 34, 376-380.

## ADDITIONAL READINGS

Hayes, S. (1981). Single case design and empirical clinical practice. Journal of Consulting and Clinical Psychology, 49, 193-211.

Kazdin, A. (1977). Artifact, bias and complexity of assessment: The ABC's of reliability. Journal of Applied Behavioral Analysis, 10, 141-150.

McReynolds, L., & Kearns, K. (1983). Single-subject experimental designs in communicative disorders. Austin, TX: Pro-ed.

Wallace, C. (1962). Research design. Berkley, CA.: Association for Advanced Training in the Behavioral Sciences.

Wolery, M., & Harris, S. (1982). Interpreting results of single-subject research designs. Physical Therapy, 62, 445-452.

# CHAPTER 8

## TOTAL HABILITATION AND LIFE-LONG MANAGEMENT

CAROL G. COHEN

*Schneier Communication Unit*
*Cerebral Palsy Center*
*Syracuse, NY*

## OBJECTIVES

- Orient and expose reader to complex physical and social barriers to effective communicative interaction.

- Provide the reader with various service delivery models and discuss problems inherent in each.

- Review multifaceted role and responsibilities of speech-language pathologist with respect to case management of individuals with severe expressive communication disorders.

- Develop an awareness of advocacy issues and the role of the speech-language pathologist with regard to local and national legislators, third-party funding agencies, school districts, and policymakers in general.

# INTRODUCTION

Despite advances in technology and attempts to disseminate knowledge more widely, persons with severe expressive communication disorders who utilize augmentative communication techniques are not integrated into the mainstream of society. Individuals with "atypical" communicative behaviors are not traditionally afforded the same educational, vocational, and recreational opportunities as their able-bodied peers. Thus, they may be handicapped well beyond their level of impairment or disability (see chapter 7). To facilitate the creation of a society that promulgates interaction with impaired speakers, barriers that preclude effective, expressive communicative exchange for individuals who use augmentative communication components must be studied and ultimately removed. Total habilitation or rehabilitation of severely speech- and writing-impaired persons refers to the mainstreaming of communicatively disabled individuals into all facets of community life by means of therapy, experiential learning, and formal education for these individuals and their potential communication partners. Total habilitation will affect the educational, recreational, and vocational planning throughout an individual's life. It involves a process of orienting, exposing, and integrating the interactive patterns and life styles of able-bodied and disabled individuals. Those who manage the severely communicatively impaired client must be cognizant of ways to maximize communicative participation in the community-at-large and recognize the need to transcend isolated environments and segregated living. To achieve societal integration of severely communicatively impaired persons, the total habilitation process must focus on client advocacy and a continuum of care from the point of initial diagnosis/assessment through life-long management of the impaired individual.

This chapter contains a discussion of barriers that inhibit interaction and offers suggestions to minimize the ramifications of expressive communication disorders. Issues related to service delivery, such as the team approach, the role of the speech-language pathologist, and a current perspective on funding, are presented. Finally, this chapter addresses integrated care plans that promote the infiltration of augmentative communication into the lives of individuals with severe expressive communication disorders and the role of advocacy in lessening the impact of handicaps on the lives of these individuals.

# BARRIERS TO EFFECTIVE COMMUNICATION

There are numerous and complex factors that serve to modify and shape the communicative styles and patterns of nonspeaking persons and affect the habilitation process (Calculator & D'Altilio, 1983; Farrier, Yorkston, Marriner, & Beukelman, 1985; Kraat, 1982). As discussed previously, communication breakdowns in message delivery can be attributed to mechanical or device-based issues, training deficiencies, attitudinal considerations, physical limitations of the client, environmental composition, and historical precedents (Cohen, 1985). These issues will be reviewed briefly below, as they relate to the ongoing process of clinical management.

## *Mechanical (Device) Issues*

Limitations imposed by the augmentative communication aid itself include the slow speed of message preparation and delivery, restricted lexicons, unique output modes, and the ease with which the aid can be used during interaction (Kraat, 1982).

Speed of message transmission has been addressed by numerous authors in this text and others (Beukelman & Yorkston, 1980; Buzolich, 1983; Harris, 1982; Yoder & Kraat, 1983). The typically slow rates of information exchange between users of augmentative communication devices and their partners contribute to the nonspeaker's passivity and lack of conversational initiation and to the domination of dialogue by unimpaired speakers. Severely speech-impaired persons learn very early that most communicative attempts result in frustration and miscommunications. Consequently, these individuals learn to be "world watchers" and to demonstrate minimal "conversational control" (Farrier et al., 1985).

The use of nonconventional symbol sets and systems, such as Blissymbolics (Bliss, 1965) or Picsyms (Carlson, 1985), can also present a barrier to effective message transmission. These lexical sets and symbol systems can preclude many opportunities for information exchange, since potential partners may be unfamiliar with the symbols and/or reluctant to learn about a new symbol set or system. Negative environmental response to symbols narrows the range of user experiences by limiting what, when, how, and with whom the client is able to communicate. Further, the client becomes increasingly reluctant to employ the symbols, especially in novel circumstances with inexperienced partners. When selecting a lexicon, the speech-language pathologist must consider how recognizable and learnable the symbol set or system is to listeners (Shane, Lipschultz, & Shane, 1982). Communication failures of retarded adults utilizing language boards have been traced in part to the design of the board itself (Calculator & D'Altilio, 1983). The authors found that a rearrangement of the layout of the client's display and a modification of vocabulary items increased the use of both the board and other modes of communication, and increased the likelihood that the individual would respond to the communication acts of others.

Typical unimpaired communicators employ a combination of output modes, including speaking, gesturing, writing, and facial expressions. It is generally agreed that spoken language allows for the richest and most varied communicative exchanges. Users of augmentative communication strategies and techniques employ unique output forms, such as sign systems, idiosyncratic gesticulation, hard copy, monitor displays, and synthesized speech. The patterns of spoken language may not be effective or appropriate for these alternate production formats. Therefore, the rules and structure of discourse may require modification to accommodate unusual primary communication patterns (Kraat, 1982). Atypical production forms may have an impact upon the nature and level of expressive language the user is capable of generating and the listeners are capable of comprehending. Therefore, users of augmentative communication devices can be at a distinct disadvantage. For example, school-aged children who use augmentative communication aids often engage in routinized and ritualistic message exchange. Their linguistic capabilities may exceed the level of actual output; however, severely speech-impaired individuals tend to repeatedly generate those words and phrases that have previously met with success (Calculator & Dollaghan, 1982). The children in Harris' study (1982) used those "communicative modes that were most accessible to them, required the least amount of physical effort, resulted in the fastest message transmission, and with which they were the most comfortable" (p. 33). This trend was also observed in large residential facilities with an adult retarded population (Shane et al., 1982).

The "approachability" factor is a psychosocial ramification of disability. The tendency in our society is to avoid persons who exhibit overt differences. Typical communication partners--particularly those individuals who have had little or no contact with severely impaired communicators--will vary their behaviors and their style of information delivery when dealing with nonspeakers. Shane and Cohen (1981) characterized the vocal behaviors of unimpaired communication partners during exchanges with nonspeaking persons; for example, individuals interacting with impaired speakers tended to overarticulate, hypergesticulate, increase the volume, and reduce the vocabulary and syntax to a less-sophisticated level. These phenomena can be compared to the patterns of discourse observed between native language speakers and speakers of a foreign tongue and between adults and children, and occurs with (unaided) manual signers and (aided) device users.

## *Educational Deficiencies*

Deficiencies in professional education at the preservice and inservice levels will affect the total habilitative process. Successful participation in educational, social, and vocational programs is dependent upon the speech-impaired individual's ability to communicate and interact with a variety of communication partners in different environments (Shane & Yoder, 1981). According to these authors, there are two primary reasons why devices are not, in many instances, being utilized and incorporated into the daily activities of the client who uses an augmentative communication aid. First, the number of personnel available to evaluate and fit persons in need of systems is insufficient. Second, there is a dearth of qualified professionals available to train individuals in the utility of aids as tools for interacting. Undergraduate and graduate curricula must respond accordingly to this gap in clinical preparation. Because augmentative communication is a relatively new area of clinical practice, it is not surprising that certain obstacles to education now exist. These obstacles include: the limited number of professional preparation programs offering courses in augmentative communication, the lack of appropriate methodologies for teaching students how to handle professional stress, and the limited information available to professionals regarding appropriate training strategies both for client instruction and for communication partners (Cohen, 1985).

*Professional education*. Members of the augmentative communication team need to "assess the degree to which existing augmentative systems truly augment communicative effectiveness; provide a system which, given appropriate client and staff training, can potentially circumvent problems not presently being addressed by the client's training program; train the client to functionally use the system to meet communication needs; familiarize others with strategies which will increase their likelihood of communicating effectively, efficiently, and satisfyingly with the client" (Calculator & D'Altilio, 1983, p. 190).

Professional education at the preservice level, then, should not only stress principles and practices in treatment, but should also orient students to a rationale and philosophy of augmentative approaches to treatment. A basis upon which sound theoretical methodologies can be implemented must be developed during the initial phases of education and not as an inservice antecedent to formal clinical training. It is suggested that students discuss with their instructors and colleagues the professional issues involved in clinical intervention for severely speech/language- and writing-impaired persons. Speech-language pathologists need to be familiar with the expertise of the other team professionals, and must demonstrate an appreciation and understanding of related disciplines and the contribution that each team member can make to the assessment, intervention, and, in effect, life-long management process. Clinical practicum experiences should encourage the speech-language pathologist to adopt a perspective about realistic decision-making with regard to intervention strategies and prescriptions for aids. Coercive tactics and technological excessiveness by team members when recommending augmentative aids and techniques should always be avoided. Above all, professionals involved with severely communicatively impaired persons must maintain an ethical and moralistic view that will guide every aspect of remediation. Since decision-making is the vital link between each level of client management, professionals working with this population need to be skilled problem-solvers.

Some of the aforementioned considerations can be translated into the following concrete instructions:

1. Students should be encouraged to form study groups to discuss issues related to the augmentative communication area.

2. Increased opportunities to work directly with parents and significant others should be provided in an effort to help them better understand the process of rejection, denial, and, ultimately, acceptance of the disability of their child or relative.

3. The nature and impact of handicapping conditions in society should be studied.

4. Students should be provided with coursework in administration and management procedures, computer technology, and counseling to prepare them for work settings that will demand this knowledge and to enable them to establish productive systems of service delivery, including integrated care plans for total habilitation.

*Professional stress.* In addition to professional training factors, problems indigenous to human services disciplines also present barriers to effective program implementation. Many facilities experience high rates of staff attrition as a result of anxiety and stress, burnout, low pay, and low esteem. In many instances, psychological issues, such as professional resistance to alternate therapeutic methods and fear of new practices, must be circumvented. It is the author's experience that many speech-language pathologists have difficulty making life-long management decisions, such as recommending specific augmentative aids and informing clients and caregivers that the client's oral language acquisition is at risk. These and other factors cause emotional overburdening. Professional anxiety and stress must be addressed early in student training programs, since it will have an impact upon the quality of treatment provided by future practitioners. Enhancement of the communicatively impaired individual's performance must be of primary concern to the team; thus, it is imperative that professionals be aware of these stress factors and how to avoid them.

*Client instruction*. Severely communicatively impaired individuals generally require intensive, environmentally based approaches to training (Cohen, 1985). Instructional strategies should be developed for those natural settings where conversation, written expression, and leisure activities are more likely to occur, such as in the home, in school, on the job, and during recreation. In this manner, individuals who use augmentative communication aids or techniques can apply interactive strategies to real experiences and can learn to manipulate and control actual communicative interchanges. Obsolete administrative dogma, professional inexperience, and/or gaps in student preparation should be eliminated so these factors do not create barriers to the effective implementation of augmentative communication interventions. Partnerships between the professional and the client in natural language settings should be encouraged to elicit more socially appropriate and acceptable communication. Providing treatment during classroom activities, promoting participation in communication groups, setting up "real" or potential dialogues, completing assignments, engaging in computer games, and encouraging peer tutoring are some strategies that will provide opportunities for communicative interactions that are analagous to real-life situations.

*Training communication partners*. For communicatively impaired persons to become an integral part of their community, the community must understand and accept them. Community training prepares potential partners, who live near or work with these individuals, to interact with them. Current and potential communication partners must be exposed to speech/language-impaired individuals of varying ages, cognitive levels, and physical capabilities. Through familiarity and education, able-bodied citizens will eventually appreciate the implications and ramifications of a severe expressive communication impairment and will become sensitized to interactive techniques that facilitate message exchange. For example, primary communication partners may need to be trained to facilitate the use of manual/gestural systems and communication devices. They may also need to be taught to recognize the intent of paralinguistic and kinesic cues (Kraat, 1982) that accompany the use of aids and techniques.

## Attitudinal Considerations

Beukelman (chapter 7) discusses how the attitudes of unimpaired individuals may handicap persons with severe speech impairments well beyond the level of their disability. Typically, these attitudes may be based upon misinformation and myth. Historically, nonspeaking persons were considered to be mentally retarded because they did not speak and did not have alternative means available with which to communicate. While the physically disabled person may by limited experientially because of neuromotor involvement, intellectual faculties can be, and often are, reasonably intact. Conversely, the expressive capabilities of mentally retarded individuals and other nonspeakers without gross physical involvement are frequently underestimated because of preconceived notions about the nature of certain handicapping conditions and connotations associated with them. Intervention programs that address attitudinal considerations provide education to unimpaired individuals and should lessen the handicaps of individuals who use augmentative aids and techniques.

## Environmental Considerations

"Environment refers to the various places where communicative behaviors occur, such as the home, the community, and the place of work" (Halpern & Fuhrer, 1984, p. 4). The environment plays an important role in shaping a person's behavior and can affect a person's interactive communicative performance. The term interaction, as it is used here, "refers to the dynamic relationship that exists between behavior and environment . . . " (Halpern & Fuhrer, 1984, p. 4). The environmental issues that must be evaluated and characterized to achieve total integration and successful interaction include: (a) the composition and constellation of communication partners in each setting; (b) the physical characteristics of each setting; (c) the activities specific to each setting; (d) the communication processes in each environment; (e) the opportunities for interaction in each environment; and (f) the expectations of the user in each environment.

The author suggests that a checklist be constructed for each environment in which the client can potentially interact and participate communicatively with speaking and nonspeaking partners. The Schneier Communication Unit in Syracuse, New York, has developed ecological checklists/surveys for this purpose. For additional information contact: Director, Adaptive Services, 1603 Court St., Syracuse, New York 13208. Formalized descriptions of environmental features will assist the professional in the assessment and program planning process. Communication aids and devices should cross environmental boundaries to promote communication with a variety of listeners.

## Historical and Developmental Barriers

The severely speech-impaired individual experiences a dearth of communicative precedents; that is, there is a history of expressive failure and reduced investigation of linguistic structure, use, and function (Kraat, 1982). Although the obstacles that confront a nonspeaker may appear to be insurmountable (whether the impairment is acquired or congenital), the professional must possess the tools to ameliorate predispositions that impede progress toward integration and total habilitation.

**SERVICE DELIVERY**

*Professional Team*

The individuals on the team responsible for the development of a client's integrated care plan include the speech-language pathologist, associated health, education, and human service professionals, the client, and the primary caregivers. The level of participation and consultation provided by each team member depends upon the particular needs of the client and the availability of the specialists. The most important question facing this team is how to successfully integrate the severely communicatively impaired client into community life so that reasonable levels of autonomy, participation, and self-fulfillment are achieved.

The integrated care profile developed by the professional team should reflect present and future communication styles, behaviors, and needs of the client. Approaches to intervention and the manner in which the client's physical, cognitive, social, emotional, vocational, and medical status will affect expectations must be addressed. The team must work together to facilitate opportunities throughout the individual's life for equal and appropriate involvement in educational, leisure, and vocational pursuits. Management of the augmentative communication program will influence the degree to which the client is able to interact in all settings and, ultimately, is accepted in society.

*Speech-language pathologist*. The ASHA Position Statement on Nonspeech Communication states that the role of the speech-language pathologist with regard to communication augmentation includes assessing, describing, and documenting communicative/interactive behaviors and needs; evaluating and assisting in the selection of the various communication techniques in order to develop an effective repertoire of communication modes; and developing speech and vocal capabilities to the fullest potential (ASHA, 1981). Executing these responsibilities requires a knowledge of how to select and apply symbols, implement and evaluate intervention procedures, and develop and integrate program plans. The professional is also expected to train interactants and to coordinate and monitor on-going treatment. A description of the specialist's responsibility with regard to the dispensing of products, including prosthetic devices, can be extrapolated from the ASHA Code of Ethics (ASHA, 1979).

There are often additional demands placed upon the speech-language pathologist who works with the severely communicatively impaired population. Traditionally, speech-language pathologists were primarily concerned with clinical issues, including assessment, prescription, treatment, and intervention followup. Successful management of nonspeaking individuals requires that the professional also administer the process (i.e., research equipment, materials, and software), educate significant others involved with the client, and advocate for the client's communication rights in the community-at-large and in future endeavors (Cohen, 1985). Students of speech-language pathology must be sensitive to the role expectations for the speech-language pathologist in the management of severely communicatively impaired persons. For example, the ASHA Position Statement on Nonspeech Communication (ASHA, 1981) states that the speech-language pathologist is the most likely candidate to coordinate service delivery for nonspeaking clients. The team coordinator is responsible for interpreting and disseminating data from the different disciplines involved, monitoring all phases of implementation, and providing a mechanism of checks and balances on the effectiveness of the augmentative aid or augmentative components selected. The speech-language pathologist must also cultivate research capabilities. Specifically, the communication professional must keep abreast of trends in relevant technology, maintain current information on the state-of-the-art in hardware and software design and availability, and be knowledgeable about operation, maintenance, component parts, and special interfacing techniques. As educator and advocate, the speech-language pathologist must provide ongoing training and orientation to the client, staff, family and friends, and other interactants in various environments. Finally, the concept of life-long management requires an awareness of local and national advocacy issues, such as pertinent legislation, public relations activities, and group or individual efforts that affect the public's perception and image of the severely speech- and writing-impaired individual in the community.

## Models of Delivery

Shane and Yoder (1981) presented three models of service delivery for children and adults with severe communication impairment: (a) Local Educational Agency; (b) Itinerant Specialty Team; and (c) Specialty Clinic Model.

The Local Educational Agency (LEA) approach utilizes specialists from the educational facility to develop and implement the components of the individual's communication plan. A sample model of a Local Educational Agency providing augmentative services can be obtained from the Non-oral Communication Center, located in the Plavan School in Fountain Valley, California (Montgomery, 1980).

The Itinerant Specialty Team (IST) model includes a group of specialists charged with evaluating, monitoring, and updating program plans for nonspeaking individuals within a designated geographic region. Information on an IST model is available from the Schneier Communication Unit of the Cerebral Palsy Center, Syracuse, New York (Cohen & Anastasio, 1985).

The Specialty Clinic Model (SCM) is usually housed in a hospital, clinic, or university setting. Comprehensive assessment, prescription, device fitting, and training are provided by the augmentative communication team; however, the team also provides support and consulting services to the professionals and other caregivers who interact with the client on a daily basis. Many of the well-known augmentative communication programs in this country are based upon this specialty clinic concept. The Communication Enhancement Clinic of Children's Hospital Medical Center in Boston is an example of an SCM. For additional information, contact Director, Communication Enhancement Clinic, 300 Longwood Ave., Boston, Massachusetts 02115

## *Scheduling*

Clinicians have traditionally treated communication disorders using either intermittent or intensive scheduling methods or a combination of the two (ASHA, 1973). Intermittent scheduling involves therapy several times weekly and intensive scheduling suggests daily treatment over an extended period. Generally, though, with either plan, intervention occurs at the same time of the day. It has been demonstrated repeatedly that traditional therapy formats, such as the individualized half-hour treatment session in isolation, are not appropriate augmentative communication training strategies.

An alternative course for remediation is flexible scheduling, previously discussed by Shane et al. (1982). In flexible scheduling services are provided at variable times throughout the day and evening in natural settings and according to the individual's communication needs, styles, and strengths. This type of treatment scheduling can be provided intermittently or intensively. The rationale for this approach is that the focus of training must extend beyond direct client contact to include other critical environmental factors that have a daily influence on the client's interactive behaviors. The current generation of speech-language pathologists will need to assume the role of "transenvironmental interventionist" in order to influence the nature and success of communicative interactions and the status of the client in the community. Human dialogue does not occur without partners, context, environmental cues, and external events. Service delivery institutions must respond accordingly.

In certain environments, such as schools, it may be difficult for the speech-language pathologist to offer flexible scheduling due to administrative and time constraints. However, flexibility is possible in communication groups and on field trips, where professionals can intervene and offer instruction in a less than traditional fashion. In residential settings, day treatment programs, and home-based environs where the client's day is less rigidly structured, the aforementioned format should prove to be very effective. Chapter 6 of this text offers a variety of instructional perspectives relating to specific training strategies that capitalize upon the concept of environmental influences and events.

## CURRENT PERSPECTIVES ON FUNDING FOR
## AUGMENTATIVE COMMUNICATION

Securing financial assistance for augmentative communication aids through third-party resources represents one of the most demanding components of the service delivery process. Often, after a thorough evaluation is completed, recommendations delineated, and a plan for implementation outlined, the family and the professionals find that they are unable to obtain funding for equipment and training. Their inability to obtain funding stems from the fact that the speech-language pathologists that coordinate assessment and treatment, as well as the individuals who care for the client, often are not experienced in the mechanics and nuances of the funding procedure and do not have the time to carefully study the process and pursue the proper procedures. It is important for augmentative communication specialists to study the funding literature and to educate themselves with regard to potential sources of funding, procedures for applying for funds, pending legislation and existing regulations related to funding, and to open lines of communication between funding agency representatives and clinical personnel.

According to Depape (1979), there are four basic steps involved in the funding process: (a) a funding coordinator is selected, (b) potential sources are identified, (c) required information is identified and then submitted and justified to the appropriate agencies, and (d) if funding is secured, final arrangements are organized and completed, including ordering, purchasing, and integrating the equipment as well as training the client, family, and professional team. This process may take weeks or even months depending upon the complexity of the system(s) and the individual client profile. Ruggles (1979) outlined a slightly different four-stage procedure to obtain funding for communication aids. Whereas Depape's process centers on the actual acquisition of monies, Ruggles concentrates to a greater extent on the needs or qualifications of the professional involved in completing the process. The first step is self-evaluation, the second step is professional education, the third is client assessment, and the final task is the actual submission of the funding requests. Self-evaluation is described as a personal inventory of knowledge bases and potential resources for funding. The funding coordinator's own skills, the agency's assertiveness in the nonspeech area, pertinent legislation, and private and public sources should be examined. Professional education provides opportunities to advocate for the provision of communication aids by creating relationships with funding agency representatives. Client assessment generates data for justifying the purchase of communication instru-

mentation and materials. The last phase provides the third-party funder with the proposal and written documentation for the communication aid.

Depape (1979) and Ruggles (1979) both provide systematic approaches for
individuals seeking funding for augmentative communication aids and techniques.
They offer common sense advice and enumerate specific activities and tasks that are
designed to facilitate the process of obtaining funding. Their recommendations and
guidelines are practical and can be implemented in most settings where severely
communicatively impaired clients are served.

Available literature primarily provides advice on securing monies for
communication aids and dealing with third-party funding agencies and regulatory
agencies. As discussed in chapter 1, funding issues extend well beyond the purchase
cost of equipment. The cost of training individuals to use communication aids and the
costs to maintain equipment are essential considerations. It is unlikely that money
used to purchase aids will be well spent unless funding to insure their successful
implementation is provided. The remainder of this section will elaborate upon four
generic levels of funding that speech-language pathologists working with nonspeaking
populations must consider.

## *Level I*

Initially, it may be necessary to purchase equipment and materials that will
enable professionals to provide diagnostic/evaluative services for nonspeaking clients.
Earlier in this chapter, three service delivery models were described, including the
local educational agency, itinerant team, and specialty clinic. This assessment center
philosophy can be established according to any of these models; however, regardless of
the structure, seed monies and start-up funds must be secured. Federal and state
rehabilitation and education service monies and research grants should be investigated
for Level I funding support. Also, the interested student or speech-language
pathologist should investigate funding through charitable foundations and
industry/corporate programs. Finally, a diagnostic/evaluation service can be
established in the same way as one would construct a capital investment-based business
venture; that is, a fee-for-service, profit-making organization. This option is becoming
increasingly popular with speech-language pathologists who are exploring ways to
provide specialized approaches to intervention.

## Level II

The second phase of funding (for a center-based model, in particular) is concerned with the assessment and training of communicatively impaired persons. Typically, this aspect of client management is treated as a "therapy" session for reimbursement purposes. Third-party funding programs generically include medical, vocational, and educational agencies. Specifically, Medicaid, Medicare, and state aid programs for physically disabled children, as well as private medical insurance, are resources that can be tapped for medically justifiable services. The Department of Vocational Rehabilitation should be approached when the client is a viable candidate for productive employment and enhanced communciation would facilitate that eventuality. The school district is another funding resource that can be explored when severely handicapped students are referred for consultation, communication evaluation, and therapeutic intervention. Of course, personal funds and family resources are a less frequent but possible source of income. School-based/educational service providers can tap a variety of different resources, such as federal and state educational funds and grants, that have been set aside for special services and children within the district. Recommendations for services and equipment incorporated into an Individualized Education Procedure will be purchased through financial aid programs for handicapped students. Sometimes, schools will contract with a specialty clinic for augmentative communication consultation. An itinerant team can also provide this service and travel considerable distances to evaluate and/or treat clients or groups of individuals.

## Level III

The third level of funding is the most problematic and cumbersome. Obtaining third-party financial assistance for the purchase of client-owned/operated aids continues to be a source of frustration because of capricious decision-making by uninformed claim reviewers, the absence of uniform legislation regulating the approval and denial process, and a pervasive disregard and lack of sensitivity for the needs and rights of the severely communicatively disabled in our society. The recommended systems must be justified according to the guidelines of the agency (e.g., the communication aid must be medically necessary, educationally indicated, or vocationally supportive). Additional avenues for attaining revenue include family funds, charitable or community groups, and parent or national organizations. The reader is referred to the *Health Insurance Manual for Speech-Language Pathologists and Audiologists* for additional guidelines (Downey, White, & Karr, 1984).

*Level IV*

The final area of consideration in the funding realm is research and development. Traditionally, government grants, charitable foundations, community special interest groups, and industry/corporate programs have supported research and development projects for the severely communicatively impaired. The student must review potential granting organizations and determine the appropriateness of the grant guidelines relative to the proposed task.

*Funding Terminology*

Perhaps the most common error made by clinicians and team members in preparing written documentation for funding augmentative communication aids is the misuse of descriptive terminology. For example, when applying to a medical funding agency, terms such as *prosthetic*, *medical necessity*, and *meeting basic medical needs* should be employed. Educational phraseology, such as *facilitate classroom integration*, *enhance academic performance*, and *proffer supportive technology* should be used only when applying to an educational funding agency. Vocational objectives, such as *communication system will lead to a more productive life*, *competitively employed citizen*, *create viable employment opportunities*, and *prepare client to be economically self-sufficient in a technological society* should be used when applying to prevocational and vocational agencies. The party responsible for preparing written justification must be aware of the idiosyncracies of the funding process, since the misuse of one term can precipitate immediate rejection.

*Conclusions*

It is important for the student to become familiar with current funding issues and the inadequacies of existing procedures. The education and sensitization of all echelons of individuals associated with severely speech- and/or writing-impaired clients, including federal legislators, will result in modifications to an often unreasonable and inequitable system.

## ADVOCACY AND TOTAL HABILITATION

### *Breaking Down Barriers Through Advocacy*

Given the nature of the barriers to effective communicative interaction addressed earlier in this chapter, there are a number of ways to approach the problem and remove some of the obstacles.  Persons with severe speech and/or writing impairments, their families, and the professionals who work with them must accept the challenge and assume their roles as advocates.  This means that the needs of this diverse population must be presented to the public, government, educators, and others, in a consistent and visible manner.  Providing life-long management and intervention for the user of augmentative communication techniques implies a level of integration into the mainstream of society that can only be achieved through systematic advocacy and planning on three primary levels.

1.  Mechanical and system-based issues can be effectively dealt with by participating, in an advisory capacity, with developers and manufacturers of communication aids and software.  Communication professionals and consumers themselves must form close alliances with the individuals designing aids if the needs of nonspeaking and nonwriting persons are to be properly met.  Manufacturers and their distributors must meet regularly to discuss standardization, safety features, technological advances affecting fabrication, and marketing tactics.  There have been some attempts to encourage interaction among the manufacturers, their representatives, and communication professionals.  Notably, there have been some efforts under the auspices of the International Society of Augmentative and Alternative Communication to form an alliance between manufacturers and professionals to discuss issues such as standardization and marketing.

2.  Public information networking can also effect change in the quality and quantity of instrumentation available.  For example, the demand of the general public for more intelligible, low-cost voice output capability has expedited research and development in the voice processing field.  Increased media attention to disability (in particular, severe communication impairment and the utilization of augmentative components) will serve to modify attitudes and eliminate myths.  A heightened sensitivity to the ramifications of handicapping conditions will shape the perspective of future generations of citizens regarding persons who are "different."

3. Government officials are in a position to bring about massive change. Laws and regulations must not only recognize the existence of individuals with severe expressive communication disorders, but must also provide the mechanisms to adequately support financial requirements. It is important to contact, by mail and by telephone, congressional representatives and local officials to apprise them of the issues. Inviting government officials to observe programs in operation and clients utilizing augmentative approaches is a viable mechanism also. There are many ways to affect public policy. The Governmental Affairs Department of the American Speech-Language-Hearing Association can provide suggestions for changing public policy. Third-party funding agencies and their employees must follow uniform, obligatory guidelines in order to serve the communicatively impaired population in this country. Once again, it is the responsibility of consumers, professionals, and families to advocate for these public, legislative, and regulatory concerns in order to promote complete habilitation over the course of a lifetime.

## *Education*

The professional, lay public, and private sectors need to be exposed to formal and informal educational agendas that are current, inclusive, and candid. Speech-language pathologists, designers and manufacturers, related disciplines, and other associated professionals require ongoing education. Persons involved in the management of severely communicatively impaired children and adults must understand the implication of total care plans that emphasize the integration of augmented expression into every facet of the user's life. Textbook theory and principles alone are insufficient. Hands-on experience, coupled with an awareness of human interaction and an appreciation of the inherent deterrents to efficient conversational control, must be part of any instructional curriculum.

## *Achieving Integration*

Mainstreaming the individual with a severe expressive communication disorder is always the ultimate management objective (Holmquist, 1984). From the point of initial referral, all of the plans, prescriptions, and interventions should be considered in terms of how they relate to furthering a client's participation in life's daily activities on a level commensurate with others in the same social setting.

Educational mainstreaming of children with disabilities has been a goal since the passage of P.L. 94-142 (Education For All Handicapped Children Act of 1975). To comply with the mandates of the law, certain features should be incorporated into the communication plan for the student for whom augmentative communication interventions are employed (Shane & Yoder, 1981). The suggested components for this communication plan include the following queries:

1. Is the system functional?

2. Does it provide for interactions with nonhandicapped peers?

3. Does it maximize participation?

4. Can it accommodate a variety of activities?

The professional must monitor selection of communication aids, training on the equipment, and training in the interactive use of augmentative techniques.

Social and recreational integration is critical to the client's well-being and image of self-worth. While it is difficult for a severely speech-impaired person to achieve equality in a world dominated by oral communicators, it can be accomplished if the aids and/or techniques are appropriate and listeners/interactants are trained accordingly. It is reasonable to expect that by using communication augmentation, individuals can enjoy recreational activities and social events, thereby achieving integration of their life style with the life styles of their associates and peers.

It appears that some of the most successful users of augmentative communication aids are those individuals who have been afforded the support and encouragement to return to the workplace or to capitalize upon vocational opportunities. We live in a society that revolves around its work force, and the value of individuals is often measured in terms of employment contributions. Professionals, clients, families, and other advocates must strive to integrate aided workers into jobs that capitalize upon individual needs, strengths, and capabilitites. Education of coworkers must be undertaken in order to establish the prerequisites for interactive communication. The importance of communication to success on the job site cannot be overestimated. Nonspeakers must be capable of meaningful and intelligible interchange with other employees in order to facilitate integration. Furthermore, augmented communicators must be able to socialize in a work setting according to the circumstances and the nature of their communication partners. The interrelationship between communication skills and work/leisure activities is complex. However, the role of interactive, meaningful dialogue, which affects both social acceptance and work productivity, is obvious.

Finally, active advocacy for the user of augmentative communication aids and techniques in all other activities of daily living is necessary to the total habilitation process. Barriers to effective communication cannot be dismantled if communication aids and techniques are not commonplace and accessible in all circumstances. Providing communication options that will change as the client and environmental needs change will challenge those working in the augmentative communication area and, ultimately, will have an effect upon the total habilitation of the client with a severe expressive communication disorder.

## SUMMARY

This chapter elaborates upon life-long management strategies for the severely communicatively impaired client. Barriers to effective communication are enumerated and described categorically (e.g., mechanical issues, attitudinal considerations, or society's preconceived notions about communicatively disabled persons, environmental factors that preclude interaction, and the influence of historical and developmental data). Service delivery is discussed in terms of the unique role of the speech-language pathologist as it pertains to the treatment of severely speech-impaired individuals. The expectations for the professional in this area are often more complex and demanding than the expectations for the speech-language pathologists dealing with other populations. Augmentative communication intervention encompasses assessment, research, monitoring, advocacy, funding, and education of other professionals and the public. The chapter offers suggestions and guidelines for integrating individuals who use communication aids and augmentative techniques into the community. Advocacy on a local and national level is considered by the author to be a way to change attitudes and obtain necessary legislative support for funding.

## STUDY QUESTIONS

1. How can the family of the client facilitate integration of augmentative aids and techniques into their community and daily activities?

2. What type of procedures can be utilized to educate the public regarding augmentative communication interventions?

3. Do you feel any of the barriers to effective communication can be removed? If so, how?

4. What do you feel is the speech-language professional's role regarding advocacy?

5. How do societal attitudes affect change and acceptance in the area of disability and habilitation?

6. In what ways can legislators, consumers and their families, and professionals have an effect upon the role of the disabled individual in the community and bring about change?

7. What seems to be the most important information the professional must possess in order to proceed with the process of obtaining funding for a personal communication aid?

## REFERENCES

American Speech-Language-Hearing Association.    (1973).    Task force report on traditional scheduling procedures in schools.  Language, Speech, and Hearing Services in Schools, 4(3), 100-109.

American Speech-Language-Hearing Association.  (1979, January).  Code of Ethics of the American Speech-Language-Hearing Association.  Asha, 22(4), 267-272.

American Speech-Language-Hearing Association.  (1981, August).  Position statement on nonspeech communication.  Asha, 23(8), 577-581.

Beukelman, D., & Yorkston, K.  (1980).  Nonvocal communication:  Performance evaluation.  Archives of Physical Medicine and Rehabilitation, 61, 272-275.

Bliss, C.  (1965).  Semantography-Blissymbolics.  Sydney, Australia:  Semantography Publications.

Buzolich, M.  (1983).  Interaction analysis of augmented and normal adult communicators.  Unpublished doctoral dissertation, University of California, San Francisco.

Calculator, S., & D'Altilio, C. (1983). Evaluating the effectiveness of a communication board training program. Journal of Speech and Hearing Disorders, 48, 185-191.

Calculator, S., & Dollaghan, C. (1982). The use of communication boards in a residential setting: An evaluation. Journal of Speech and Hearing Disorders, 47, 281-287.

Carlson, F. (1985). Picsyms categorical dictionary. Lawrence, KS: Baggeboda Press.

Cohen, C. (1985). Augmentative communication: A state-of-the-art. Paper presented at the University of Wisconsin Continuing Education Workshop, Madison.

Cohen, C., & Anastasio, J. (1985). Itinerant specialty team model. Unpublished excerpts from a grant prepared for United Cerebral Palsy Center, Syracuse, NY

Depape, D. (1979). Guidelines for seeking funding for communication aids. Madison, WI: Trace Research and Development Center.

Downey, J., White, S., & Karr, S. (1984). Health insurance manual for speech-language pathologists and audiologists. Rockville, MD: American Speech-Language-Hearing Association.

Farrier, L., Yorkston, K., Marriner, N., & Beukelman, D. (1985). Conversational control in nonimpaired speakers using an augmentative communication system. Augmentative and Alternative Communication, 1, 65-73.

Harris, D. (1982). Communication interaction processes involving nonvocal physically handicapped children. Topics in Language Disorders, 2, 21-37.

Halpern, A., & Fuhrer, M. (Eds.). (1984). Introduction. Functional assessment in rehabilitation. Baltimore: Brooks Publishing.

Holmquist, E. (1984). I am my own person. Conversations with non-speaking people. Toronto: Canadian Rehabilitation Council for the Disabled.

Kraat, A. (1982). Special considerations in augmentative communication use. Paper presented at First International Conference of Augmentative and Alternative Communication, Toronto, Canada.

Montgomery, J.   (1980).   <u>Non-oral communication:   A training guide for the child</u> <u>without speech</u>.  Fountain Valley, CA:  Fountain Valley School District, Plavan School.

Ruggles, V. (1979).   <u>Funding of non-vocal communication aids:   Current issues and</u> <u>strategies</u>.  New York:  Muscular Dystrophy Association.

Shane, H., &  Cohen, C. (1981).   A discussion of communicative strategies and patterns by nonspeaking persons.  <u>Language, Speech, and Hearing Services in Schools</u>, <u>12</u>, 201-215.

Shane,  H., Lipschultz, R.,  &  Shane,  C.   (1982).   Facilitating the communicative interaction of nonspeaking persons in large residential settings.   <u>Topics in</u> <u>Langugage Disorders</u>, <u>2</u>, 73-84.

Shane, H., & Yoder, D. (1981).  Delivery of augmentative communication services:  The role of the speech-language pathologist.   <u>Language, Speech, and Hearing</u> <u>Services in the Schools</u>, <u>12</u>, 211-215.

Yoder, D., & Kraat, A. (1983).  Intervention issues in nonspeech communication.  In J. Miller, D. Yoder, & R. Schiefelbusch (Eds.), <u>Contemporary issues in language</u> <u>intervention</u> (pp. 27-51).  <u>ASHA Reports</u>, <u>12</u>.

## ADDITIONAL READINGS

Beukelman, D., Yorkston, K., & Dowden, P.  (1985).  <u>Communication augmentation:  A</u> <u>casebook of clinical management</u>.  San Diego:  College-Hill Press.

Fishman, S., Timler, G., & Yoder, D.  (1985).  Strategies for the prevention of communication breakdown in interactions with communication board users. <u>Augmentative and Alternative Communication</u>, <u>1</u>, 38-51.

Hoffman, A. (1983-1986).  <u>The many faces of funding</u>.  Mill Valley, CA:  Phonic Ear, Inc.

Johnson-Martin, N., Porter, P., & Goolsgy, E. (1984).  Service delivery models in rural settings:   The North Carolina experience.   <u>Abstracts from the Third</u> <u>International Conference of Augmentative and Alternative Communication</u>, Boston, MA.  Toronto, Canada:  ISAAC.

Odle, S., Wethered, C., & Selph, S. (1982). Communication skills. In J. Greer, R. Anderson, & S. Odle (Eds.), <u>Strategies for helping severe and multiply handicapped citizens</u>. Baltimore: University Park Press.

Yoder, D. (1982). Foreword. <u>Topics in Language Disorders</u>, <u>2</u>.

# CHAPTER 9

## FUTURE NEEDS AND DIRECTIONS

PAMELA MATHY-LAIKKO

*Department of Communicative Disorders*
*University of Wisconsin - Madison*


DAVID E. YODER

*Department of Medical Allied Health Professions*
*University of North Carolina at Chapel Hill*

## OBJECTIVES


- Discuss the research/knowledge base in augmentative communication.

- Discuss the influence of assumptions (models, theories) about communication on current methods of measuring the effectiveness of augmentative communication components.

- Discuss the need for a unified theory of communication to guide future research in human communication sciences and disorders.

- Introduce human factors/ergonomics and discuss ways that future research in augmentative communication could be enhanced by research results and principles in that field.

- Discuss considerations for interpreting the results of research that examines face-to-face interactions of individuals who use augmentative aids and techiques and their speaking partners, and suggest directions for future research.

- Discuss directions for future research with regard to examining the effects of implementing aided or unaided techniques with individuals who are cognitively impaired.

- Discuss appropriate designs for future research in augmentative communication.

## INTRODUCTION

The preceding chapters of this book have described many accomplishments and innovations in technology, assessment, training, and service delivery in augmentative communication that have expanded the potential for social interactions for persons with severe expressive communication disorders. To continue these advances and to provide guidelines for future developments in this area, however, requires that these past accomplishments be critically evaluated. It is essential that we develop a valid means of assessing the effects of augmentative communication components on the communication process, because this will enable us to determine if advances in this area are having a positive impact on the abilities/skills of persons with severe expressive communication disorders. From this point, future developments would be guided by a clear understanding of past successes and failures.

This chapter focuses on current research in, and our assumptions about, augmentative communication, and presents challenges for future research to develop valid measures of the impact of augmentative components on the communication process.

## CURRENT RESEARCH CONSIDERATIONS

### Lack of Empirical Data

In any science, the literature can be divided into at least two broad categories: primary sources (e.g., research reports), and secondary sources (e.g., textbooks, book chapters, review articles, etc.) (Kuhn, 1970). Literature in the augmentative communication area requires an additional category, i.e., descriptive reports of intervention approaches and technological applications. Such reports "characterize the probable" (Beukelman, 1985, p. 55); they describe potentially useful hardware and software and/or treatment or diagnostic techniques. These reports do not, however, supply empirical data supporting the efficacy or efficiency of proposed interventions. Beukelman (1985) issued the following criticism:

> Reports of technological and educational approaches have been introduced and comments about how these approaches would probably be successful with nonspeaking individuals have been published . . . . While visionary writing about the probable is necessary as a guide, without empirical reports these statements of the probable are of limited usefulness. (p. 56)

In an attempt to categorize the more than 300 entries in the augmentative communication literature, Villarruel, Mathy-Laikko, Ratcliff, and Yoder (1985) found that roughly one-third of the entries are descriptive reports, one-third are books and review articles, and one-third are research reports. Unfortunately, the empirically based sources measure the impact of augmentative interventions according to a relatively narrow range of dependent variables. These often include the number of symbols learned or the speed of message transmission over time in words per minute. Clearly, the data available for answering important questions in the area of augmentative communication is limited, thus making it difficult to answer such questions as: (a) which augmentative components provide for optimal communicative competence, particularly for individuals who have physical and cognitive impairments? and (b) which training materials and strategies are most useful when implementing augmentative communication aids and techniques across communicative contexts?

### *Human Factors Engineering*

Human factors engineering, or ergonomics, addresses questions that are analogous to those facing professionals in the augmentative communication area. The goal of human factors research is to design machines that accommodate the limits of the human user (Wickens, 1984). Obviously, the successful use of any tool designed to assist individuals to communicate is affected by human limitations. Ergonomics deals with both human physical limitations (e.g., range of motion for easy reach of controls, fatigue levels, etc.) as well as machine designs that are compatible with the information-processing capacities of the brain (e.g., perceptual processing, attention, working memory, etc.) (Wickens, 1984). The scope of human factors research is vast, touching every conceivable type of interaction between humans and machines. For example, topics covered in the proceedings of two recent ergonomics/human factors conferences (Eberts & Eberts, 1985; Mital, 1984) include attention and vigilance, human-computer interaction, human performance and cognitive processes, work-station designs, training, and motor learning.

Future research in augmentative communication could benefit from the work being done in the human factors field.  For example, studies such as those outlined above could provide initial guidelines for designing and modifying augmentative communication aids and selection techniques.  More importantly, augmentative communication research would benefit from adopting human factors principles, which take a systems approach to the study of person-machine-environment relationships (Meister, 1976).  The development of new augmentative communication aids and techniques should be guided by an understanding of the principles of human factors and of person-machine concepts (Goodenough-Trepagnier & Rosen, 1982; Meister, 1976).

Face-to-face communication between an augmentative communication user and an unimpaired speaker can be viewed as a person-machine or a person-technique system.  As such, it too is affected by changes in human components (learning, fatigue) and the machine or technique's components.  In other words, the study of aided and unaided techniques to increase communicative competence can be considered a form of human factors research.  Guided by human factors principles, future research in augmentative communication should be directed toward comparing features of augmentative communication components (e.g., symbol sets, selection and production techniques, output modes).  Further, these comparisons must be made within and across communicative contexts to fill the various communication needs (face-to-face conversation, written communication, telephone communication, and so on) of severely speech- and/or writing-impaired individuals.

## COMPONENT MODEL[1] OF COMMUNICATION AND ITS EFFECTS ON CURRENT RESEARCH

The field of human communication sciences and disorders began with a restricted view of communication, focusing primarily on the speech signal (articulation).  In recent years it has undergone many changes.  The fields of behavioral and cognitive psychology, linguistics, sociolinguistics, child development,and others have had an impact on communication sciences and disorders.

---

[1]In this chapter, the term model is intended to be synonymous with diagram or outline.  It does not denote theory (cf. Brodbeck, 1959).

This is evident in the inclusion of developmental theory and language (syntax, morphology, phonology, semantics, pragmatics) in the study of speech and hearing disorders. With each new development in the knowledge base, new assessments and treatment techniques were added, influencing training and rehabilitation/habilitation practices.

The field of human communication sciences and disorders has not been guided by a unified theory of communication. However, over the years a model of communication has been constructed. Our working theory of communication reflects a "component model." During a typical communication assessment each component (speech, hearing, and language) is evaluated and a differential diagnosis is made. For example, if a person's language comprehension is within normal limits on standardized tests but speech is unintelligible, the primary communication disorder is their inability to use speech to convey message elements (words, phrases, sentences, etc.). Thus, the focus of habilitation/rehabilitation is to develop the most effective means of augmenting speech. This diagnostic process is useful in planning intervention goals; however, it does not address how deficits in one or more components actually affect an individual's ability to communicate in everyday contexts.

The study of augmentative communication reveals serious problems with the component model, particularly as it is applied to conversation. Communicative behavior is not merely a sum of its components; it should be viewed as a dynamic system of inseparable, interrelated, and interdependent parts (see chapter 3; Kirchner & Skarakis-Doyle, 1983; Watzlawick, Beavin, & Jackson, 1967). Examination of the interaction characteristics between individuals who use augmentative communication aids and techniques and their partners has shown that merely providing a way to convey message elements (e.g., a communication aid) does not solve the expressive communication problems of these persons (Kraat, 1985). Therefore, a future need is to replace the component model with a unified theory of communication that accounts for more than observable speech behaviors and enables a clear understanding of the impact of communication augmentation components on the communication process. This perspective on the study of communication intervention is also in line with the systems orientation of the human factors field (Meister, 1976).

## *Effects of the Component Model on Current Research*

Previous chapters have discussed the dependent variables that are most often considered in measuring the effectiveness of communication aids or techniques. Among these are *speed, flexibility,* and *independence* (see chapter 3). Although no empirical research directly compares the flexibility and independence of augmentative communication components, strategies for increasing speed of communication (i.e., rate measured in accurate words per minute--[wpm]) have been developed and evaluated.  Unfortunately, these strategies, which include manipulation of (a) message units (phonemes, words, sentences) and (b) selection techniques in conjunction with message units, are often implemented without considering how they will affect the overall process of communication.

*Manipulation of message units*.  Strategies for increasing the effectiveness of augmentative communication techniques have focused on constructing optimal message units to reduce the number of moves (selections) required per word/message (e.g., Baker, 1982; Beukelman & Yorkston, 1982, 1984; Goodenough-Trepagnier, Tarry, & Prather, 1982).  For example, Goodenough-Trepagnier et al. (1982) have generated sets of frequent phoneme (SPEEC) and letter (WRITE) sequences based on an analysis of a word frequency list for spoken English.  They presented data for one individual who, using a 400-phoneme SPEEC board, was able to increase his wpm rate by 30 percent over the rate for his alphabetic printer.  However, when individuals use an alphabetic printer, their partners can predict and often guess words, thus reducing the need to spell each word and, in effect, speeding up the rate of message exchange.  Predictive guessing may be more difficult, if not impossible, when the SPEEC or WRITE system is employed.  Thus, while systems such as SPEEC or WRITE may increase wpm rate for some communication purposes (e.g., writing), their effect on conversation may differ.  Research comparing SPEEC and WRITE to alphabet/word boards during conversation is needed to confirm this hypothesis.  Another strategy for manipulating message units to enhance communicative effectiveness (rate) involves the use of computer prediction programs (see Beukelman & Yorkston, 1984) or abbreviation expansion programs (Vanderheiden, 1984a).  The goal of these programs is to reduce the number of moves (key strokes) required to complete a message.  Although prediction and abbreviation expansion strategies result in increases in wpm rate, their overall speed when compared to letter-by-letter techniques during conversation and in other communicative contexts has not been examined.

In addition to modification at the phoneme, letter, and word level, it has also been suggested that preprogramming augmentative communication aids with frequently used phrases would greatly reduce the number of selections required per message unit and would increase speed (measured in wpm) (Baker, 1982; Beukelman & Yorkston, 1982).  To examine the potential for use of this strategy, Beukelman and Yorkston (1982) collected communication samples over a 14-day period from Canon Communicator (Canon USA, Canon Plaza, Lake Success, NY) users.  Ninety-two percent of the messages were unique from other messages in the sample.  Beukelman and Yorkston interpreted these findings to suggest that clinicians and system developers must be alerted "to the compromise that must be struck between message content uniqueness and speed (rate) enhancement through message retrieval.  Some individual users may tolerate reduced uniqueness in order to increase communication speed.  However, others may desire a high degree of uniqueness and may be willing to sacrifice communicative speed to obtain it" (p. 3).

Examining the construction of conversations during social interaction indicates that "message uniqueness" on the part of any participant is a product of preserving the conversational and social relevance of one's contribution to ongoing talk (Brown & Levinson, 1978; Maynard & Zimmerman, 1984; Sacks, Schegloff, & Jefferson, 1974). Given this, it would seem probable that the use of preprogrammed phrases during conversations entails the risks of confusing the listener. Semantic compaction (Baker, 1982) would be subject to similar limitations.

Nevertheless, many communication aids allow the user to store phrases. Future research, therefore, should explore the use of preprogrammed messages for managing conversation and for training communicative skills. For example, preprogrammed phrases may be used to accomplish specific communicative goals (e.g., bank transactions, store communications, ordering in a restaurant) (Goossens' & Kraat, 1985). To determine which phrases are needed for use in such contexts, environmental observations can be made to collect inventories of the communication expectations (Brown et al., 1980). When the requirements of a context are known in advance, needed phrases may be easier to predict and thus to plan (Garfinkel, 1967).

It has also been suggested that preprogramming phrases that frequently serve to mark disjuncture and/or transitions during conversation (e.g., "What's new," "I have something to say about that," "Speaking of . . .") may affect the conversational management of users of augmentative communication techniques (Beukelman & Yorkston, 1984; Higginbotham, Mathy-Laikko, & Yoder, in press). Examination of research (e.g., Atkinson & Heritage, 1984) on how unimpaired speakers mark disjuncture during conversation may be a useful starting point for designing studies that compare the ability of individuals to manage conversations with and without the use of preprogrammed phrases.

The mode of output also seems to affect communication effectiveness. Two recent studies using micro- and macroanalyses examined interaction between augmentative communication users and unimpaired speakers (Buzolich, 1983; Mathy-Laikko & Coxson, 1984). In Buzolich's study (1983), conversations between two dyads were analyzed. Each dyad consisted of an unimpaired speaker and a person who was an experienced user of the Handi-Voice 120 (HC Electronics, Mill Valley, CA) and a nonelectronic alphabet board. The microanalysis of rate of turn exchange indicated that the nonelectronic alphabet board allowed for greater participation during message construction on the part of the unimpaired speaker and was found to be faster in mean duration of turn exchanges. In the macroanalysis, all subjects rated the alphabet speller as faster because it allowed the unimpaired speaker to guess and predict the message. Unimpaired speakers expressed feelings of impatience and discomfort during the long silent encoding periods when the Handi-Voice was used. The macroanalysis suggested that subjects in the study made positive evaluations of the nonelectronic aid because of their active participation in the message construction.

Mathy-Laikko and Coxson (1984) also analyzed listener perceptions of the output mode and corroborated Buzolich's (1983) results. Their results show that output mode may affect listeners' attitudes toward persons using communication augmentation. Naive listeners (persons defined as having little or no experience with handicapped persons) and sensitized listeners (persons who had taken a minimum of one course in special education or communicative disorders) were asked to evaluate three output modes: synthesized speech, visual nonretrievable, and printed output. In the speech condition, each word or letter was spoken immediately after it was selected. During the print condition, the printer was activated after each message was completed. The listener groups rated the printed output as being slower than speech and visual nonretrievable output. Interestingly, the actual rate of word selection did not differ across conditions. But, during the speech and the visual nonretrievable conditions, listeners had to pay more careful attention during message construction. They were less aware of "waiting" for the message to be completed than they were during the print condition. The authors suggest that listener attitudes must be considered in measuring the effectiveness of augmentative communication components.

*Manipulation of selection techniques*. Another way to improve rate of conversational communication is to manipulate the transmission technique in order to determine which technique or combination of techniques provides the fastest selection rate given the user's physical limitations. To expedite this process, a number of researchers (e.g., Goodenough-Trepagnier & Rosen, 1982; Vanderheiden, 1984b) have attempted to develop computer models for assessing and comparing selection techniques. Unfortunately, measurements in wpm are usually obtained during transcription tasks (e.g., Vanderheiden, 1984b) and there are at least two problems associated with using transcription to measure effectiveness of communication expression. First, as discussed above, valid assessments require that measurements of augmentative components be made in the context within which they are designed to be used. Second, using transcription tasks for comparing augmentative aids and techniques does not take into account the fact that familiarity with a particular expressive mode will have a greater effect on communicative expression rate than on transcription rate. For example, several studies (using unimpaired persons) have compared decrements in wpm rates during transcription and communicative expression tasks when handwriting or typing modes are used (Chapanis, Parrish, Ochsman, & Weeks, 1972, 1977; Weeks, Kelly, & Chapanis, 1974). Results suggest that differences do exist and seem to reflect the subject's familiarity with the expressive mode. One study compared the typing rate of experienced typists (pretest >40 wpm transcription rate) during an expressive task and found that typing rates decreased to less than 20 wpm (Chapanis et al., 1972). In contrast, comparison of expression versus transcription rates using handwriting have shown very small to nonexistent wpm rate decrements (Chapanis et al., 1972). Foulds (1980) suggested that these differential effects may be related to familiarity. Cursive writing was the usual means for these subjects to transfer their ideas to paper, while typing was used primarily for transcription (e.g., to type final drafts of term papers, reports, etc.). Foulds (1980) predicted that the decrement between transcription and expression could be significantly reduced for persons who are experienced in creative expression on the typewriter (e.g., newspaper reporters, authors, etc.). The implications for augmentative interventions are that research methodologies that utilize transcription to predict rate of communicative expression must be reconsidered.

In summary, the dependent measures used to evaluate effectiveness, such as rate, are influenced by our assumptions about communication as a component model. We have largely ignored the impact of communication aids, special symbols, strategies, and techniques on the overall process of communication. Thus, the validity of our measurements is questionable. Future research is needed to develop valid measures for comparing the effect of variations in features of the aid or technique on the communication process. This research should examine interaction with the goal of discovering how the constraints of the augmentative aids and techniques are overcome during conversations. This will necessitate abandoning the goal of expecting conversational interactions to conform to the standards of communication shaped by modeling augmentative communication on the speech component.

## TOWARD A UNIFIED THEORY OF COMMUNICATION--PRELIMINARY CONSIDERATIONS

Higginbotham and Yoder (1982) provide a comprehensive discussion of the components of communication within natural conversational interaction (i.e., their coordination and interrelationships). They proposed that more than the ability to produce and comprehend words, communicative competence is dependent on:

1. knowledge of certain social conventions;

2. communication of culturally relevant nonverbal signals; and

3. ways in which these signals are exchanged (p. 1).

Because communication is so complex and involves the strategic employment of highly interrelated (both structurally and functionally) verbal and nonverbal components, research corroboration from a number of theoretical perspectives is needed to gain an understanding of normal and disordered conversation (Higginbotham et al., in press; Van Kleek, 1984). A unified theory of communication must be able to account for conversational interaction:

A back-and-forth series of verbal and nonverbal exchanges between two or more participants who observe certain rules and also violate them in an irregular flow of speaker's and listener's turns, acceptable and unacceptable simultaneous activities, acoustic and visual pauses, and a number of other positive and negative behaviors within each turn, differently oriented between speakers and listeners or among listeners, and conditioned by personality, situational context, and cultural background. (Poyotos, 1982, p. 156)

Future research in human communication sciences and disorders should be guided by a unified theory of communication.  Such a theory will require a systems approach, and does not mean finding yet another component to add to the ever expanding collection.  To be of value for research as well as heuristic purposes, the theory must be able to generate hypotheses that can be tested.

Recognizing the limitations of measures such as words per minute for evaluating the effectiveness of augmentative communication, researchers have begun to examine the face-to-face interactions of individuals who use augmentative techniques and their speaking partners (see chapters 4, 5, 6, 7; Higginbotham et al., in press; Kraat, 1985).  Such research has provided insight regarding the impact of augmentative aids, symbols, and techniques on the communication process.  Basically, a negative picture of the communication aid user's abilities has been presented.  That is, they most frequently communicate in one word turns and are seen as respondents rather than as sharing conversational control.

Our current understanding, however, is shaped by the analyses techniques employed.  Higginbotham et al. (in press) have argued for a reconsideration of results of interaction studies from two perspectives:  (a) the validity of the communication samples collected for these studies; and (b) the appropriateness of the data analyses employed.  Generally, the data used in interaction studies is collected in "one-shot" videotaped sessions ranging from 10 minutes to 30 minutes in length (see chapter 7; Beukelman & Yorkston, 1980; Calculator & Luchko, 1983; Lossing, Yorkston, & Beukelman, 1985).  The rationale for this type of communication sampling is based on expressive language analysis techniques.  The assumptions are that a sample of communication in one context is sufficient as a measure of communication competency and will predict communicative behaviors in other contexts.  Both assumptions have been questioned.  For example, opportunities (or sufficient motivation) to use particular skills or communicative functions may not occur during the sampling period.  Also, data collection equipment (video and audio) and observers are likely to affect the behavior of subjects in experimental settings, causing them to behave differently than they would normally in non-experimental settings (see Higginbotham & Mathy-Laikko, 1984; Kazdin, 1982a).  In these ways, generalizations from the sample context to other contexts may be invalid because of the sampling conditions, as described (see also chapter 5).

The data coding and analyses procedures employed to study face-to-face interactions of these dyads have also been criticized (Higginbotham et al., in press). Coding protocols are often based on research from mother-child interaction (e.g., Dore, 1977; Halliday, 1975; McKirdy & Blank, 1982) and their application may be inappropriate for two reasons. Taxonomies from mother-child research are limited to capturing and describing the communicative functions in adult-child interactions (Higginbotham et al., in press). In addition, coding schemes from mother-child research reflect the study of the speech component (i.e., verbal/vocal communication) and do not incorporate other communication modes. Another problem is that by adopting such analyses schemes the researcher may inadvertently import the research questions that such coding schemes were designed to address (e.g., the effect of maternal language input on child language development) to the study of conversations between unimpaired speakers and users of augmentative communication aids and techniques.

The outcomes of interaction analysis using frequency counts or percentage of occurrences of communicative functions (e.g., question, request for information, request for clarification, response, etc.) reduces communication to "amounts of behavior that are affected by other amounts of behavior" (the component model) instead of preserving the phenomenon being studied (Higginbotham et al., in press). Since conversation is organized on a turn-by-turn basis, with each succeeding turn directly influencing the next turn (Sacks, et al., 1974), valid analyses must find a way to study conversation without destroying its sequential structure and be able to capture its collaborative nature (i.e., how both participants contribute to the outcome).

Research results and methods within the fields of human communication (e.g., Gottman & Notarius, 1978; Gottman & Ringland, 1981; Sackett, Gluck, & Ruppenthal, 1978; Scherer & Ekman, 1982), sociolinguistics (e.g., Ervin-Tripp, 1969; Goffman, 1983; Hymes, 1974), and conversation analysis (within sociology) (e.g., Atkinson & Heritage, 1984; Heritage, 1984; Psathas, 1979) may help to answer some of the issues that have been raised. For example, in the study of topical talk by unimpaired individuals, Maynard (1980) and Maynard and Zimmerman (1984) found that topic change in conversation can be accomplished in a variety of ways, including a series of minimal responses (e.g., "um hum," "yea") and/or a series of silences by the listener. These methods regularly resulted in the introduction of new topics. Viewed from the perspective of conversational control, these results suggest that silences and minimal responses are resources available to participants to exert control in conversation. Higginbotham et al., (in press) indicate that similar strategies may be utilized by impaired speakers as a means of control during conversations with unimpaired speakers, but that our current analyses have missed them. For example, in a study of face-to-face interaction between a 56-year-old man who used an alphabet/word board and a 26-year-old unimpaired woman, Mathy-Laikko and Maynard (1985) reported that when the communication aid user did not attempt to take his turn, but instead was silent and gazed at the unimpaired speaker, the unimpaired speaker regularly responded by rephrasing her previous open ended question to provide narrow options (e.g., yes/no or multiple choice). In effect, the communication aid user's silences "controlled" the number and type of the speaker's questions.

## ADVANCES IN TECHNOLOGY--IMPACT ON AUGMENTATIVE COMMUNICATION

Advances in technology have opened many communication, vocational, and educational opportunities for persons who have cognitive, sensory, physical and/or communicative disabilities (Brandenberg, Bingston & Vanderheiden, in press a,b,c; Browning & Nave, 1983). Further, new developments in technology and computer science are occurring at an accelerating pace (Nilsson, 1985). Many of these new developments may be of direct or indirect benefit to persons with disabilities. The one area of computer science that is likely to have the most impact on augmentative communication is artificial intelligence.

Artificial intelligence is the branch of computer science "that is concerned with designing intelligent systems, that exhibit the characteristics that we associate with intelligence in human behavior--understanding, language, learning, reasoning, solving problems, and so on" (Mulsant & Servan-Schreiber, 1985, p. 143). The subfields within artificial intelligence include systems and language, problem solving, theorem proving, automatic programming, person-machine communications, and expert systems (Mulsant & Servan-Schreiber, 1985). Discussion of all of these areas is beyond the scope of this chapter (see Mulsand & Servan-Schreiber, 1985). Instead we will briefly describe the areas of person-machine communications and expert systems and suggest how advances in these fields may have an impact on augmentative communication.

Person-machine communication is concerned with the development of computer systems that will process spoken and written material and will produce spoken output (Mulsant & Servan-Schreiber, 1985). The "machine" will recognize and process the human voice in the same way it now uses information from the keyboard. For persons with physical disabilities who are unable to use a keyboard, such systems could be used for word processing and environmental control. At present, the ability to reliably recognize speech that falls outside the range of normal intelligibility is limited. Further, this technology is expensive and the number of vocabulary items it can learn to recognize is limited (Dabbagh & Damper, 1985). However, because computers with speech recognition ability are of great value to many fields (e.g., industry, medicine) (Kurzweil, 1986; Mulsant & Servan-Schreiber, 1985), rapid advances in such capabilities are foreseeable in the near future (Kurzweil, 1986).

"An expert system is a computerized model of the reasoning process of an expert" (Yager, 1983, p. 252). An expert is someone who can scan a vast amount of material in their area of expertise and quickly make useful decisions (Mulsant & Servan-Schreiber, 1985). Development of expert system has involved attempts to model the reasoning processes of persons in geology, physics, and other fields. Applied to augmentative communication, expert systems could be developed using data from the unimpaired speaker as an "expert" in communicative decision making. This information could be used in the development of software for communication aids and computers. For example, the program might be able to predict the most likely next word, phrase, and so forth given the previous communicative exchange, thus speeding up the individual's rate of communication in words per minute.

Other technological advances that will benefit augmentative communication are: (a) increased availability of digitized speech hardware and software; (b) improvements in intelligibility and a reduction in the size of speech synthesizers; (c) a reduction in size of microprocessors and peripherals; and (d) the expansion of memory capacity. As a result of these developments, more portable and more versatile augmentative communication components will be available at reduced costs (Rodgers, 1984).

Valid measurement tools that are based on a clear understanding of the communicative process are needed to assess the impact of these and future technologies on the communicative competencies of individuals who use augmentative aids and techniques. Human factors principles should be applied to determine the cost-benefit ratio of modifying current augmentative components.

Finally, it is unlikely that technology will be able to develop a true speech prosthesis that is identical to the unimpaired speech-communication system in every respect. Therefore, research in augmentative communication should continue to be oriented toward determining the most effective compensatory means for overcoming the constraints on the communication process imposed by an individual's communication impairment and the augmentative communication components.

## CONSIDERATIONS FOR FUTURE RESEARCH

To evaluate the effects of these interventions and set future goals in the augmentative communication area, valid methods are needed to measure the impact of augmentative communication aids and techniques as they are employed in specific communicative contexts for specific purposes. Two basic questions should be addressed in this research:

1. How are individuals who use augmentative communication techniques managing to successfully fulfill communication goals in spite of the constraints placed on them by their communication impairment and disability (including the constraints of the augmentative communication aids and techniques)?

2. What effects do manipulations of augmentative components (ouput mode, selection techniques, vocabulary, conversational strategies, etc.) have on the communication process?

Another area that should be studied in the future relates to the effect of implementing aided or unaided techniques on a particular group or groups of individuals (see chapters 1, 2, and 6). Behaviorist and developmentalist theories have contributed to our understanding of the application of communication aids with individuals who are cognitively impaired. Proponents of the behaviorist position consider the task of language learning to be qualitatively different for persons with severe/profound cognitive impairments than it is for nonhandicapped individuals. Therefore, they reject language training programs that are based on normal developmental theory in favor of special techniques hypothesized to accommodate specific language learning deficits of this population. The argument is that certain input characteristics and response demands of aided and unaided augmentative communication techniques (and symbol sets) may simplify the task of language learning for persons with cognitive impairments (Karlan, Lloyd, & Fristoe, 1983) and facilitate language learning. For example, beginning in the early 1970s (e.g., Bricker 1972), behaviorists began to examine the effects on language learning of training persons with severe/profound cognitive/linguistic deficits to communicate using gestures and manual signs (e.g., ASL) or graphic symbols (e.g., Blissymbols). This work was inspired by research in which primates were trained to use signs and symbol codes. Recently, attempts have been made to isolate the relative contributions of the features of aided and unaided symbol sets (e.g., iconicity, abstractness, response demands, vocabulary) that have been hypothesized to contribute to the language learning process (see Doherty, 1985). However, the contributions of such features to language development remains an empirical question.

A different perspective has been adopted by researchers within the developmental tradition. They have examined the abilities that the learner brings to the task of language learning (especially cognitive and linguistic) in order to predict the impact of training aided or unaided symbols on language development. This view is reflected in a number of decision/assessment schemes for determining if and when to implement communication augmentation. Such schemes indicate, among other things, that appropriate candidates are those persons with production delays related to cognitive level and not to chronological age (see chapter 2; Chapman & Miller, 1980; Owens & House, 1984; Shane & Bashir, 1980). Support for this position is based on a cognitive theory of language development. According to this theory, certain cognitive attainments appear to be necessary, but are not sufficient, for the development of language. For example, in their review of 43 communication training studies with severely/profoundly mentally retarded and autistic persons, Bryen and Joyce (1985) found that among the factors that differentiated studies that reported successful outcomes was the tendency to take into account cognitive abilities in subject selection. While these results do not resolve the question of how to best view the relationship between implementation of augmentative communication components (i.e., from a behaviorist or a developmental perspective), they suggest that future empirical studies should be conducted to examine these issues.

Future studies will probably provide support for the elements of both the behavioral and developmental perspectives. For example, evidence for information processing differences (slower than normal) in Down's syndrome individuals (Lincoln, Courchesne, Kilman, & Galambos, 1985) suggests that prolonging the duration of language input may have an impact on language processing. Another issue involves individual learner differences. In addition to primary cognitive deficits, mentally retarded persons have a higher incidence of sensory motor, perceptual, and other deficits. Further, as suggested above, they may vary in their abilities to process information. Thus, future research in this area must attempt to assess the impact of augmentative components on persons with different learning strengths and weakenesses. Moreover, because group designs tend to mask individual differences within and between subjects (Kazdin, 1982b), the employment of single-subject designs to address these issues is advocated.

## Selecting the Most Appropriate Research Designs

According to Bauer (1985), single-subject designs are important for the scientific investigation of communication disorders because "they open complex human speech and interactional disorders to exploration, discovery, and clinical accounting" (p. 68). Further, because persons with severe expressive communication disorders comprise a low-incidence, heterogeneous population, the assumptions for parametric analysis may be difficult, if not impossible, to meet. Another advantage of single-subject designs is that they provide a way to examine the effects of individual differences because the subjects act as their own controls. Single-subject design methodologies have also been suggested as the most efficient way for clinicians to organize treatment of their communicatively disordered clients (Vetter, 1985). Contributions to our knowledge base, through carefully planned and analyzed treatment of individual cases by the clinician-researcher, could have an important impact on future advances in our understanding of augmentative communication (Beukelman, 1985).

## *Assumptions and First Steps*

Augmentative communication aids and techniques must be regarded as augmenting communication, and not just substituting for speech. To examine their impact on the communication process from a perspective of a unified model of communication, baseline measures must be collected on the current communication behaviors of persons who have severe expressive communication disorders in target contexts. The effects of aids and techniques on the accomplishment of communicative goals within designated contexts should then be measured.

This type of research goes against the grain of our current emphasis on developing tools to analyze communication in the clinical setting. Examining communication in natural settings has always been a problem because of the enormous time demands inherent in this process. However, as illustrated in this chapter, current methods have not provided needed information on the communication process. This is partly due to the fact that we have not clearly defined what we expect from augmentative communication techniques, users of augmentative communication techniques, and the communicative context. Such definitions are needed to determine the unit(s) of analysis that is sensitive to change (improvement) in communicative ability. Words per minute, for example, may be a valid measure of motor learning for keyboard use, but it tells us very little about the effects of an augmentative communication technique on an individual's ability to use it strategically for communication in natural contexts (e.g., making a bank transaction, initiating conversation with a stranger).

Communicative behavior can be divided into any number of units (e.g., phonemes, words, wpm, communicative functions, episodes) (Van Kleek, 1984). But if the unit does not reflect the research question, it is of little value. The area of augmentative communication (and the field of communication disorders as a whole) suffers from the lack of valid measures of communicative ability. Given this, a first step for future research in augmentative communication is to momentarily put aside efforts to predict (measure) augmentative communication success using dependent variables (such as the number of questions asked unimpaired, speakers, increases in wpm, or the intelligibility of one speech synthesis program over another). Instead, a more valid unit to start with is the successful accomplishment of specific communicative goals within daily living contexts. For instance, a specific goal within a grocery store context is to use communicative skills in strategic ways in an effort to find and purchase one's groceries. Initial analysis of the impact of a particular augmentative communication component on this goal, then, would involve measuring the success or lack of success in meeting it. If the user is unsuccessful (e.g., does not manage to purchase the groceries), then we can go back and look at the strategic employment of all components within the target context to determine the source of the communication breakdown. For example, was the primary problem due to the lack of an effective means of obtaining the grocery clerk's attention, the grocery clerk's inability to understand or refusal to communicate with the user of augmentative communication techniques, or the user's lack of knowledge of the social conventions for how to ask for help? When the goal is met, we can try to determine the factors that lead to its successful accomplishment. It will also be important to examine user effects, as well as effects of the technique within and across target contexts, to understand what abilities certain users of augmentative communication techniques possess that make them more effective communicators than others. As we continue to examine conversations between communication aid users and their unimpaired partners, the units of analysis could be modified to look at how users of augmentative communication techniques employ them to persuade, protest, control the topic, and so forth. With this information, the next step is to analyze how modifications of augmentative components and training in interaction strategies affect the communication process for individuals who use communication augmentation.

## CONCLUDING REMARKS

Throughout this text other important goals for the future have been proposed. One that bears repeating here is advocacy (see chapter 8). Continued research documenting the existence and needs of persons with severe expressive communicative disorders is necessary to convince legislators, third-party payers, and university training programs of the need to develop funding sources for augmentative aids and services and for preservice and inservice course work in the evaluation and treatment of persons with severe expressive communication disorders (Matas, Mathy-Laikko, Beukelman & Legresley, 1985). Augmentative communication interventions must continue to be improved in order to enable users of augmentative communication techniques to become their own highly visible and very communicative advocates. We have certainly come a great distance toward this goal, but to paraphrase Robert Frost, ". . . *the woods are lovely dark and deep, but we've got promises to keep and miles to go before we sleep, and miles to go before we sleep.*"

## STUDY QUESTIONS

1. Discuss the major weaknesses of the research that has measured the impact of augmentative communication interventions.

2. Design a research project that you believe addresses a current need in augmentative communication.

3. Present a rationale for the unit of analysis you have selected in the above research project.

4. Considering the issues in this chapter, how should professionals in the augmentative communication area evaluate new developments in and applications of communication technologies?

## REFERENCES

Atkinson, J.M., & Heritage, J. (1984). Structures of social action: Studies in conversational analysis. New York: Cambridge University Press.

Baker, B. (1982). A semantic compaction system that makes self-expression easier for communicatively disabled individuals. Byte, 7, 186-202.

Bauer, H. (1985). Single-subject research designs in communicative interaction and disorders. Seminars in Speech and Language, 6, 67-101.

Beukelman, D. (1985). The weakest ink is better than the strongest memory [Letter to the editor]. Augmentative and Alternative Communication, 1, 55-57.

Beukelman, D., & Yorkston, K.M. (1980). Nonvocal communication: Performance evaluation. Archives of Physical Medical Rehabilitation, 61, 142-149.

Beukelman, D., & Yorkston, K. (1982). Communication interaction of adult communication augmentation system use. Topics in Language Disorders, 2, 39-54.

Beukelman, D., & Yorkston, K. (1984). Computer enhancement of message formulation and presentation for communication augmentation system users. Seminars in Speech and Language, 5, 1-10.

Brandenberg, S., Bingston, D., & Vanderheiden, G. (in press, a). Rehabilitation resource book series - Book 1: Communication aids. San Diego: College-Hill Press.

Brandenberg, S., Bingston, D., & Vanderheiden, G. (in press, b). Rehabilitation resource book series - Book 2: Switches, training, and environmental control. San Diego: College-Hill Press.

Brandenberg, S., Bingston, D., & Vanderheiden, G. (in press, c). Rehabilitation resource book series - Book 3: Software and hardware for individuals with sensory and physical disabilities. San Diego: College-Hill Press.

Bricker, D. (1972). Imitative sign training as a facilitator of word-object association with low functioning children. American Journal of Mental Deficiency, 26, 509-516.

Brodbeck, M. (1959). Models, meaning, and theories. In L. Gross (Ed.), Symposium on Sociological Theory (pp. 372-403). Evanston, IL: Row, Peterson & Co.

Brown, L., Falvey, M., Vincent, L., Kaye, N., Johnson, F., Ferrara-Parrish, P., & Gruenwald, L. (1980). Strategies for generating comprehensive longitudinal and chronological age appropriate individual education programs for adolescent and young adult severely handicapped students. Journal of Special Education, 14, 199-215.

Brown, P., & Levinson, S. (1978). Universals in language usage: Politeness phenomena. In E. Goody (Ed.), Questions and politeness (pp. 56-289). New York: Cambridge University Press.

Browning, P., & Nave, G. (1983). Computer technology for the handicapped: A literature profile. The Computing Teacher, February, 56-59.

Bryen, D., & Joyce, D. (1985). Language intervention with the severely handicapped: A decade of research. Journal of Special Education Research, 19, 7-39.

Buzolich, M. (1983). Interaction analysis of augmented and normal adult communicators. Unpublished doctoral dissertation, University of California, San Francisco.

Calculator, S., & Luchko, C. (1983). Evaluating the effectiveness of a communication board training program. Journal of Speech and Hearing Disorders, 48, 185-199.

Chapanis, A., Ochsman, R., Parrish, R., & Weeks, G. (1972). Studies of interactive communication: I-The effects of four communication modes on the behavior of teams during cooperative problem solving. Human Factors, 14, 487-509.

Chapanis, A., Parrish, R., Ochsman, R., & Weeks, G. (1977). Studies in interactive communication: II. The effects of four communication modes on the linguistic performance of teams during cooperative problem solving. Human Factors, 19, 101-126.

Chapman, R., & Miller, J. (1980). Analyzing language and communication in the child. In R.L. Schiefelbusch (Ed.), Nonspeech language and communication: Analysis and intervention (pp. 159-196). Baltimore: University Park Press.

Dabbagh, H. & Damper, R. (1985). Text composition by voice: Design issues and implementations. Augmentative and Alternative Communication, 1, 84-93.

Doherty, J. (1985). The effects of sign characteristics on sign acquisition and retention: An intergrative review of the literature. Augmentative and Alternative Communication, 1, 108-121.

Dore, J. (1977). "Oh them sherriff": A pragmatic analysis of children's responses to questions. In S. Ervin-Tripp & C. Mitchell-Kernan (Eds.), Child discourse (pp. 139-163). New York: Academic Press.

Eberts, R., & Eberts, C. (Eds.). (1985). Trends in ergonomics/Human factors II. New York: Elsevier Science Publishing Co.

Ervin-Tripp, S. (1969). Sociolinguistics. In Berkowitz (Ed.), Advances in experimental social psychology (pp. 91-127). Baltimore: Academic Press.

Foulds, R. (1980). Communication rates for nonspeech expression as a function of manual tasks and linguistic constraints. Proceedings of the Third International Conference on Rehabilitation Engineering. Washington, DC: RESNA.

Garfinkel, H. (1967). Studies in ethnomethodology. Englewood Cliffs, NJ: Prentice-Hall.

Goffman, E. (1983). Forms of talk. Philadelphia: University of Pennsylvania.

Goodenough-Trepagnier, C., & Rosen, M. (1982). An analytical framework for optimizing design and selection of nonvocal communication techniques. Proceedings of the International Federation of Automatic Control Aspects of Prosthetics and Orthodics (pp. 63-78).

Goodenough-Trepagnier, C., Tarry, E., & Prather, P. (1982). Derivation of an efficient nonvocal communication system. Human Factors, 24, 163-172.

Goossens', C., & Kraat, A. (1985). Technology as a tool for conversation and language learning for the physically disabled. Topics in Language Disorders, 6, 56-70.

Gottman, J. & Notarius, C. (1978). Sequential analysis of observational data using markov chains. In T. Kratochwill (Ed.), Single subject research: Strategies for evaluating change (pp. 237-284). New York: Academic Press.

Gottman, J., & Ringland, J. (1981). The analysis of dominance and bidirectionality in social development. Child Development, 52, 393-412.

Halliday, M. (1975). Learning how to mean: Explorations in the development of language. New York: Elsevier-North Holland.

Heritage, J. (1984). Garfinkel and ethnomethodology. Cambridge: Polity Press.

Higginbotham, D., & Mathy-Laikko, P. (1984, October). The application of videotape recording for the collection and analysis of communicative behavior data. Paper presented at the Third International Conference on Augmentative and Alternative Communication, MIT, Boston, MA.

Higginbotham, D., Mathy-Laikko, P., & Yoder, D. (in press). Studying conversations augmentative communication system users. In L. Bernstein (Ed.), The vocally impaired. New York: Academic Press.

Higginbotham, D., & Yoder, D. (1982). Communication within natural conversational interaction: Implications for severe communicatively impaired persons. Topics in Language Disorders, 2, 1-19.

Hymes, D. (1974). Foundations in sociolinguistics: An ethnographic approach. Philadelphia: University of Pennsylvania Press.

Karlan, G., Lloyd, L., & Fristoe, M. (1983). The effects of presentation modality upon learning in a comprehension task using oral, manual, and dual mode stimulus cues. Journal of Speech and Hearing Research, 26, 436-443.

Kazdin, A. (1982a). Observer effects: Reactivity of direct observation. New Directions for Methodology of Social and Behavioral Science Series, 14, 5-20.

Kazdin, A. (1982b). Single-case research designs: Methods for clinical and applied settings. New York: Oxford Press.

Kirchner, D., & Skarakis-Doyle, E. (1983). Developmental language disorders: A theoretical perspective. In T. Gallagher & C. Prutting (Eds.), Pragmatic assessment and intervention issues in language (pp 215-246). San Diego: College-Hill Press.

Kraat, A. (1985). Communication interaction between aided and natural speakers: A state of the art report. Toronto: Canadian Rehabilitation Council for the Disabled.

Kuhn, T. (1970). The structure of scientific revolutions. Chicago: University of Chicago Press.

Kurzweil, R. (1986). The technology of the Kurzweil voice writer. Byte, March, 177-186.

Lincoln, A., Courchesne, E., Kilman, B., & Galambos, R. (1985). Neuropsychological correlates of information-processing by children with Down's Syndrome. American Journal of Mental Deficiency, 89, 403-414.

Lossing, C., Yorkston, K., & Beukelman, D. (1985). Communication augmentation systems: Quantification in natural settings. Archives of Physical Medicine and Rehabilitation, 66, 380-384.

Matas, J., Mathy-Laikko, P., Beukelman, D., & Legresley, K. (1985). Identifying the nonspeaking population: A demographic study. Augmentative and Alternative Communication, 1, 17-31.

Mathy-Laikko, P., & Coxson, L. (1984, November). Listener reactions to augmentative communication system ouput mode. Paper presented at the American Speech-Language-Hearing Association, San Francisco.

Mathy-Laikko, P., & Maynard, D. (1985). Topical talk between a natural speaking interactant and an augmentative communication system user. Unpublished manuscript, University of Wisconsin-Madison.

Maynard, D. (1980). Placement of topic changes in conversation. Semiotica, 30, 263-290.

Maynard, D., & Zimmerman, D. (1984). Topical talk, ritual and the social organization of relationships. Social Psychology Quarterly, 47, 301-316.

McKirdy, L., & Blank, M. (1982). Dialogue in deaf and hearing preschoolers. Journal of Speech and Hearing Research, 25, 487-499.

Meister, D. (1976). Behavioral foundations of system development. New York: John Wiley & Sons.

Mital, A. (Ed.). (1984). Trends in ergonomics/Human factors. New York: North-Holland.

Mulsant, B. & Servan-Schreiber, D. (1985). Toward a new paradigm of health care: Artificial intelligence and medical management. Human Systems Management, 5, 137-147.

Nilsson, N. (1985). Artificial intelligence, employment, and income. Human Systems Management, 5, 123-135.

Owens, R., & House, L. (1984). Decision-making processes in augmentative communication. Journal of Speech and Hearing Disorders, 49, 18-25.

Poyotos, F. (1982). Language and nonverbal behavior in the structure of social conversation. Language Sciences, 4, 155-185.

Psathas, G. (1979). Everyday language: Studies in ethnomethodology. New York: Irvington Publishers.

Rodgers, B. (1984). The holistic application of high technology for conversation, writing, and computer access aid systems. In C. Smith (Ed.), Proceedings of Discovery 84: Technology for Disabled Persons. Menomine, WI: UW-Stout Vocational Rehabilitation Institute.

Sackett, G., Gluck, J., & Ruppenthal, G. (1978). Introduction: An overview of methodological and statistical problems in observational research. In G. Sackett (Ed.), Observing behavior volume II: Data collection and analysis methods (pp. 1-14). Baltimore: University Park Press.

Sacks, H., Schegloff, E., & Jefferson, G. (1974). A simplist systematics for the organization of turntaking for conversation. Language, 50, 696-735.

Scherer, K. & Ekman, P. (1982). Handbook of methods in nonverbal behavior research. Cambridge: Cambridge University Press.

Shane, H., & Bashir, A. (1980). Election criteria for the adoption of an augmentative communication system: Preliminary considerations. Journal of Speech and Hearing Disorders, 45, 408-415.

Vanderheiden, G. (1984a). A high-efficiency flexible keyboard input accelerating technique: Speedkey. Proceedings of the Second Annual International Conference on Rehabilitation Engineering. Washington, DC: RESNA.

Vanderheiden, G. (1984b). A unified quantitative modeling approach for selection-based augmentative communication systems. Unpublished doctoral dissertation, University of Wisconsin-Madison.

Van Kleek, A. (1984, June). Perspectives in social interaction research: A model, philosophy, and methodology. Invited Paper, Fifth Annual Wisconsin Symposium on Research in Child Language Disorders, Department of Communciative Disorders, University of Wisconsin-Madison.

Vetter, D. (1985). Evaluation of clinical intervention: Accountability. Seminars in Speech and Language, 6, 55-65.

Villarruel, F., Mathy-Laikko, P., Ratcliff, A.E., & Yoder, D.E. (1985). Alternative and augmentative communicative bibliography. (Available from Trace Research and Development Center, S-151, Reprint Service, University of Wisconsin-Madison, 1500 Highland Avenue, Madison, WI 53705-2280).

Watzlawick, P., Beavin, J., & Jackson, D. (1967). Pragmatics of human communication: A study of interactional patterns, pathologies and paradoxes. New York: W.W. Norton & Co.

Weeks, G., Kelly, M., & Chapanis, A. (1974). Studies in interactive communication: V. Cooperative problem solving by skilled and unskilled typists in a typewriter mode. Journal of Applied Psychology, 59, 665-674.

Wickens, C. (1984). Engineering psychology and human performance. Columbus, OH: Charles E. Merrill.

Yager, R. (1983). An introduction to applications of possibility theory. Human Systems Management, 3, 246-269.

# GLOSSARY

**abbreviation expansion program:** an augmentative technique in which words, phrases, or entire sentences are coded and recalled by the user using a short abbreviation. This technique can be used with all unaided and aided techniques that include an alphabet in their selection vocabulary.

**adaptive positioning:** the provision of supports and adaptive equipment to optimize the functional abilities of individuals with physical impairments.

**agglutination:** a process of combining symbols to represent new concepts.

**aid:** a physical object or device that is helpful. Augmentative communication aids include any type of language or communication board, book, chart, or mechanical or electrical device.

**alternative communication:** term used in conjunction with *augmentative communication* to address the needs of individuals without any speech. It is rarely used in this text, for even the most severely speech/language-impaired and vocally impaired individuals may produce meaningful vocalizations under some conditions.

**American Sign Language (ASL):** a manual, gestural communication system used by the severely hearing impaired/deaf. Each sign in this system performs a linguistic function; for example, a sign may signal a letter of the alphabet, or a word or a phrase, or may convey morphological or syntactic information.

**amyotrophic lateral sclerosis (ALS):** a disease that causes degeneration of upper and lower motor neurons. Individuals with ALS may require augmentative and, ultimately, alternative communication interventions.

**anarthria:** without speech; severe dysarthria resulting in speechlessness.

**aphasia:** acquired neurologic loss of the ability to use and/or understand language; for persons with aphasia, the ability to speak, listen, read, or write may be impaired. Adults with aphasia need intervention procedures targeted toward the reacquisition of language skills concurrent with the optimization of their communication functioning.

**apraxia** (verbal/oral): developmental or acquired condition associated with a neurological disorder, characterized by a deficit in the ability to carry out coordinated movements of the respiratory, laryngeal, and oral muscles for articulation in the absence of paralysis. Augmentative techniques may facilitate and/or compensate for apraxic speech.

**assistive device:** mechanical and/or electrical equipment designed to increase an individual's ability to interact with the environment. Assistive devices include communication aids, amplification devices, and environmental controls.

**athetoid cerebral palsy:** a congenital or early-acquired motor impairment characterized by frequent, involuntary, writhing movements. Individuals with athetoid cerebral palsy often have dysarthric speech. Nonverbal communication and writing may also be impaired as a result of problems with muscle tone, posture, and involuntary movements.

**augmentative communication:** all communication that supplements or augments speech. Augmentative communication represents an area of clinical practice that attempts to compensate for the impairment and disability patterns of individuals with severe expressive communication disorders through the use of both special and standard augmentative components (see below).

**augmentative components (of a communication system):** standard and/or special aids, techniques, symbols, and strategies that are required to enhance or augment the speech of severely speech/language-impaired individuals. *Standard augmentative components* are used by able-bodied persons to supplement speech and include ordinary gestures, facial expression, writing, and so on. *Special augmentative components* include symbols, aids, techniques, and strategies that have been specially developed or refined for use by individuals with severe communication disorders. They include the use of special gestures, graphic symbols, communication aids, signs, and special selection techniques, such as scanning, encoding, and direct selection. Augmentative communication components are recommended/prescribed and taught in an effort to provide, to the greatest extent possible, a functional communication system that addresses the particular communication needs of an individual.

**autism:** a condition of the early years of life, characterized by (a) the inability (failure) to relate in the ordinary way to people and situations, (b) repetitive activities, (c) developmental language disorders, and (d) marked inability to adjust socially.

**Blissymbols:** a symbol system adopted for communication in nonreading, disabled populations that utilizes a consistent set of symbols (e.g., pictographs, ideographs, arbitrary, and mixed symbols) to represent common meanings. It permits agglutination.

**brain stem lesions:** any pathological or traumatic discontinuity of tissue or loss of function within the brain stem. If damage occurs to areas that control speech, a locked-in syndrome may result that requires augmentative interventions.

**capability profiling:** a comprehensive approach to assessment that involves identification of an individual's maximum level of performance across critical areas of interest.

**chronemics:** the study of temporal aspects of communication; for example, the rate of communication exchanges, timing between responses, and the amount of time it takes to express ideas.

**communication:** the process by which information, ideas, and messages are exchanged between individuals through verbal and nonverbal behaviors.

**communication aid:** a physical object or device that helps an individual carry on a conversation, write, make basic needs known, and so on. Communication aids are commercially available or can be individually constructed boards, charts, and mechanical or electrical devices, among others.

**communication breakdown:** a communication failure between partners during conversation. Such breakdowns occur frequently during interactions between severely speech/language-impaired individuals and their partners.

**communication repair:** the ability to compensate for or fix a conversation after a communication breakdown has occurred. Individuals using augmentative components and their communication partners learn compensatory strategies that will repair misunderstandings, confusions, and ambiguities when they occur and will permit communication to continue.

**communication system (multi-component):** a dynamic and integrated network comprised of speech and a collection of techniques, aids, symbols, strategies, and skills that an individual uses to communicate. Note: Provision of an *augmentative communication system* includes training in the use of speech (if possible), as well as the most effective use of appropriate augmentative components (symbols, aids, techniques, skills, and strategies) in varying situations and environments.

**communicative competence**: the knowledge and skills necessary to exchange messages and information adequately for a stipulated purpose.

**conversational competence**: the knowledge and skills necessary to exchange messages and information adequately for conversation.

**conversational control**: obtaining and maintaining a turn during conversations (e.g., "um hum," "yea," silence, gaze, questions). Unimpaired speakers generally exhibit a disproportionate amount of control during conversations with severely speech/language-impaired individuals. Strategies employed by individuals who use augmentative communication aids and techniques to maintain conversational control are often nonverbal (e.g., vocalizations, silence, gazing toward the speaking partner).

**cosmesis**: a term used to measure the overall attractiveness or appearance of a communication aid. It directly affects the acceptability of the aid to the user and to others in the environment.

**criteria-based profiling**: an approach to assessment that identifies whether a client meets or exceeds the minimal levels of performance necessary for successful use of a specific aid or technique. This approach is used for screening and expediting assessment. It is based on a series of branching decisions that allows the assessment team to exclude a large number of possible questions and proceed to critical decisions.

**dactylogy**: movement of the hand and fingers as a means of communication between individuals; in this instance, it refers to the use of a finger alphabet.

**deixis**: direct indexing of a referent.

**direct selection**: a selection-based technique that involves pointing to objects, pictographs, words, and so on, as a means of message transmission.

**disability**: aspect of a communication disorder that refers to the reduced ability of a individuals to meet daily communication needs. The nature and degree of a disability is dependent on many factors, including the severity of the impairment, the communication life style of the individual, and the extent of an individual's compensation for the impairment through self-learning, specialized instruction, or prosthetic intervention.

**disjuncture**: transition during conversation.

**dynamic symbols:** symbols that have their meanings conveyed by change, transition, and/or movement and, therefore, cannot be considered permanent and enduring. Gestures, manual sign, and speech (natural and synthetic) are dynamic in nature.

**dysarthria:** a collective name for a group of speech disorders resulting from paralysis, weakness, or incoordination of the speech musculature due to damage of the central or peripheral nervous system. As the severity of a dysarthria increases, clinical management may require augmentative interventions.

**echolalic (echopraxic):** the inappropriate repetition of words, phrases, or sentences previously spoken by others.

**elicitation techniques:** techniques that are used in training to increase the likelihood that certain behaviors will occur (e.g., modeling, expansion, prompting, and questioning).

**encoding:** message transmision technique wherein an individual gives multiple signals that, taken together, specify the desired item from the individual's selection vocabulary. The signals may consist of a pattern or code, which may be memorized (memory-based) or referred to on a chart (chart-based).

**Exacttalk:** novel, spontaneous, and unpredictable mesages.

**Fitzgerald key:** an organizing format for communication aid displays.

**gestures:** a "natural" form of communication used to express concrete and referential concepts. Culture has a strong influence on gestures. Gestural modes require no instrumentation, only patterned muscle movements.

**glossectomy:** surgical removal of all or part of the tongue that may result in the need for augmentative communication aids and techniques..

**Guillain-Barré:** a rare acute neurological disorder of unknown cause, occurring after certain viral infections or vaccinations and involving partial paralysis of several muscle groups, including in some cases, those involved in speech.

**habilitation:** the mainstreaming of, in this case, communicatively handicapped individuals into all facets of community life by means of therapy, experiential learning, and formal education. Total habilitation, which impacts upon the educational, recreational, and vocational planning throughout an individual's life, involves a process of orienting, exposing, and integrating the interactive patterns and life styles of able-bodied and disabled individuals.

**handicap**:    refers to societal disadvantages resulting from an impairment and subsequent communication disability.    The extent of an individual's communication handicap depends upon the type of disability and the attitudes and biases of those who are in contact with the disabled individual.

**hypertonic**:  increased muscle tone.

**hypotonic**:  decreased muscle tone.

**iconicity**:    the relationship between a symbol and its meaning, ranging somewhere between *transparent* (symbols that are readily understandable) and *opaque* (symbols that are not understandable even when both the symbol and its meaning are provided to the learner).    *Translucency* falls between transparency and opaqueness on the iconicity continuum.    With *translucent* signs or symbols, the relationship between the symbol and its meaning is understandable only when both are provided.

**ideographs**:  graphic symbols used to represent ideas.

**idiosyncratic codes**:    ways of encoding words and/or messages with eye blinks, gestures, and/or vocalizations (of different quality, sound, and/or duration). While idiosyncratic codes may be useful, they are not understandable by most communication partners.

**impairment**:    refers to any loss or abnormality of psychological, physiological, or anatomical structure or function.    For the severely communicatively disordered individual, the impairment may be reflected in the loss or abnormal function of those aspects of the body responsible for speech and/or language.

**interdisciplinary team**:    a group of individuals that possesses expertise in widely divergent areas. The team makes decisions as a whole based upon shared information.    Augmentative communication assessment teams often function as interdisciplinary teams when making decisions about the selection and implementation of augmentative communication system components.

**joystick**:  A physical device used to control an electronic device.  With communication aids, joysticks usually are designed to activate two to eight switches when pushed off center in a specific direction.  Some joysticks use a gating scheme, which helps to guide the vertical stick to the desired switch when the stick is pushed.  Joystick operation needs to be coordinated with adequate seating and positioning.

**kinesics:** the study of the communicative information exchanged through body movements, facial expressions, and eye contact.

**laryngectomy:** surgical removal of all or part of the larynx that may result in the need for speech aids (e.g., electrolarnyx) or other augmentative communication aids and techniques.

**lexicon:** a special vocabulary that is used within a profession. In this case, *lexicon* may refer to the vocabulary displayed on a language/communication aid and/or a particular set of signs.

**logogram:** an abstract symbol or letter representing an entire word (e.g., $ for dollars).

**macroglossia:** oversize of the tongue.

**mental retardation:** (as defined by the American Association on Mental Deficiency) cognitive deficits with an onset that occurs during the developmental period. To be considered mentally retarded, persons must score at least two standard deviations below the average for his or her age group on a standardized intelligence test and show significant impairment in adaptive behavior.

**microglossia:** undersize of the tongue.

**mixed cerebral palsy:** congenital or early acquired motor impairment with both athetoid and spastic characteristics. As with other types of cerebral palsy, individuals may have dysarthric speech and experience difficulty with writing and nonverbal communication.

**mode:** distinguishes between the major channels or forms of communication, such as speech, gesture, and writing.

**nonverbal communication:** communication that does not involve the use of words in any form (spoken, written, or signed). Examples include communicative information exchanged through body movements, facial expressions, and eye contact (*kinesics*); vocal sounds accompanying verbal messages (*paralinguistics*); positioning in relation to other persons (*proxemics*); and the time it takes to express an idea (*chronemics*).

**opaque symbols:** see iconicity.

**orthography:**   symbolic representation of the sounds of language by letters or characters; the area of language study dealing with letters and their sequences in words.

**paralinguistics:**   vocal sounds accompanying verbal messages; includes vocalization to communicate ideas.

**pedagogical signs:**   a symbol set that is used to provide an easy transition to written English or to speech; related to "manually coded English" (MCE).

**pictogram:**   a pictorial representation of numerical data or relationships.

**pictograph:**   a pictorial representation of a thing or concept.

**polysemic symbols:**   little pictographs; used as a code to recall prestored phrases and sentences (e.g, the Minspeak semantic encoding approach).

**positioning for communication:**   see adaptive positioning.

**prediction:**   strategies that can be used with aided and unaided augmentative communication techniques for manipulating message units to enhance the speed of communication (word-per-minute rate).   Familiar communication partners often predict messages when provided with only minimal information from individuals who use augmentative aids and techniques (e.g., general topic area, initial letter of a word, etc.)  In addition, software is available that reduces the number of moves (key strokes) required to complete a message.  For example, in letter prediction schemes, the last letters selected are examined by the program; then, based upon frequency information, the letters that are most likely to follow are placed on the individual's scanning panel.  With this technique, the individual's scanning panel changes after each letter is selected.

**predictive profiling:**   a method of assessing the capabilities of a communicatively impaired individual on a number of carefully constructed tasks prior to selecting a communication aid or device for that individual.

**production-based techniques:**   message transmission techniques in which the individual actually produces the symbols used for communication.   Most production-based techniques are the same as those used by unimpaired individuals.

**prosody:**   study of the metrical structure of verse.

**proxemics:**   the way individuals position themselves in relation to other people.

**psycholinguistics**: study of the interaction between psychological factors and linguistic behavior.

**psychometric**: measurement of psychological variables, such as intelligence, aptitude, and emotional disturbance.

**Quicktalk**: prestored, predictable, or often-used messages.

**rebus symbols**: predominantly pictographic symbols (i.e., line drawings that represent whole words or parts of words). Rebuses can have phonological, morphological, or semantic significance. A rebus may consist of (a) a single drawing, (b) several drawings, or (c) a combination of letters of the alphabet and drawings.

**scanning**: a message transmission technique in which items are presented one at a time to the user. For example, in *linear* scanning, item choices are presented one at a time until the desired item is selected by an individual. The scanning array may be presented by a communication partner or via an electronic communication aid. Other scanning techniques include *row-column* scanning and *directed* scanning.

**selection-based techniques**: message transmission techniques that involve directly selecting or indicating desired symbols from a preformed set of symbols rather than physically producing symbols.

**skill**: great ability or proficiency, usually developed over time through training and practice.

**sociolinguistics**: the study of linguistic behavior as influenced by social and cultural factors.

**spastic cerebral palsy**: a congenital or early acquired motor impairment characterized by limited movements. Individuals with spastic cerebral palsy may have dysarthric speech and difficulty writing. Nonverbal communication may also be impaired as a result of problems with muscle tone, posture, and lack of movements.

**special augmentative components**: see augmentative components.

**speed**: an important dimension used to judge the advantages of a specific technique in meeting the requirements of a multi-component communication system; involves rate and efficiency of message transmission.

**standard augmentative components**: see augmentative components.

**static symbols:** symbols that do not require any change or movement to express meaning (e.g., graphic symbols and objects that are permanent and enduring).

**strategy:** a specific way of using augmentative aids or techniques more effectively for specific purposes. A strategy, taught to an individual or self-discovered, is a plan that can improve one's performance.

**switches:** a physical device used to control assistive devices and computers (e.g., touch panels, membrane keyboards, paddle switch, eyebrow switch, pneumatic switch, voice activated switch, etc.). Switch operation needs to be coordinated with adequate seating and positioning.

**symbols:** symbols/signs suggest, or stand for, something else by reason of relationship or convention. Visual signs that singly or in combination can function as symbols include photographs; gestures; manual signs; picto-ideographs such as Picsyms, rebuses, and Yerkes lexigrams; printed words; and tokens. Auditory signs that can serve this function include both phoneme sequences and noise sequences. Tactile signs include the raised-dot configurations of the Braille alphabet.

**synthesized speech:** speech produced with a computer using various technologies. Synthesized and digitized speech are available features on many augmentative communication aids.

**system:** an integrated group of components that work together as a whole.

**Tadoma codes (and other vibrotactile codes):** a vibrotactile technique that allows reception of speech by deaf individuals. With this technique, an individual places his hand on the speaker's jaw and lips in such a way that he can simultaneously feel the breath from the speaker's nose, the movement of the speaker's lips and jaws, and the vibration from the speaker's throat.

**technique:** a particular method for doing something. In this text, the term refers to different methods for transmitting ideas. Linear scanning, row-column scanning, two-movement encoding, signing, and common gestures are examples of different transmission techniques.

**telegraphic:** utterances that consist of key words rather than complete sentences/phrases. The use of telegraphic utterances is used as a strategy during augmentative interventions to increase the speed of message transmission.

**translucent symbols:** see iconicity.

**transparent symbols:** see iconicity.

**unaided communication technique:** a technique that does not require a physical aid. Gesture, sign, facial expressions, and oral speaking are considered unaided communication techniques.

**unaided symbols (and unaided symbol systems):** symbols that do not require aids or devices for production. Production of unaided symbols requires only the sender's face, head, hands, arms, and other parts of the body. These symbols (most of which may be thought of as dynamic) are frequently referred to as manual, although speech is included in this category.

**user interface:** any device that is used by an individual to access a communication aid (e.g., switches, touch panels, joysticks, lightbeams and sensors, or other physical means). To "interface" an individual means to find the anatomical site and control mechanism or technique that the individual can use most effectively to operate an aid or device.

**variable depth techniques:** techniques that have shorter selection times for some items and longer selection times for others; all scanning techniques are variable depth techniques. Encoding techniques that have variable length codes are in general faster and more efficient than fixed length encoding schemes. Morse code is an example of a variable depth encoding technique.

**verbal:** verbal communication refers to communication through spoken, written, or signed.

**vibrotactile codes:** see Tadoma codes.